T0226438

Cutaneous Lymphoma

Editor

ELISE A. OLSEN

DERMATOLOGIC CLINICS

www.derm.theclinics.com

Consulting Editor
BRUCE H. THIERS

October 2015 • Volume 33 • Number 4

ELSEVIER

1600 John F. Kennedy Boulevard • Suite 1800 • Philadelphia, Pennsylvania, 19103-2899

http://www.theclinics.com

DERMATOLOGIC CLINICS Volume 33, Number 4
October 2015 ISSN 0733-8635, ISBN-13: 978-0-323-40082-4

Editor: Jessica McCool
Developmental Editor: Alison Swety

Dermatologic Clinics (ISSN 0733-8635) is published quarterly by Elsevier Inc., 360 Park Avenue South, New York, NY 10010-1710. Months of publication are January, April, July, and October. Business and editorial offices: 1600 John F. Kennedy Blvd., Suite 1800, Philadelphia, PA 19103-2899. Customer service office: 11830 Westline Drive, St. Louis, MO 63146. Periodicals postage paid at New York, NY, and additional mailing offices. Subscription prices are USD 365.00 per year for US individuals, USD 559.00 per year for US institutions, USD 425.00 per year for Canadian individuals, USD 681.00 per year for Canadian institutions, USD 495.00 per year for international individuals, USD 681.00 per year for international institutions, USD 165.00 per year for US students/residents, and USD 240.00 per year for Canadian and international students/residents. International air speed delivery is included in all *Clinics* subscription prices. All prices are subject to change without notice. **POSTMASTER:** Send address changes to *Dermatologic Clinics*, Elsevier Health Sciences Division, Subscription Customer Service, 3251 Riverport Lane, Maryland Heights, MO 63043. **Customer Service: 1-800-654-2452 (U.S. and Canada); 314-447-8871 (outside U.S. and Canada). Fax: 314-447-8029. E-mail: journalscustomerservice-usa@elsevier.com (for print support); journalsonlinesupport-usa@elsevier.com (for online support).**

Reprints. For copies of 100 or more, of articles in this publication, please contact the Commercial Reprints Department, Elsevier Inc., 360 Park Avenue South, New York, New York 10010-1710. Tel.: 212-633-3874; Fax: 212-633-3820; Email: reprints@elsevier.com.

The *Dermatologic Clinics* is covered in *MEDLINE/PubMed (Index Medicus), Current Contents/Clinical Medicine, Excerpta Medica, Chemical Abstracts,* and *ISI/BIOMED.*

Contributors

CONSULTING EDITOR

BRUCE H. THIERS, MD
Professor and Chairman, Department of
Dermatology and Dermatologic Surgery,
Medical University of South Carolina,
Charleston, South Carolina

EDITOR

ELISE A. OLSEN, MD, FAAD
Professor of Dermatology and Medicine,
Director, Cutaneous Lymphoma Research and
Treatment Center, Director,
Dermatopharmacology Study Center, Duke
University Medical Center, Durham, North
Carolina

AUTHORS

KIMBERLY A. BOHJANEN, MD
Associate Professor, Department of
Dermatology, University of Minnesota,
Minneapolis, Minnesota

CATHERINE G. CHUNG, MD
Assistant Professor of Dermatology and
Pathology, Penn State Hershey Medical
Center, Hershey, Pennsylvania

OANA CRACIUNESCU, PhD
Associate Professor of Radiation Oncology,
Department of Radiation Oncology, Duke
University Medical Center, Durham, North
Carolina

MADELEINE DUVIC, MD
Professor of Medicine and Dermatology,
Division of Internal Medicine, Deputy
Chairman, Department of Dermatology,
Blanche Bender Professor in Cancer Research,
University of Texas MD Anderson Cancer
Center, Houston, Texas

LARISA J. GESKIN, MD, FAAD
Associate Professor of Dermatology and
Medicine, Director of Comprehensive
Cutaneous Oncology Center, Department of
Dermatology, Columbia University, New York,
New York

EMMILIA HODAK, MD
Department of Dermatology, Rabin Medical
Center, Beilinson Hospital, Sackler Faculty
Medicine, Tel Aviv University, Petah Tikva,
Israel

AURIS O. HUEN, PharmD, MD
Resident in Dermatology, Department of
Dermatology, Perelman School of Medicine,
University of Pennsylvania, Philadelphia,
Pennsylvania

LAUREN C. HUGHEY, MD
Associate Professor of Dermatology,
University of Alabama at Birmingham,
Birmingham, Alabama

CHRIS R. KELSEY, MD
Associate Professor of Radiation Oncology, Department of Radiation Oncology, Duke University Medical Center, Durham, North Carolina

WERNER KEMPF, MD
Kempf und Pfaltz Histologische Diagnostik; Department of Dermatology, University Hospital Zürich, Zürich, Switzerland

ELLEN J. KIM, MD
Sandra J. Lazarus Associate Professor of Dermatology, Department of Dermatology, Perelman School of Medicine, University of Pennsylvania, Philadelphia, Pennsylvania

CHRISTINA MITTELDORF, MD
Department of Dermatology, HELIOS Kliniken GmbH, Hildesheim, Germany

PATRICIA L. MYSKOWSKI, MD
Dermatology Service, Department of Medicine, Memorial Sloan Kettering Cancer Center, New York, New York

CUONG V. NGUYEN, MD
Department of Dermatology, University of Minnesota, Minneapolis, Minnesota

ELISE A. OLSEN, MD, FAAD
Professor of Dermatology and Medicine, Director, Cutaneous Lymphoma Research and Treatment Center, Director, Dermatopharmacology Study Center, Duke University Medical Center, Durham, North Carolina

LEV PAVLOVSKY, MD, PhD
Department of Dermatology, Rabin Medical Center, Beilinson Hospital, Sackler Faculty Medicine, Tel Aviv University, Petah Tikva, Israel

LAUREN C. PINTER-BROWN, MD, FACP
Health Sciences Professor of Medicine, Department of Internal Medicine, Division of Hematology-Oncology, Geffen School of Medicine, University of California, Los Angeles, Santa Monica, California

BRIAN POLIGONE, MD, PhD
Director of Cutaneous Lymphomas, James P. Wilmot Cancer Center, University of Rochester School of Medicine, Rochester, New York

CHRISTIANE QUERFELD, MD, PhD
Director, Cutaneous Lymphoma Program, Department of Hematology/Hematopoietic Cell Transplantation, Department of Pathology, City of Hope Comprehensive Cancer Center, Duarte, California; Memorial Sloan Kettering Cancer Center, New York, New York

ALAIN H. ROOK, MD
Department of Dermatology, Hospital of the University of Pennsylvania, Philadelphia, Pennsylvania

STEVEN T. ROSEN, MD, FACP
Provost, Chief Scientific Officer, Director, City of Hope Cancer Center and Beckman Research Institute, Department of Hematology/Hematopoietic Cell Transplantation, City of Hope Comprehensive Cancer Center, Duarte, California

NATALIE SPACCARELLI, MD
Department of Dermatology, Hospital of the University of Pennsylvania, Philadelphia, Pennsylvania

DANIEL J. TANDBERG, MD
Resident, Department of Radiation Oncology, Duke University Medical Center, Durham, North Carolina

POOJA VIRMANI, MBBS, MD
Research Fellow, Dermatology Service, Department of Medicine, Memorial Sloan Kettering Cancer Center, New York, New York

GARY S. WOOD, MD
Johnson Professor and Chair, Department of Dermatology, University of Wisconsin and VA Medical Center, Madison, Wisconsin

JIANQIANG WU, MD, PhD
Associate Scientist, Department of Dermatology, University of Wisconsin and VA Medical Center, Madison, Wisconsin

JASMINE ZAIN, MD
Director, T-cell Lymphoma, Department of Hematology/Hematopoietic Cell Transplantation, City of Hope Comprehensive Cancer Center, Duarte, California

JOHN A. ZIC, MD
Associate Professor of Medicine/Dermatology, Division of Dermatology, Vanderbilt University School of Medicine, Nashville, Tennessee

Contents

Primary cutaneous lymphomas (PCLs) are an extremely heterogeneous group of non-Hodgkin lymphomas that manifest in the skin. Their diagnosis is complex and based on clinical lesion type and evaluation of findings on light microscopic examination, immunohistochemistry, and molecular analysis of representative skin biopsies. The evaluation, classification, and staging system is unique for mycosis fungoides (MF) and Sézary syndrome (SS), the most common subtypes of cutaneous T-cell lymphoma (CTCL) versus the other subtypes of Non-MF/Non-SS CTCL and the subtypes of cutaneous B-cell lymphoma (CBCL). Since current treatment is stage-based, it is particularly important that the correct diagnosis and stage be ascertained initially. The purpose of this article is to review the current evaluation, diagnosis, classification, staging, assessment techniques, and response criteria for the various types of both T-cell and B-cell PCLs.

Primary cutaneous lymphomas comprise a prognostically heterogeneous group of lymphocytic skin neoplasms, which display a broad spectrum of clinical, histologic, immunophenotypic, and genetic features. The histopathological examination plays an essential role and is often the starting point in the diagnostic workup of cutaneous lymphomas. In most cases, the histopathological and the phenotypic analysis alone are limited to provide a list of differential diagnoses. As a consequence of overlapping clinical, histologic, phenotypic, and genetic features among several entities of cutaneous lymphomas, the clinicopathological correlation is of utmost importance to achieve the final diagnosis.

Early stage mycosis fungoides represents the most common clinical presentation of cutaneous lymphoma, with skin-directed therapies long established in its treatment. These therapies continue to change as new treatment regimens emerge. Other skin-directed treatments include light and radiation therapy. Therapies with higher levels of evidence and less systemic toxicity are usually preferred as first-line treatment. However, even these established therapies, like topical corticosteroids and carmustine, lack randomized clinical trials to establish their efficacy. Research is also needed to further define the role of combination topical therapies and how skin-directed therapies can be used as adjuvants to systemic medications.

Therapies based on ultraviolet light have long been established in mycosis fungoides (MF). They have traditionally included whole-body ultraviolet light B, both broad-band and narrow-band, and psoralen plus ultraviolet A. Phototherapy may be applied alone in early stage MF or in combination with systemic therapy in refractory early stage MF and advanced MF. This article reviews the most frequently used forms of phototherapy for MF with emphasis on efficacy, safety, and practical considerations.

Radiation therapy is an extraordinarily effective skin-directed therapy for cutaneous T-cell lymphomas. Lymphocytes are extremely sensitive to radiation and a complete response is generally achieved even with low doses. Radiation therapy has several important roles in the management of mycosis fungoides. For the rare patient with unilesional disease, radiation therapy alone is potentially curative. For patients with more advanced cutaneous disease, radiation therapy to local lesions or to the entire skin can effectively palliate symptomatic disease and provide local disease control. Compared with other skin-directed therapies, radiation therapy is particularly advantageous because it can effectively penetrate and treat thicker plaques and tumors.

Retinoids are natural and synthetic vitamin A analogs with effects on cell proliferation, differentiation, and apoptosis. They have significant activity in hematologic malignancies and have been studied extensively in cutaneous T-cell lymphoma. Retinoids bind to nuclear receptors and exert their effects through moderation of gene expression. Retinoic acid receptor and retinoic X receptor exert regulatory activity in vivo, binding to distinct ligands. Studies investigating systemic retinoids as monotherapy and in combination with other agents active against cutaneous lymphoma are reviewed. Side effects associated with retinoids include teratogenicity, dyslipidemias, and hypothyroidism, which should be carefully monitored in patients receiving treatment.

Interferons are polypeptides that naturally occur in the human body as a part of the innate immune response. By harnessing these immunomodulatory functions, synthetic interferons have shown efficacy in combating various diseases including cutaneous T-cell lymphoma. This article closely examines the qualities of interferon alfa and interferon gamma and the evidence behind their use in the 2 most common types of cutaneous T-cell lymphomas, namely, mycosis fungoides and Sézary syndrome.

This article reviews methotrexate and the more potent, related compound, pralatrexate, for the treatment of cutaneous T-cell lymphomas, including mycosis fungoides,

Sézary syndrome, and CD30+ lymphoproliferative disorders. Although these folate antagonists are traditionally viewed as antiproliferative cell cycle inhibitors, it is recognized that they inhibit DNA methylation, providing a rationale for their use as epigenetic regulators and cell proliferation inhibitors. The underlying mechanisms are outlined and key supporting data are presented, followed by a brief mention of recent mathematical modeling supporting the general superiority of combination therapy. Several novel examples involving folate antagonists are proposed.

Cutaneous T-cell lymphomas (CTCLs) are non-Hodgkin's T-cell lymphomas that present as skin lesions. Mycosis fungoides with large cell transformation has a 5-year overall survival of 32% with involved skin and 7% with extracutaneous involvement. Failure to cure advanced MF with large cell transformation and peripheral T-cell lymphoma has resulted in a search for novel targeted agents including antibodies and gene modulators. Histone deacetylase inhibitors are small molecules that seem to be particularly active for T-cell lymphoma.

Extracorporeal photopheresis (ECP) is an immunomodulating procedure that leads to an expansion of peripheral blood dendritic cell populations and an enhanced TH1 immune response in cutaneous T-cell lymphoma (CTCL). Because of its excellent side effect profile and moderate efficacy, ECP is considered first-line therapy for erythrodermic mycosis fungoides (MF) and Sézary syndrome. Patients with a measurable but low blood tumor burden are most likely to respond to ECP, and the addition of adjunctive immunostimulatory agents may also increase response rates. There may be a role for ECP in the treatment of refractory early stage MF, but data are limited.

Use of monoclonal antibodies (mAbs) has revolutionized cancer therapy. Approaches targeting specific cellular targets on the malignant cells and in tumor microenvironment have proven to be successful in hematologic malignancies, including cutaneous lymphomas. mAb-based therapy for cutaneous T-cell lymphoma has demonstrated high response rates and a favorable toxicity profile in clinical trials. Several antibodies and antibody-based conjugates are approved for use in clinical practice, and many more are in ongoing and planned clinical trials. In addition, these safe and effective drugs can be used as pillars for sequential therapies in a rational stepwise manner.

Traditional chemotherapies, interleukins, phosphorylase inhibitors, and proteasome inhibitors are important therapies available to patients with cutaneous T-cell lymphoma (CTCL). Traditional chemotherapies, both in combination and as single agents, are commonly used in relapsed, refractory CTCLs that behave in an aggressive manner. Interleukins, phosphorylase inhibitors, and proteasome inhibitors are less commonly used but data support a role in patients with more refractory disease.

Mycosis fungoides (MF) and Sézary syndrome (SS) are common types of primary cutaneous T-cell lymphoma. Early-stage MF has a favorable prognosis and responds well to skin-directed regimens. Patients with advanced-stage MF, transformed MF, and SS are treated with combined systemic and skin-directed therapies. However, the disease is incurable with standard regimens, and frequent relapses are common. Owing to the lack of improvement in overall survival with standard regimens, hematopoietic stem cell transplant (HSCT) has been explored as a potential curative option. This article reviews the role of HSCT in MF/SS and discusses data regarding conditioning regimens, treatment-related complications, and outcomes.

Primary cutaneous CD30⁺ lymphoproliferative disorders (LPDs) account for approximately 25% of cutaneous lymphomas. Although these LPDs are clinically heterogeneous, they can be indistinguishable histologically. Lymphomatoid papulosis rarely requires systemic treatment; however, multifocal primary cutaneous anaplastic large cell cutaneous lymphoma and large cell transformation of mycosis fungoides are typically treated systemically. As CD30⁺ LPDs are rare, there is little published evidence to support a specific treatment algorithm. Most studies are case reports, small case series, or retrospective reviews. This article discusses various treatment choices for each of the CD30⁺ disorders and offers practical pearls to aid in choosing an appropriate regimen.

The diagnosis of primary cutaneous B-cell lymphoma (CBCL) requires that the search for a more widespread lymphoma has been negative. The clinical presentation, outlook, and treatment options of the common types of CBCLs, with emphasis on differences or similarities to their nodal counterparts, are discussed. Treatment may range from observation to topical therapies to systemic therapies, depending on the histology, degree and area of skin involvement, patient performance, and comorbidities. Rare lymphomas, such as intravascular large B-cell lymphoma and Epstein-Barr virus–positive cutaneous lymphoproliferations that are associated with immunodeficiency, are also briefly described.

DERMATOLOGIC CLINICS

Erratum

Errors were made in the July 2015 issue of *Dermatologic Clinics* (Volume 33, Issue 3) on page iv of the "Contributors" section. Lisa A. Drage was incorrectly identified as a Fellow; her correct academic title is Associate Professor of Dermatology. Her Fellow, Tania M. Gonzalez-Santiago, was incorrectly identified as an Associate Professor of Dermatology.

Dermatol Clin 33 (2015) xi
http://dx.doi.org/10.1016/j.det.2015.08.008
0733-8635/15/$ – see front matter © 2015 Elsevier Inc. All rights reserved.

Erratum

Errors were made in the July 2015 issue of Dermatologic Clinics (Volume 33, Issue 3) on page iv of the "Contributors" section. Lisa A. Drage was incorrectly identified as a Fellow; her correct academic title is Associate Professor of Dermatology. Her Fellow, Tania M. Gonzalez-Santiago, was incorrectly identified as an Associate Professor of Dermatology.

Dermatol Clin 33 (2015) xi
http://dx.doi.org/10.1016/j.det.2015.08.005
0733-8635/15/$ – see front matter © 2015 Elsevier Inc. All rights reserved.

Preface
Cutaneous Lymphoma

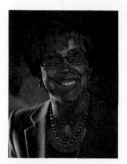

Elise A. Olsen, MD, FAAD
Editor

The cutaneous lymphomas are a heterogeneous group of B-cell and T-cell non-Hodgkin lymphomas that are considered rare cancers. Even the most common subtype of cutaneous T-cell lymphoma, mycosis fungoides (MF) (along with its leukemic counterpart Sézary syndrome [SS]), has an incidence of only about 6 to 7 per million persons by the SEER data. There has been considerable change in the past 10 years in terms of defining the various subtypes of cutaneous lymphoma, developing new standards for diagnosis, classification, staging, and response criteria, and introducing new FDA-approved treatments and a new approach to effective management of MF/SS that is not necessarily chemotherapy dependent. It is important for both dermatologists and oncologists to understand how to diagnose and manage these patients using these advances, particularly as none of these cutaneous lymphomas currently has a curative treatment and all have considerable impact on the quality of life and a potential adverse effect on survival of affected patients.

This issue brings together the experience of not only physician authors with direct expertise in the management of patients with cutaneous lymphoma but also those who have contributed to the recent advances in this area. Taken together, these articles cover the evaluation, diagnostic elements from both clinical and pathologic assessment, and staging/classification of all types of B-cell and T-cell cutaneous lymphoma. The entire spectrum of treatments utilized for MF and SS is given in individual articles, and separate articles on the treatment of the CD30+ lymphoproliferative disorders and cutaneous B-cell lymphoma give an overview on these other common types of cutaneous lymphoma.

On behalf of my coauthors, I hope that the information provided in this issue will accomplish several goals, the first of which is to update physicians on the advances in this area in the last decade. Since all current treatment for cutaneous lymphoma, regardless of subtype, is stage-based, it is important that those initially seeing these patients are aware of the nuances involved in staging and classification. In addition, this issue can serve as a ready resource of all the current treatment options for cutaneous lymphoma, particularly MF, including efficacy and safety information germane to clinical practice. In summary, if this is accomplished, then the lives of those with cutaneous lymphoma will be advanced.

Elise A. Olsen, MD, FAAD
Cutaneous Lymphoma Research
and Treatment Center
Dermatopharmacology Study Center
Duke University Medical Center
Durham, NC, USA

E-mail address:
Elise.olsen@dm.duke.edu

Dermatol Clin 33 (2015) xiii
http://dx.doi.org/10.1016/j.det.2015.07.001
0733-8635/15/$ – see front matter © 2015 Published by Elsevier Inc.

Evaluation, Diagnosis, and Staging of Cutaneous Lymphoma

Elise A. Olsen, MD

KEYWORDS

- Primary cutaneous lymphoma (PCL) • Cutaneous T-cell lymphoma (CTCL)
- Cutaneous B-cell lymphoma (CBCL) • Mycosis fungoides • Sézary syndrome

KEY POINTS

- The unique features of the diagnosis, evaluation, classification and staging of mycosis fungoides and Sézary syndrome.
- The evaluation, classification and staging of the nonMF/nonSS CTCLs and the most common subtypes of CBCLs.
- The response criteria for evaluation of therapeutic efficacy for all subtypes of cutaneous lymphoma.

INTRODUCTION

Cutaneous lymphomas are an extremely heterogeneous group of non-Hodgkin lymphomas (NHLs) that manifest in the skin.[1,2] Although most patients do not have evidence by traditional screening methods of extracutaneous disease at the time of presentation (and, hence, fit the classic definition of primary cutaneous lymphoma [PCL]), those with certain clinical or histologic subtypes commonly have, or will, develop nodal, visceral, and/or blood involvement. The prognosis and survival of patients varies not only on the type of cutaneous lymphoma but the stage as well; each lymphoma has its own best treatments to date, which are primarily stage based. Because there is no cure for any of these cutaneous lymphomas, but treatment can be life saving and insure quality of life, the overall prognosis for any given patient begins with the correct diagnosis and staging. It is the purpose of this article to discuss the evaluation, diagnosis, and staging of the 3 main subcategories of cutaneous lymphoma.

SUBTYPES AND EPIDEMIOLOGY OF CUTANEOUS LYMPHOMA

The annual incidence of PCLs is estimated at 10.0 to 10.7 per million person-years,[3,4] and they account for 19% of cases of extranodal lymphomas.[4] The World Health Organization–European Organization for Research and Treatment of Cancer (WHO-EORTC) have classified the cutaneous lymphomas with primary cutaneous manifestations into cutaneous T-cell lymphomas (CTCLs) and cutaneous B-cell lymphomas (CBCLs) (**Box 1**).[5,6] The CBCLs are the least common of the PCLs, estimated at 3.1 per million person-years in an assessment of the National Cancer Institute's Surveillance, Epidemiology, and End Results (SEER) registry for 2001 to 2005 but making up 29% of all PCLs.[4] The annual incidence rate of CBCLs steadily increased to an annual rate of 3.92 between 2006 and 2010.[7] The age-adjusted incidence of all types of CTCLs, based on 2 different sets of SEER, ranged from 6.4 to 7.7 million person-years.[4,8] What is clear is that the incidence

Potential conflicts of interest: none.
Department of Dermatology, Trent & Erwin Roads, Duke University Medical Center, Durham, NC 27710, USA
E-mail address: elise.olsen@dm.duke.edu

Dermatol Clin 33 (2015) 643–654
http://dx.doi.org/10.1016/j.det.2015.06.001

derm.theclinics.com

Box 1
WHO/EORTC classification of cutaneous lymphomas

CTCLs and cutaneous NK-cell lymphomas

Mycosis fungoides (MF)

MF variants and subtypes

Folliculotropic MF

Pagetoid reticulosis

Granulomatous slack skin

Sézary syndrome

Adult T-cell leukemia/lymphoma

Primary cutaneous CD30+ lymphoproliferative disorders

Primary cutaneous anaplastic large cell lymphoma

Lymphomatoid papulosis

Subcutaneous panniculitis-like T-cell lymphoma

Extranodal NK/T-cell lymphoma, nasal type

Primary cutaneous peripheral T-cell lymphoma, unspecified

Primary cutaneous aggressive epidermotropic CD8+ T-cell lymphoma (provisional)

Cutaneous γ/δ T-cell lymphoma

Primary cutaneous CD4+ small/medium-sized pleomorphic T-cell lymphoproliferative disorder (provisional)

Primary cutaneous acral CD8+ T cell lymphoma (provisional)

CBCLs

Primary cutaneous marginal zone lymphoma

Primary cutaneous follicle center lymphoma

Primary cutaneous diffuse large B-cell lymphoma, leg type

Primary cutaneous diffuse large B-cell lymphoma, other

Intravascular large B-cell lymphoma

EBV+diffuse large B-cell lymphoma of the elderly (provisional)

Precursor hematologic neoplasm

Blastic plasmacytoid dendritic cell neoplasm

Abbreviations: MF, mycosis fungoides; NK, natural killer.
Adapted from Willemze R, Jaffe E, Burg G, et al. WHO-EORTC classification for cutaneous lymphomas. Blood 2005;105:3769; with permission.

of both CBCLs and CTCLs has continued to increase dramatically and consistently over the past 3 decades,[4] CTCL by 2.9 per million per decade.[8] Based on the numbers available, there are over 3000 new patients with the diagnosis of PCL each year.

Mycosis fungoides (MF) is the most common type of CTCL, comprising 53–54%[4,9] to 73%[8] of cases of CTCL in various SEER reviews. Sézary syndrome (SS) is classified as a separate entity from MF by the WHO-EORTC[10] but shares the same histologic criteria and staging as MF and often evolves from MF.[1] SS accounted for 2.5% of the cases of CTCL in the report by Criscione and Weinstock.[8] The prevalence of MF is likely more than 50,000 based on survival curves, but this number is unsubstantiated without a formal registry. The 10-year survival of patients with MF with tumor or nodal involvement is compromised (42% and 20% respectively),[5] and the 5-year survival of patients with SS (who have blood and may also have node involvement) is 24% in one report.[5] Although these patients with tumor or node stage MF or leukemic blood involvement are the minority of patients with MF, they represent the potential progression for which treatments used in those with lesser disease strive to prevent. There is no current cure for MF or SS; patients living with MF or SS endure the chronic symptoms and signs of their disease and the constant time, cost, and potential side effects of treatment to prevent progression. Although there are general clinical characteristics, such as skin (T) stage, or histologic features, such as large cell transformation (LCT), that are able to identify those with a worse prognosis in certain situations, there is great heterogeneity in these subclasses of PCL and no treatment available that targets the trigger for the final unremitting growth of the lymphoma that occurs in some patients. In addition, no genetic markers are currently available that would help identify subsets of patients more likely to respond to certain treatments.

Short of a long-term national registry of patients with cutaneous lymphoma and clear documentation of the effect on overall prognosis and survival of the various treatments used and the potential for clinical, histologic, and genetic factors to influence the outcome or choice of treatment, physicians are unable to make the kind of advances necessary to move toward a curative treatment of MF and SS. The same issues are present in the other types of CTCLs and CBCLs, none of which currently have curative treatment and, because of their relative small numbers, would benefit greatly from a national registry.

What follows in this article is the consensus approach of the International Society for Cutaneous Lymphomas (ISCLC), the EORTC Cutaneous Lymphoma Taskforce, and the United States Cutaneous Lymphoma Consortium (USCLC) on the diagnosis and staging of both the CTCLs and CBCLs. Given that there are certain nuances of MF and SS, including type of skin lesions, node histology, and potential blood involvement, that separates these cancers from the other cutaneous lymphomas, a separate and distinct staging system exists for MF and SS from that of the non-MF/non-SS CTCLs and the CBCLs.

MYCOSIS FUNGOIDES AND SÉZARY SYNDROME
Diagnosis

Classically, the lesions of MF are described as patches, plaques, or tumors.[1] Patches are flat but may be scaly or have textural change. Plaques are defined as slightly raised lesions and can be smooth, scaly, crusted, or ulcerated. A tumor is defined as a lesion at least 1 cm in diameter that has vertical growth or depth. Most of these lesion subtypes are erythematous on presentation but can be hyperpigmented. When the presentation involves diffuse scaling or confluence of patch or plaque lesions and covers 80% or greater body surface area (BSA), this meets the criteria for the term erythroderma.[1] There are other clinical presentations of MF including poikiloderma (a relatively specific finding for MF), hypopigmented macules and patches, follicular plugging, alopecia, keratoderma, blisters, and redundant skin within the axillary or inguinal folds.

The diagnosis of MF or SS is one that requires clinicopathologic correlation but starts with a representative skin biopsy suggestive of MF. Because the type of lesion may affect both the hematoxylin and eosin (H&E) and immunophenotyping results and the potential to find a clone of the T-cell receptor (TCR) gene rearrangement (GR), the choice of skin lesion for biopsy is critical. The most indurated lesion should be biopsied and if various types of lesions are present, a biopsy of each type of lesion should be taken: this is important to help identify clinical and histologic prognostic factors as well as to help differentiate between the types of CTCL. For example, a biopsy of a patch of alopecia may indicate that a patient has a folliculotropic form of MF in which the base of the abnormal lymphocytic infiltrate is far deeper than one would expect with a typical patch lesion. In general, H&E as well as immunophenotyping with various T-cell surface markers, including at

a minimum CD3, CD4, CD8, CD7, and CD30, and one B-cell marker, such as CD20, are used to assess the infiltrate. The lymphocytic infiltrate may be affected by topical steroids or other topical or systemic immunosuppressive agents, so it is important for patients to be off of these, if possible, for at least the 2 weeks before the skin biopsy; this is especially true for patch stage lesions. The specifics of the histologic criteria for the diagnosis of MF/SS are covered in Dr Kempf's article in this issue.

The evaluation for a clonal TCR GR in the skin is a necessary part of the evaluation as the presence of a positive clone is supportive evidence of MF: both gamma and beta testing should be explored before making a final conclusion as to whether positive. However, it is important to keep in mind that a TCR GR clone may be present in benign skin conditions as well, so the presence of a clone is not a *sine qua non* of malignancy. The specifics of testing for clonality are key, with the BIOMED-2 method currently favored. A biopsy collected on saline is preferred for clonality testing as the yield will be increased; but it is clear that, with thick plaques and tumors, this clonality testing can be performed on formalin fixed tissue.

Multiple skin biopsies may be necessary for the diagnosis in cases of erythroderma where the percentage of inflammatory cells is high and the tumor cells low; in such cases in which the skin biopsy remains suggestive but not diagnostic of lymphoma, a lymph node biopsy or blood studies indicative of lymphoma may enable a diagnosis of MF or SS to be made. One must also keep in mind that a MF-like histology in the skin can be a manifestation of a drug reaction: most of these cases typically do not demonstrate clonality of the TCR GR. When suspected, the potentially offending drug should be discontinued for at least 2 to 3 months before ascribing the condition to lymphoma.

A useful algorithm focusing on clinicopathologic correlation was developed by the ISCL in 2005 for the diagnosis of early MF (**Table 1**).[11] This algorithm is a point scoring system that includes points for clinical, histologic, molecular, and clonality findings with an overall point score of 4 indicating probable MF. This point scoring was not meant to be used for the diagnosis of hypopigmented MF (although it seems to have validity) or for SS.

Evaluation and Staging

Clinical assessment
A full physical examination is important for evaluation with emphasis on the skin and lymph nodes.

Table 1
Clinicopathologic algorithm for the diagnosis of early MF

Criteria	Major (2 Points)	Minor (1 Point Each)
Clinical Persistent and/or progressive patches/ thin plaques plus 1. Non–sun-exposed location 2. Size/shape variation 3. Poikiloderma	Any two	Any one
Histopathologic Superficial lymphoid infiltrate plus 1. Epidermotropism 2. Atypia	Both	Either
Molecular/biological Clonal TCR gene rearrangement	—	Any
Immunopathologic 1. <50% CD2$^+$, 3$^+$, 5$^+$ T cells 2. <10% CD7$^+$ T cells 3. Epidermal/dermal discordance of CD2, CD3, CD5 or CD7	—	Any one

Adapted from Pimpinelli N, Olsen EA, Santucci M, et al. Defining early mycosis fungoides. J Am Acad Dermatol 2005;53:1054.

The type of skin lesions and percent BSA covered by the skin lesions should be noted and will establish the T stage (**Table 2**). The T stage has independent prognostic significance[12,13] as does patch versus plaque lesions.[14] All peripheral or central lymph node groups should be assessed for any that are enlarged or abnormal (firm or fixed), and any lymph node 1.5 cm or greater on examination should be further assessed by imaging and biopsy.

Blood work

The basic blood tests to perform in suspected MF/SS include a complete blood count (CBC) with differential, complete metabolic panel and lactate dehydrogenase (LDH). In addition, there are several disease-specific tests to help determine whether there is any significant blood tumor burden. A Sézary cell prep includes determining the percentage of Sézary cells in the buffy coat of the CBC. Sézary cells are lymphocytes with hyperconvoluted nuclei that may also be larger than normal lymphocytes; they are not specific to MF or SS and can be seen in small numbers in healthy individuals or patients with inflammatory skin

disease.[15,16] Although a subjective test, the Sézary cell prep is, nonetheless, useful as there are situations where the typical cell surface markers are lacking on the malignant lymphocytes and the abnormal cell population would otherwise be missed on flow cytometry. Flow cytometry offers an objective test of potential blood involvement and is particularly useful when focused on those parameters that have been found to be associated with blood involvement in MF and SS (ie, CD4/CD8 ratio, CD4+CD26− and CD4+CD7− lymphocytes).

The percentage and absolute numbers of both Sézary cells and abnormal cells by flow cytometry are used to determine blood staging, which is divided into B_0, B_1, and B_2 (**Table 2**). B_0 is essentially normal, and B_2 indicates a significant blood tumor burden that moves a patient to a stage equal to nodal lymphoma. The absolute number of abnormal lymphocytes is a mathematical computation of the absolute number of lymphocytes multiplied by either the percent of Sézary cells/100 or the percent abnormal cells by flow cytometry/100.

A blood TCR GR clonality study is important to perform to help assess B status. B_2 blood involvement, according to the ISCL/EORTC consensus criteria, must also include a clone of the TCR GR in the blood. Although the guidelines did not specifically require the clone in the blood to match that of the skin, this is more or less understood that it should. Left unsaid is what to do when a patient has a high Sézary cell count or abnormal cells on flow cytometry but a different clone in the blood than in the skin. There are T-cell clones seen in the blood that increase with age and would not be expected to match the malignant clone in the skin. The author's personal approach is to note B_0-B_2 based on the total abnormal lymphocyte number and separate notation for clonality for all B ratings including +/+ for a positive clone in the blood that matches the same clone as in skin, +/− for a positive clone in the blood but a different or absent clone in the skin, −/+ for no clone in the blood and a positive clone in the skin, and −/− for no clone in either blood or skin. The same method of testing for clonality in the blood should be done as that performed in the skin.

The specific designation of SS, as noted by the ISCL and USCLC,[17] implies that a patient has erythroderma and B_2 blood involvement with a positive clone.

Radiology

In cases when the skin examination would be characterized as T_1, there are no abnormal

Table 2
ISCL/EORTC/USCLC revisions to the TNMB classification of MF/SS

TNMB Classification	Description of TNMB
Skin	
T_1	Limited patches, papules, and/or plaques covering <10% of the skin surface; may further stratify into T_{1a} (patch only) vs T_{1b} (plaque +/− patch)
T_2	Patches, papules, or plaques covering ≥10% of the skin surface; may further stratify into T_{2a} (patch only) vs T_{2b} (plaque +/− patch)
T_3	One or more tumors (≥1 cm diameter)
T_4	Confluence of erythema covering ≥80% BSA
Node	
N_0	No clinically abnormal peripheral or central lymph nodes; biopsy not required
N_1	Clinically abnormal peripheral or central lymph nodes; histopathology Dutch grade 1 or NCI LN_{0-2}
N_{1a}	Clone negative
N_{1b}	Clone positive
N_2	Clinically abnormal peripheral or central lymph nodes; histopathology Dutch grade 2 or NCI LN_3
N_{2a}	Clone negative
N_{2b}	Clone positive
N_3	Clinically abnormal peripheral or central lymph nodes; histopathology Dutch grade 3–4 or NCI LN_4 Clone positive or negative
N_x	Clinically abnormal peripheral or central lymph nodes, no histologic confirmation
Visceral	
M_0	No visceral organ involvement
M_1	Visceral involvement (must have pathology confirmation, and organ involved should be specified)
Blood	
B_0	Absence of significant blood involvement: ≤5% of peripheral blood lymphocytes are atypical (Sézary cells); <15% CD4+CD7− or CD4+CD26− cells; or <250/ul Sézary cells, CD4+CD7− or CD4+CD26− cells
B_{0a}	Clone negative
B_{0b}	Clone positive
B_1	Low blood tumor burden: >5% of peripheral blood lymphocytes are atypical (Sézary) cells greater than B_0 criteria but does not meet the criteria of B_2
B_{1a}	Clone negative
B_{1b}	Clone positive
B_2	High blood tumor burden: >1000/uL Sézary cells, CD4+CD7− or CD4+CD26− cells; or >40% CD4+CD7-cells; or >30% CD4+CD26- cells; or CD4/CD8 >10; with positive clone

Adapted from Olsen EA, Whittaker S, Kim YH, et al. Clinical endpoints and response criteria in mycosis fungoides and Sézary syndrome: a consensus statement of the International Society for Cutaneous Lymphomas (ISCL), the United States Cutaneous Lymphoma Consortium (USCLC), and the Cutaneous Lymphoma Task Force of the European Organization of Research and Treatment of Cancer (EORTC). J Clin Oncol 2011;29:2598–607; and *From* Olsen E, Vonderheid E, Pimpinelli N, et al. Revisions of the staging and classification of mycosis fungoides and Sézary syndrome: a proposal of the International Society for Cutaneous Lymphomas (ISCL) and the Cutaneous Lymphoma Task Force of the European Organization of Research and Treatment of Cancer (EORTC). Blood 2007;110:1715.

nodes on physical examination and the blood staging is B_0, only a chest radiograph is recommended to screen for visceral disease. For all other cases, imaging is recommended to complete staging. Computed tomography (CT) scans of the chest, abdomen, and pelvis +/− neck are recommended to assess visceral and nodal disease: contrast enhances the ability to size the nodes and is preferred unless there is renal impairment or contrast allergy. PET scans are not specifically recommended in MF/SS, although some reports suggest they add staging accuracy.[18] MRI may be used instead of CT but is usually reserved for cases where there is a history of contrast allergy.

Biopsies

Liver and spleen involvement can usually be designated as lymphoma by imaging studies alone, but other solid organs require a biopsy for confirmation. Bone marrow (BM) biopsy in MF is not generally recommended unless there is an unexplained hematologic abnormality exclusive of the abnormal lymphocytic population; if performed, a positive BM biopsy would not be considered visceral involvement if B_2 blood involvement already exists.

Any lymph node that is 1.5 cm or greater in the short axis would be considered suspicious of lymphoma and an excisional biopsy versus a core biopsy or fine-needle aspirate (FNA) recommended. In contradistinction to the other cutaneous lymphomas, there is a gradation of involvement histologically in the lymph node of MF or SS that falls short of lymphoma (so-called dermatopathic lymph node, LN1–LN3), which depends on the architectural features of the lymph node, features that cannot be discriminated from frank lymphoma by core biopsy or FNA. The lymph node or N staging is detailed in **Table 2**. The exception to an excisional biopsy is if the only lymph node that is enlarged is a central one that would require significant surgical risk to remove or if there is only

Table 3
ISCL/EORTC revisions to the staging of MF/SS

Stage	T	N	M	B
IA	1	0	0	0, 1
IB	2	0	0	0, 1
IIA	1–2	1, 2	0	0, 1
IIB	3	0–2	0	0, 1
IIIA	4	0–2	0	0
IIIB	4	0–2	0	1
IVA$_1$	1–4	0–2	0	2
IVA$_2$	1–4	3	0	0–2
IVB	1–4	0–3	1	0–2

From Olsen E, Vonderheid E, Pimpinelli N, et al. Revisions to the staging and classification of mycosis fungoides and Sézary syndrome: a proposal of the International Society for Cutaneous Lymphomas (ISCL) and the Cutaneous Lymphoma Task Force of the European Organization of Research and Treatment of Cancer (EORTC). Blood 2007;110:1719.

Table 4
Modified severity weighted assessment tool

Body Region (% BSA)	Patch[a]	Plaque[b]	Tumor[c]
Head (7%)			
Neck (2%)			
Anterior trunk (13%)			
Arms (8%)			
Forearms (6%)			
Hands (5%)			
Posterior trunk (13%)			
Buttocks (5%)			
Thighs (19%)			
Legs (14%)			
Feet (7%)			
Groin (1%)			
Subtotal of lesion BSA			
Weighting factor	1	2	4
Subtotal lesion BSA × weighting factor			
mSWAT score = summation of each column line in final row above			

[a] Patch = any size lesion without significant elevation above the surrounding uninvolved skin or induration;
[b] plaque = any size lesion that is elevated or indurated;
[c] tumor = any solid or nodular lesion ≥1 cm in diameter with evidence of deep infiltration in the skin and/or vertical growth.
From Olsen EA, Whittaker S, Kim YH, et al. Clinical endpoints and response criteria in mycosis fungoides and Sézary syndrome: a consensus statement of the International Society for Cutaneous Lymphomas (ISCL), the United States Cutaneous Lymphoma Consortium (USCLC), and the Cutaneous Lymphoma Task Force of the European Organization of Research and Treatment of Cancer (EORTC). J Clin Oncol 2011;29:2598–607.

a need to establish a similar process to that in the skin or blood; in that case, a core biopsy with flow cytometry and clonal TCR GR studies may suffice. If any enlarged nodes are not biopsied, the designation in staging should be Nx.

Staging

Once the individual classification of TNMB has been determined, then these can be rolled into the staging system for MF and SS (**Table 3**). In a departure from how the term staging is used with other NHLs, the TNMB characterization of stage in MF/SS can be noted as initial as well as maximum and current stage. It is not uncommon for patients with MF to present with $T_2N_0M_0B_0$ (stage IB) disease, progress to $T_3N_0M_0B_0$ (stage IIB) disease, be treated, and then currently have $T_1N_0M_0B_0$ (stage IA) disease. Without the communication of all these TNMB classifications (stages), especially in consideration of a clinical trial, a given patient's risk for progressive disease would not be fully communicated or information generated to help determine best treatments.

Response Assessment

It is important to note how the response to a given treatment is assessed as most papers in this issue relate to treatment. The methods in clinical trials of MF/SS since 2001 have used either the Severity Weighted Assessment Tool (SWAT) or modified SWAT (mSWAT) score, which involves determining the percentage BSA covered by patch, plaque, or tumor of MF/SS, then multiplying each lesion BSA by a factor that gives gradations of weight to patch versus plaque versus tumor and summing these scores (**Table 4**).[19,20] The change in SWAT or mSWAT from the beginning of treatment can be used to assess overall response. Complete response (CR) in the skin is defined as complete clinical clearing, partial response (PR) as 50% to 99% clearing, and objective response (OR) as the combination of CR and PR (**Table 5**).[20] There are scoring systems to assess local response in the skin to agents applied to limited BSAs, but agents used in this manner are not able to prevent new lesions from occurring outside the treated areas. There is a global scoring system that addresses the entire TMNB spectrum (**Table 6**) which is heavily weighted to the response in skin[20]; this has only recently been developed, and most treatment studies in the past have only addressed the response in the skin.

Table 5 Response in skin in MF and SS	
Complete response	100% clearance of skin lesions. If there is any question of postInflammatory changes or xerotic skin vs residual disease, confirmation of clearing is also necessary in a representative biopsy or biopsies. If a biopsy of questionable residual disease is positive (meets the criteria of early MF[9]), then the response should be labeled as partial response.
Partial response	50%–99% clearance of skin disease from baseline without new tumors (T_3) in patients with T_1, T_2 or T_4 only skin disease.
Stable disease	<25% increase to <50% clearance in skin disease from baseline without new tumors (T_3) in patients with T_1, T_2 or T_4 only skin disease.
Progressive disease	≥25% increase in skin disease from baseline or new tumors (T_3) in patients with T_1, T_2, or T_4 only skin disease.
Relapse	Any disease recurrence in those with complete response

From Olsen EA, Whittaker S, Kim YH, et al. Clinical endpoints and response criteria in mycosis fungoides and Sézary syndrome: a consensus statement of the International Society for Cutaneous Lymphomas (ISCL), the United States Cutaneous Lymphoma Consortium (USCLC), and the Cutaneous Lymphoma Task Force of the European Organization of Research and Treatment of Cancer (EORTC). J Clin Oncol 2011;29:2598–607.

Table 6 Global response score for MF and SS				
Global	Skin	Nodes	Blood	Viscera
CR	CR	All categories have CR/NI.		
PR	CR	All categories do not have a CR/NI, and no category has a PD.		
PR	PR	No category has a PD and if any category is involved at baseline, at least one has a CR or PR.		
SD	PR	No category has a PD and if any category is involved at baseline, no CR or PR in any.		
SD	SD	CR, PR, SD in any category and no category has a PD.		
PD	PD in any category.			
Relapse	Relapse in any category.			

Abbreviations: NI, noninvolved; PD, progressive disease; SD, stable disease.

From Olsen EA, Whittaker S, Kim YH, et al. Clinical endpoints and response criteria in mycosis fungoides and Sézary syndrome: a consensus statement of the International Society for Cutaneous Lymphomas (ISCL), the United States Cutaneous Lymphoma Consortium (USCLC), and the Cutaneous Lymphoma Task Force of the European Organization of Research and Treatment of Cancer (EORTC). J Clin Oncol 2011;29:2598–607.

NON-MYCOSIS FUNGOIDES AND NON-SÉZARY SYNDROME CUTANEOUS T-CELL LYMPHOMAS

Incidence and Prognosis

The most common types of the non-MF/non-SS CTCLs are the two CD30+ lymphoproliferative disorders (LPDs) (ie, primary cutaneous anaplastic large cell lymphoma [PCALCL] and lymphomatoid papulosis [LyP]). These CD30+ LPDs represent the most common differential diagnosis for MF. The prognosis for PCALCL, which, by its definition, excludes any extracutaneous disease at diagnosis, is excellent with treatment but like MF/SS, there is no cure currently, and continued treatment and vigilance must be used to prevent internal spread. The prognosis for LyP is excellent, with the potential for any internal spread being extremely rare.[21] LyP not uncommonly occurs with MF/SS and is discriminated from MF by its presentation (usually papules of a self-remitting nature) and biopsy findings consistent with one of 5 subtypes (see the article by Kempf in this issue).

The other types of non-MF/non-SS CTCLs are rare and also much more concerning in their prognosis compared with the CD30+ LPDs. Many present with tumors with the main differential being other primary CTCLs, primary CBCLs, systemic T- or B-cell lymphomas with skin metastasis, or even pseudolymphomas. Histologic methods for assessing these other subtypes are discussed further in Dr Kempf's article in this issue. Readers are directed to publications on each of these cutaneous T-cell tumor subtypes for further specifics on prognosis and treatment.

Diagnosis

Like MF/SS, diagnosis of the CD30+ LPDs begins with a skin biopsy; but even more importantly than in MF, the clinical history is key to the final diagnosis. Both PCALCL and LyP are characterized histologically by CD30+ T cells (typically CD4+) that have at least 25% of the lymphocyte population defined as large cells.[21] The latter may also be seen in patients with MF with so-called LCT, usually in patients with tumor stage disease. In this case, the diagnosis of MF with LCT versus PCALCL is made by the type of other lesions present: patients with MF typically also have patches/plaques that have classic histology for MF, which is absent in PCALCL. LyP lesions are small and self-remitting, whereas MF does not spontaneously improve; PCALC lesions are generally larger than LyP lesions and more persistent. However, when the percentage of large cells exceeds 75%, the diagnosis is more likely PCALCL than MF.[21] The histologic findings and clinical

parameters of PCALCL and LyP are discussed further in articles by Drs Kempf and Hughey in this issue.

Evaluation

Clinical assessment

Like MF and SS, a full physical examination of patients with possible non-MF/non-SS CTCL is important at baseline. Unlike MF/SS, any lymph node that is 1 cm or greater would be of concern in these patients. Peripheral or central lymph nodes can be further evaluated by core biopsy or FNA with flow and TCR GR clonality studies, because, in contradistinction to that in MF and SS, there is no equivalent to dermatopathic nodes in these other CTCLs which would require an excisional biopsy to differentiate from frank lymphoma.

Blood work

The basic blood tests to perform in suspected non-MF/non-SS CTCL include a CBC with differential, complete metabolic panel, and LDH. Because there is no blood tumor burden with these conditions, the only reason to do a Sézary cell prep or blood flow cytometry would be to exclude MF/SS in cases where the diagnosis is hazy. BM biopsy is not recommended in LyP, and guidelines on its use in the other CTCLs are not clear.

Radiology

PET/CT is recommended for the assessment of the non-MF and non-SS CTCLs and all CBCLs.

Biopsies

Any abnormality noted on imaging should be further assessed, and either a core biopsy or FNA of lymph nodes or visceral organs suspected of lymphoma should suffice. If there is any confirmation of extracutaneous disease, these CTCLs would no longer be classified as primary cutaneous but rather as a systemic lymphoma. However, in a confusing area, the literature allows for patients with PCALCL and a single regional lymph node to remain characterized as PCALCL.

Staging

The staging of non-MF/non-SS CTCLs is different than MF and SS and is the same as the primary CBCLs (**Table 7, Fig. 1**). The major difference from MF/SS relates to the characterization of the skin lesions according to size and location relative to lymph node drainage regions versus the type of skin lesions and percentage BSA covered used to classify MF/SS. The staging of LyP defies capture by current staging systems as the lesions are in a constant state of flux and occur diffusely over the body surface.

Table 7
ISCL/EORTC TNM classification of cutaneous lymphomas other than MF/SS

Classification		Description
Skin (T)	T1	Solitary skin involvement
	T1a	Solitary lesion <5 cm diameter
	T1b	Solitary lesion ≥5 cm diameter
	T2	Regional skin involvement: multiple lesions limited to 1 body region or 2 contiguous body regions
	T2a	All disease encompassing a <15 cm diameter circular area
	T2b	All disease encompassing a 15 to ≤30 cm diameter circular area
	T2c	All disease encompassing a ≥30 cm diameter circular area
	T3	Generalized skin involvement
	T3a	Multiple lesions involving 2 noncontiguous body regions
	T3b	Multiple lesions involving ≥3 body regions
Lymph nodes (N)	N0	No clinical or pathologic lymph node involvement
	N1	Involvement of one peripheral or central lymph node region that drains an area of current or prior skin involvement
	N2	Involvement of ≥2 peripheral or central lymph node regions or involvement of any lymph node region that does not drain in an area of current or prior skin involvement
	N3	Involvement of central lymph nodes
Viscera (M)	M0	No evidence of extracutaneous non–lymph node disease
	M1	Extracutaneous non–lymph node disease present

T= any type of skin lesion.
Adapted from Kim YH, Willemze R, Pimpinelli N, et al. TNM classification system for primary cutaneous lymphomas other than mycosis fungoides and Sézary syndrome: a proposal of the International Society for Cutaneous Lymphomas (ISCL) and the Cutaneous Lymphoma Task Force of the European Organization of Research and Treatment of Cancer (EORTC). Blood 2007;110(2):480.

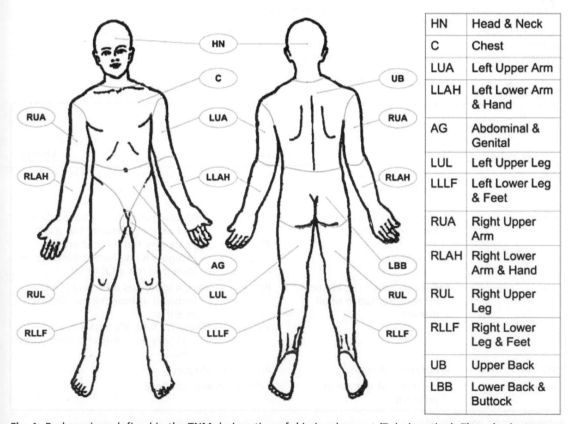

HN	Head & Neck
C	Chest
LUA	Left Upper Arm
LLAH	Left Lower Arm & Hand
AG	Abdominal & Genital
LUL	Left Upper Leg
LLLF	Left Lower Leg & Feet
RUA	Right Upper Arm
RLAH	Right Lower Arm & Hand
RUL	Right Upper Leg
RLLF	Right Lower Leg & Feet
UB	Upper Back
LBB	Lower Back & Buttock

Fig. 1. Body regions defined in the TNM designation of skin involvement (T designation). These body areas are based on regional lymph node drainage patterns. (*From* Kim YH, Willemze R, Pimpinelli N, et al. TNM classification system for primary cutaneous lymphomas other than mycosis fungoides and Sézary syndrome: a proposal of the International Society for Cutaneous Lymphomas (ISCL) and the Cutaneous Lymphoma Task Force of the European Organization of Research and Treatment of Cancer (EORTC). Blood 2007;110(2):479–84.)

Response Assessment

There is no mSWAT equivalent for the non-MF/non-SS CTCLs, although in many cases, the mSWAT for skin would suffice. CR, PR, and OR in the skin are as defined for MF/SS. A global scoring system has been published for LyP (**Table 8**) and PCALCL (**Table 9**) with potential for the latter to be used for other non-MF/non-SS PCLs.

Table 8
LyP response in skin

CR	100% clearance of skin lesions
PR	50%–99% clearance of skin disease from baseline without new larger and persistent nodules/tumors[b] in those with papular disease only
SD	<50% increase to <50% clearance in skin disease from baseline without new larger and persistent nodules/tumors in those with papular disease only
IDA[a]	>50% increase in skin disease from baseline without larger and persistent nodules/tumors[b]
PD[c]	1. Occurrence of larger and persistent nodules/tumors if not present before 2. Extracutaneous spread
Relapse	Any disease recurrence in those with CR

Persistent lesions are defined as lesions that do not show spontaneous regression after 12 weeks.
Abbreviations: IDA, increased disease activity; PD, progressive disease; SD, stable disease.
[a] The term *increased disease activity* indicates an increased number of papulonodular lesions (<2 cm), which do not imply impaired prognosis.
[b] Larger lesions are defined as greater than 2 cm in diameter.
[c] Whichever criterion appears first.
Adapted from Kempf W, Pfaltz K, Vermeer MH, et al. EORTC, ISCL, and USCLC consensus recommendations for the treatment of primary cutaneous CD30-positive lymphoproliferative disorders: lymphomatoid papulosis and primary cutaneous anaplastic large-cell lymphoma. Blood 2011;118(15):4024–35.

Table 9
Global disease response score in PCALCL

Global Score	Definition	Skin	Nodes	Viscera
CR	Complete disappearance of all clinical evidence of disease	CR	Both categories have CR or NI.	
PR	Partial response of measurable disease	CR	Both categories do not have a CR/NI, and neither category has a PD.	
		PR	No category has a PD; if either category is involved at baseline, at least one has a CR or PR.	
SD	Failure to attain CR, PR, or PD representative of all disease	PR	No category has a PD and if either involved at baseline, no CR or PR in either.	
		SD	There is CR/NI, PR, or SD in any category and neither category has a PD.	
PD	Progressive disease	PD in any category		
Relapse	Recurrence of disease in prior CR	Relapse in any category		

Abbreviation: NI, noninvolved.
Adapted from Kempf W, Pfaltz K, Vermeer MH, et al. EORTC, ISCL, and USCLC consensus recommendations for the treatment of primary cutaneous CD30-positive lymphoproliferative disorders: lymphomatoid papulosis and primary cutaneous anaplastic large-cell lymphoma. Blood 2011;118(15):4024–35.

CUTANEOUS B-CELL LYMPHOMAS
Incidence

There are 3 main types of primary CBCL (ie, primary cutaneous marginal zone lymphoma [MZL], follicular center cell lymphoma (FCCL), and diffuse large B-cell lymphoma, leg type). Each usually presents with infiltrated plaques, nodules, or tumors but each subtype has its own histology, typical location, potential for progression, and current treatment algorithm. This is discussed in greater detail in the articles by Drs Kempf and Pinter-Brown elsewhere in this issue.

Diagnosis

Like the CTCLs, the CBCLs can be diagnosed by a combination of H&E, immunophenotyping, and B-cell clonality studies (immunoglobulin heavy or light chain rearrangement) performed on representative skin lesions. The diagnosis hinges much more on positive clonality than the T-cell lymphomas, and there may be difficulty in distinguishing these from pseudolymphomas, which also typically present clinically with thick plaques or tumors. The presence of an abnormal lymph node may lead to a final diagnosis: however if positive for lymphoma, patients would be viewed as having a systemic lymphoma with skin manifestations versus a PCL.

Evaluation

Clinical assessment

A full physical examination is necessary with any lymph node that is 1 cm or greater In diameter considered abnormal.

Blood work

The basic blood tests to perform in primary CBCL include a CBC with differential, complete metabolic panel, and LDH. There is no leukemic counterpart to the CBCLs as there is with MF/SS. An evaluation for paraprotein may be done in PCMZL.

Radiology

PET/CT is recommended for assessment of all CBCLs.

Biopsies

Any abnormality should be further assessed and either a core biopsy or FNA for suspected lymph nodes or visceral involvement would suffice. BM biopsy is required in diffuse large B-cell lymphoma, leg type, should be considered in PCFCCL and is not required in PCMZL. If there is any confirmation of extracutaneous disease, patients would no longer be classified as having a primary CBCL but rather as having a systemic B-cell lymphoma.

Staging

The staging of CBCLs is as with the non-MF/non-SS CTCLs (see **Table 7**) with emphasis on the characterization of the skin lesions according to size and location relative to the lymph node drainage regions.

Response Assessment

CR, PR, and OR in the skin are as previously noted. A global scoring system has been devised but not yet published although the one used for PCALCL could be utilized in the interim.

SUMMARY

The cutaneous lymphomas are a heterogeneous group of NHLs that are concerning for multiple reasons: (1) the incidence is on the rise, (2) there is no cure with current existing therapies, (3) they often require life-long treatment with systemic medications in order to prevent progression and to maintain quality of life and (4) some types and some stages of all types of cutaneous lymphoma have a very poor prognosis. The prognosis may be best related to maximum TNM or TNMB classification and treatment ideally planned based on both maximum and current TNM(B) classification; this is not currently considered in treatment algorithms and is something a registry will be able to sort out. The collective efforts of investigators in the clinical and basic research realm and a national registry of all patients with cutaneous lymphoma give patients the best chance of finding a cure for these rare and uncommon cancers.

REFERENCES

1. Olsen E, Vonderheid E, Pimpinelli N, et al. Revisions of the staging and classification of mycosis fungoides and Sézary syndrome: a proposal of the International Society for Cutaneous Lymphomas (ISCL) and the Cutaneous Lymphoma Task Force of the European Organization of Research and Treatment of Cancer (EORTC). Blood 2007;110: 1713–22.

2. Hwang S, Janik JE, Jaffe ES, et al. Mycosis fungoides and Sézary syndrome. Lancet 2008;371: 945–57.

3. Groves FD, Linet MS, Travis LB, et al. Cancer surveillance series: non-Hodgkin's lymphoma incidence by histologic subtype in the US from 1978 through 1995. J Natl Cancer Inst 2000;92:1240–51.

4. Bradford PT, Sevesa SS, Anderson WF, et al. Cutaneous lymphoma incidence patterns in the United States: a population-based study of 3884 cases. Blood 2009;113:5064–73.

5. Willemze R, Jaffe E, Burg G, et al. WHO-EORTC classification for cutaneous lymphomas. Blood 2005;105:3768–85.

6. Campo E, Swerdlow SH, Harris NL, et al. The 2008 WHO classification of lymphoid neoplasms and beyond: evolving concepts and practical applications. Blood 2011;117:5019–32.

7. Korgavkar K, Weinstock MA. Changing incidence trends of cutaneous B-cell lymphoma. J Invest Dermatol 2014;134:840–2.

8. Criscione VD, Weinstock MA. Incidence of cutaneous T-cell lymphoma in the United States, 1973–2002. Arch Dermatol 2007;143:854–9.

9. Wilson LD, Hinds GA, Yu JB. Age, race, sex, stage and incidence of cutaneous lymphoma. Clin Lymphoma Myeloma Leuk 2012;12:291–6.

10. Burg G, Kempf W, Cozzio A, et al. WHO/EORTC classification of cutaneous lymphomas 2008: histological and molecular aspects. J Cutan Pathol 2005;32:647–74.

11. Pimpinelli N, Olsen EA, Santucci M, et al. Defining early mycosis fungoides. J Am Acad Dermatol 2005;53:1053–63.

12. Kim YH, Willemze R, Pimpinelli N, et al. TNM classification system for primary cutaneous lymphomas other than mycosis fungoides and Sézary syndrome: a proposal of the International Society for Cutaneous Lymphomas (ISCL) and the Cutaneous Lymphoma Task Force of the European Organization of Research and Treatment of Cancer (EORTC). Blood 2007;110:479–84.

13. Zackheim HS, Amin S, Kashani-Sabet M, et al. Prognosis in cutaneous T-cell lymphoma by skin stage: long-term survival in 489 patients. J Am Acad Dermatol 1999;40:418–25.

14. Talpur R, Singh L, Daulat S, et al. Long term outcomes of 1263 patients with mycosis fungoides and Sézary syndrome from 1982–2009. Clin Cancer Res 2012;18(18):10.

15. Vonderheid EC, Bernengo MG, Burg G, et al. Update on erythrodermic cutaneous T-cell lymphoma: report of the International Society for Cutaneous Lymphomas. J Am Acad Dermatol 2002;46:95–106.

16. Vonderheid EC, Pena J, Nowell P. Sézary cell counts in erythrodermic cutaneous T-cell lymphoma: implications for prognosis and staging. Leuk Lymphoma 2006;47:1841–56.

17. Olsen EA, Rook AH, Zic J, et al. Sézary syndrome: evaluation, immunopathogenesis, literature review of therapeutic options and recommendations for therapy by the United States Cutaneous Lymphoma Consortium (USCLC). J Am Acad Dermatol 2011; 64(2):352–404.

18. Tsai EY, Taur A, Espinosa L, et al. Staging accuracy in mycosis fungoides and Sézary syndrome using integrated positron emission tomography and computed tomography. Arch Dermatol 2006;142: 577–84.

19. Olsen E, Duvic M, Frankel A, et al. Pivotal phase III trial of two dose levels of DAB389IL-2 (Ontak™) for the treatment of cutaneous T-cell lymphoma. J Clin Oncol 2001;19:376–88.

20. Olsen EA, Whittaker S, Kim YH, et al. Clinical endpoints and response criteria in mycosis fungoides and Sézary syndrome: a consensus statement of the International Society for Cutaneous Lymphomas (ISCL), the United States Cutaneous Lymphoma Consortium (USCLC), and the Cutaneous Lymphoma Task Force of the European Organization of Research and Treatment of Cancer (EORTC). J Clin Oncol 2011;29:2598–607.

21. Kempf W, Pfaltz K, Vermeer MH, et al. European Organization of Research and Treatment of Cancer (EORTC), International Society for Cutaneous Lymphomas (ISCL), and the United States Cutaneous Lymphoma Consortium consensus recommendations for the treatment of primary cutaneous CD30 positive lymphoproliferative disorders: lymphomatoid papulosis and primary cutaneous anaplastic large-cell lymphoma. Blood 2011;118(15):4024–35.

Pathologic Diagnosis of Cutaneous Lymphomas

Werner Kempf, MD[a,b,*], Christina Mitteldorf, MD[c]

KEYWORDS

- Lymphoma • Lymphoproliferative • Cutaneous • Skin • Diagnosis • Clinicopathological correlation
- T cell • B cell

KEY POINTS

- Clinicopathologic correlation is an essential element in the diagnostic approach to cutaneous lymphomas.
- Cutaneous lymphomas show overlapping histologic and immunophenotypic features, but can differ significantly in their course and prognosis.
- Monoclonality does not necessarily indicate malignancy. Lack of monoclonality does not exclude the diagnosis of cutaneous lymphoma.

INTRODUCTION

Primary cutaneous lymphomas (CLs) comprise a heterogeneous group of lymphocytic neoplasms with a broad spectrum of clinical, histologic, immunophenotypical, and genetic features (**Box 1**).[1–3] The histopathological examination plays an essential role and is often the starting point in the diagnostic workup of CLs. The classification of CLs follows the current World Health Organization (WHO) classification (4th edition, 2008), which is widely accepted by hematopathologists and dermatopathologists.[3] The WHO classification of the tumors of hematopoietic and lymphoid tissues follows the multiparameter approach by defining lymphomas according to their clinical, histopathological, immunophenotypic, and genetic features as well as the side of primary manifestation, which was originally introduced by the Revised European-American Lymphoma classification (REAL).[4,5]

This aim of this review is to provide an approach based on the growth patterns, cytomorphology, phenotypic, and genetic features for primary CLs and to emphasize the impact of clinicopathological correlation.

Pathologic Approach

Histopathologically, various *growth patterns* can be distinguished. Some are more prevalent in certain forms of CLs, whereas others are found throughout the entire spectrum of CLs. The growth patterns and cytomorphology provide first diagnostic hints. For example, epidermotropic infiltrates of small to medium-sized lymphocytes are most commonly found in cutaneous T-cell lymphomas (CTCLs), whereas dense dermal lymphocytic infiltrates, of variable size and cytomorphology, are commonly present in cutaneous B-cell lymphomas (CBCLs).

For practical reasons, 6 major patterns can be distinguished in CLs: epidermotropic, nodular, diffuse, subcutaneous, angiocentric/angiodestructive, and intravascular. Among each growth pattern, additional histopathological features may

---

Disclosure Statement: The authors have no conflicts of interest and no source of funding in the article to declare.

a Kempf und Pfaltz Histologische Diagnostik, Seminarstrasse 1, Zürich CH-8042, Switzerland; b Department of Dermatology, University Hospital Zürich, Gloriastrasse 31 Zürich CH-8091, Switzerland; c Department of Dermatology, HELIOS Kliniken GmbH, Senator-Brawn-Allee 33, 31135 Hildesheim, Germany
* Corresponding author. Kempf und Pfaltz Histologische Diagnostik, Seminarstrasse 1, Zürich CH-8042, Switzerland.
E-mail address: werner.kempf@kempf-pfaltz.ch

Dermatol Clin 33 (2015) 655–681
http://dx.doi.org/10.1016/j.det.2015.05.002
0733-8635/15/$ – see front matter © 2015 Elsevier Inc. All rights reserved.

Box 1
World Health Organization classification for lymphoid neoplasms

MATURE T-CELL AND NK-CELL NEOPLASMS

Mycosis fungoides (MF)

   MF variants and subtypes:

      Folliculotropic MF

      Pagetoid reticulosis

      Granulomatous slack skin

Sézary syndrome

Adult T-cell leukemia/lymphoma

Primary cutaneous CD30+ T-cell lymphoproliferative disorders

   Primary cutaneous anaplastic large cell lymphoma

   Lymphomatoid papulosis

Subcutaneous panniculitis-like T-cell lymphoma

Extranodal NK-/T-cell lymphoma, nasal type

Primary cutaneous peripheral T-cell lymphoma

   Rare subtypes:

- Primary cutaneous CD8+ aggressive epidermotropic cytotoxic T-cell lymphoma (provisional)
- Primary cutaneous γ/δ T-cell lymphoma
- Primary cutaneous CD4+ small/medium T-cell lymphoma (provisional entity)

   Primary cutaneous peripheral T-cell lymphoma, unspecified

MATURE B-CELL NEOPLASMS

Extranodal marginal zone lymphoma of mucosa-associated lymphoid tissue (MALT lymphoma)

Primary cutaneous follicle center lymphoma

Diffuse large B-cell lymphoma, NOS

   Primary cutaneous diffuse large B-cell lymphoma, leg type

   Primary cutaneous diffuse large B-cell lymphoma, others

Intravascular large B-cell lymphoma

Note: This list is mainly limited to cutaneous lymphomas in the WHO classification.
Data from Swerdlow SH, Campo E, Harris NL, et al. WHO classification of tumours of haematopoietic and lymphoid tissues. 4th edition. Lyon (France): IARC Press; 2008.

---

be identified, such as folliculotropic and syringo-tropic infiltrates or granulomatous features.

- Epidermotropic infiltrates are most commonly found in CTCLs, particularly in their initial disease stage (eg, mycosis fungoides [MF], patch, and plaque stage), throughout the entire disease evolution like in Sézary syndrome (SS), or in cutaneous CD8[+] aggressive epidermotropic cytotoxic T-cell lymphoma (AETCL).
- Nodular and diffuse infiltrates are a hallmark of progressive forms of CTCLs (eg, MF tumor stage; peripheral T-cell lymphoma [PTCL] unspecified) as well as CBCLs.

- The subcutaneous growth pattern is typically found in subcutaneous lymphomas, including the subcutaneous panniculitis-like T-cell lymphoma (SPTCL) with expression of T-cell receptor (TCR) α/β and the subcutaneous form of γ/δ T-cell lymphoma, but may rarely be observed as rare variants in other CTCL and CBCL forms.
- Angiocentric and angiodestructive (ie, angioinvasive) infiltrates are characteristic for aggressive T- and T-/natural killer (NK)-cell lymphomas, such as extranodal T-/NK-cell lymphoma, nasal type, and cutaneous γ/δ T-cell lymphoma. Exceptions to the rule are indolent or low-malignant forms of CD30+ T-cell lymphoproliferations as lymphomatoid

papulosis (LyP) type E and the angioinvasive variant of primary cutaneous anaplastic large-cell lymphoma (PCALCL).

- The intravascular growth pattern is pathognomonic for intravascular T- and B-cell lymphoma.

Cytomorphologically, small, medium-sized, and large lymphocytes can be distinguished with variable degrees of nuclear pleomorphism. In B-cell lymphomas, small lymphocytes with lymphoplasmacytoid differentiation, monozytoid B cells, as well as tumor cells with centrocyte-like differentiation can be distinguished from tumor cells resembling centroblast, immunoblasts, and plasmablasts. Noteworthy, an immunoblastic differentiation can also be seen in some form of CTCLs, especially in PCALCL, MF tumor stage, and cutaneous PTCLs, unspecified.

Phenotyping

Immunohistochemistry allows assigning the tumor cells to distinct subsets of T, B, NK/T, or NK cells, including their functional subsets (eg, follicular helper T cells or regulatory T cells). For some forms of CLs, the phenotypic features represent essential diagnostic criteria. For example, in SPTCLs, by definition, the tumor cells require expression of the α/β chain of the TCR. Certain phenotypic and genetic markers not only are of diagnostic importance but also have a prognostic implication (eg, loss of 9p21 in diffuse large B-cell lymphoma, leg-type) or represent therapeutic targets (eg, CD30, anaplastic lymphoma kinase [ALK]/p80). These markers should be specifically mentioned in the pathology report.

Genotyping

CLs are considered to represent monoclonal proliferation of T or B cells displaying identical rearrangement of TCR genes or the genes of the heavy chain of immunoglobulins (IgH). Therefore, clonality assays are mostly based on polymerase chain reaction (PCR) or Southern blot analysis, which can serve as an adjunctive diagnostic marker for CLs. It has, however, to be emphasized that the detection of a clonal T- or B-cell population by itself per se is not proving the diagnosis of lymphoma, because clonal lymphocyte populations can also be found in a subset of inflammatory skin disorders like eczematous reactions or lichenoid skin disorders.[6] Apart from clonality assays, additional genetic analysis allows the identification of genetic alterations, which are characteristic for certain CL entities.

Almost all phenotypic and genetic analyses can nowadays be examined on archival (ie,

formalin-fixed and paraffin-embedded) tissue. Because a detailed characterization of a lymphocytic infiltrate requires analyzing several phenotypic factors and, in many cases, also genetic alterations and clonality studies, biopsies or excisions of sufficient size are mandatory. In practical terms, a punch biopsy of 4 to 6 mm diameter or ideally a spindle-shaped excision with an axis length of 1 cm should be taken and immediately transferred to buffered 10% formalin at room temperature. Considering the rapid evolution of new and emerging prognostic and therapeutic markers, a tissue bank is recommended in which access to archived tissue is preserved: additional fresh tissue can be stored in liquid nitrogen at $-80°C$ or transferred to special fixatives that preserve RNA, DNA, and proteins for future examinations.

In most cases, the histopathological and the phenotypic analyses alone are limited to provide a list of differential diagnoses. As outlined earlier, CLs display overlapping clinical, histologic, immunophenotypic, and genetic features. As a consequence, clinicopathological correlation is of utmost importance to achieve the final diagnosis. Thereby, the terminology should follow the nomenclature of CLs as given in the current WHO classification for hematopoietic and lymphoid tissues to facilitate communication between clinicians and pathologists.[3]

In the following, the diagnostic criteria, the differential diagnoses, and the impact of immunophenotypical and genetic analysis for the diagnostic workup are discussed in an entity-based approach.

CUTANEOUS T-CELL LYMPHOMAS
Mycosis Fungoides

This CTCL accounts for approximately 40% to 50% of all CLs and represents therefore the most common form. The WHO classification defines the disease by its classical presentation with an evolution of 3 stages: patches, plaques, and tumors.[1-3] The disease shows a broad spectrum of clinical, histologic, and phenotypic variants. Some of these variants do not clinically follow the classic presentation with patches, plaques, and tumors, but rather exhibit unusual features such as the papular variant of MF. The papular variant, which can also be found in follicular MF and other rare clinical variants, has not been considered in the current WHO classification.

Histology
The histologic findings in early MF are subtle, and therefore, histologic diagnosis is challenging. There is a perivascular infiltrate in the upper

dermis, which contains mostly small lymphocytes, eosinophils, and a few plasma cells. The lymphocytes show subtle nuclear atypia and may be arranged along the junctional zone (lining-up) and single-cell epidermotropism (**Fig. 1**). Occasionally, vacuolization along the junctional zone can be seen. Pautrier microabscesses, which are a hallmark of plaque stage, are found in less than 20% of the cases in the patch stage.[7] In MF plaque stage, a denser bandlike infiltrate in the upper and middermis with a prominent epidermotropism of small to medium-sized atypical lymphocytes with nuclear pleomorphism and formation of Pautrier microabscesses is usually found. MF tumor stage is characterized by a dense dermal infiltrate extending into the upper parts of the subcutis, which is composed of pleomorphic tumor cells of variable size. Thereby, transformation is defined by the presence of at least 25% of large tumor cells. Usually an admixture of eosinophils, plasma cells, and histiocytes can be seen. Ulceration commonly occurs. The epidermotropism of tumor cells, as is seen in patch and plaque stage of MF, can get lost in tumor stage of the disease.

Immunophenotype and clonality
Various phenotypes can be observed in MF with a CD4+- T-helper phenotype being the most common one. Other phenotypes include CD8+, CD30+, CD56+, as well as CD4/CD8-double-positive or CD4/CD8 double-negative variants.[8,9] None of these phenotypes were shown to have a prognostic impact in MF patch or plaque stage.[10] However, cases of early MF with CD30 expression in early disease stage and a high proliferation rate particularly in the dermal component of the infiltrate have been found to be more aggressive in one study.[11] Loss of markers, particularly CD7, can be observed in MF, but also in inflammatory dermatosis. Expression of CD7 by less than 10% of the lymphocytes was proposed as a diagnostic criterion for early MF.[12] Nevertheless, the loss of this marker has little diagnostic impact, because expression of CD7 by less than 10% of the infiltrating lymphocytes is a rare finding. In addition, an increased CD4:CD8 ratio (more than 8:1) may be a hint for MF. Recently, the expression of thymocyte selection associated HMG-box (TOX) was found in a high number of early MF lesions by immunohistochemistry, but is rarely observed in chronic dermatosis.[13] Thus, this marker may be useful in the distinction, but further studies are needed to confirm this observation. Some phenotypes are more commonly associated with unusual clinical features such as CD8+ MF, which often presents with hyperpigmented or hypopigmented patches and plaques, whereas CD4/CD8 double-negative phenotype may be associated with annular lesions.[14,15]

In tumor stage, loss of T-cell markers may occur and variable expression of CD30 can be seen. Expression of CD30 in tumor stage was shown to be an independent marker for a better disease-related survival.[16] The expression of programmed cell death 1 (PD-1) can occur in all stages of MF and is not a helpful marker in the differentiation from other forms of CLs.

Because monoclonal rearrangement of TCR genes can only be found in half of the early MF cases, clonality studies are of limited value in the diagnosis of early MF.

Genetics
Inactivation of the CDKN2A-CDKN2B was shown to be associated with shorter survival in patients with transformed MF demonstrating deletion of this locus.[17]

Differential diagnosis
The history and the clinicopathologic correlation are essential to distinguish early MF from chronic eczema, psoriasis, actinic reticulosis, as well as so-called lymphomatoid drug eruptions and lymphomatoid contact dermatitis. Among lymphomas, early MF needs to be distinguished from LyP (type B and D), epidermotropic forms of cutaneous γ/δ T-cell lymphoma, SS, and adult T-cell lymphoma/leukemia (ATLL). The differential diagnosis includes, depending on the cell size of the tumor cells, a primary cutaneous CD4-positive small/medium-sized T-cell lymphoma (CD4+- SMTL), which, however, clinically usually presents with a solitary nodule and not with patches and plaques as MF. Moreover, epidermotropism is only focally present or entirely absent in CD4+- SMTL. The distinction of MF tumor stage from PCALCL may be impossible in individual cases on histologic grounds alone. Recently, the expression of

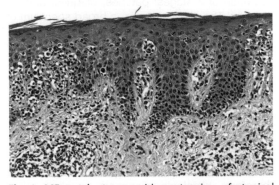

Fig. 1. MF, patch stage: epidermotropism of atypical lymphocytes. HE, ×100.

5-hydroxymethylcytosine (5-hMC) was shown to be a useful marker in the distinction. However, the most important differentiation criterion is the presence of patches and plaques preceding the evolution of tumors in MF, whereas PCALCL presents with rapidly growing solitary or grouped nodules without preceding patches and plaques.

Variants

Particularly, MF variants linked to an impaired prognosis deserve special attention. Those variants include the follicular (synonym folliculotropic) as well as the granulomatous form of the disease. Follicular (synonym folliculotropic) MF is characterized by a perifollicular dense infiltrate of mostly small to medium-sized atypical lymphocytes with prominent folliculotropism (**Fig. 2**). Epidermotropism into the interfollicular epidermis, which is a useful diagnostic finding for MF, is absent in 40% to 60% of folliculotropic MF.[18] The latter may be accompanied by mucinous degeneration of the hair follicle epithelia in half of the cases. Distinction from idiopathic follicular mucinosis is challenging. The detection of significant nuclear atypia, an elevated CD4/CD8 ratio, the presence of numerous CD30+- cells, and monoclonal rearrangement of TCR genes as well as the clinical features with multiple alopecic patches and patches or papular lesions indicate MF, whereas the occurrence of a solitary lesion in a young patient, particularly in children, and lack of nuclear atypia argue for idiopathic follicular mucinosis.[19] In addition, other forms of CTCLs such as follicular LyP and ATLL, which can manifest with folliculotropic infiltrates and accompanying follicular mucinosis, have to be distinguished from folliculotropic MF.[20,21] Folliculotropic MF and granulomatous MF carry an impaired prognosis of approximately

60% to 70% 5-year survival rate.[22,23] Therefore, the recognition and intense therapy are essential.

Remarkably, the presence of a syringotropic component, which may accompany folliculotropic infiltrates or occur exclusively without a folliculotropic component, does not show an impaired prognosis compared with the classic type of MF.[24]

The granulomatous variant of MF presents in most cases with sarcoid-like granulomas, occasionally with granuloma anulare-like features (**Fig. 3**).[25,26] The nuclear atypia of the mostly small lymphocytes is rather subtle. In addition, epidermotropism is absent in half of the cases. Distinction from sarcoidosis and other granulomatous diseases is challenging and often results in a delay in diagnosing granulomatous MF. Detection of clonal T cells is a useful adjunctive diagnostic marker to separate granulomatous MF from sarcoidosis.[27,28]

Pagetoid reticulosis is a rare unilesional MF subtype presenting with a solitary psoriasiform or hyperkeratotic lesion often at acral sites.[29] Histologically, a prominent epidermotropism and nuclear pleomorphism of the epidermotropic atypical lymphocytes are seen. Various phenotypes have been identified in pagetoid reticulosis. Therefore, the differential diagnosis is broad and includes CD4+, CD8+, CD30+, as well as CD56+ epidermotropic infiltrates. Pagetoid reticulosis shows the same excellent prognosis as other forms of unilesional MF.[30]

Sézary Syndrome

This rare CTCL form accounts for 2% to 3% of all CLs. SS carries the phenotype of central memory T cells, whereas MF phenotypically corresponds to effector memory T cells.[31] Because the histologic features are nonspecific in up to 40% of the biopsies, the characteristic clinical presentation

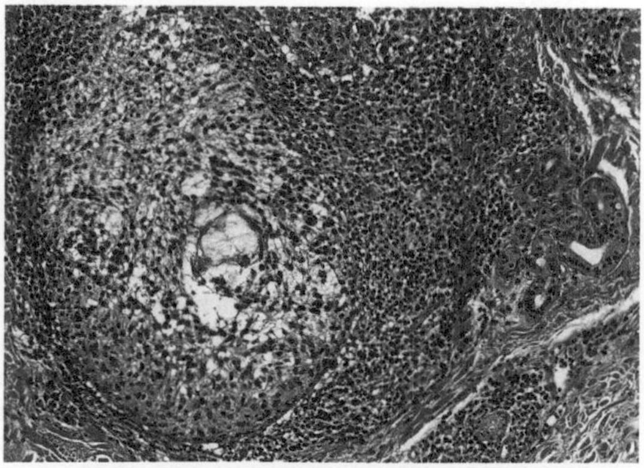

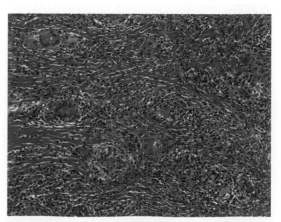

Fig. 2. Follicular MF: folliculotropic infiltrates of small to medium-sized lymphocytes with nuclear atypia. Note mucinous degeneration of the hair follicle epithelium (follicular mucinosis). HE, ×200.

Fig. 3. Granulomatous MF: sarcoidlike granulomas with admixture of small lymphocytes with subtle nuclear atypia. HE, ×100.

with erythroderma, palmoplantar hyperkeratosis, enlarged lymph nodes, and particularly, the detection of more than a thousand cerebriform large tumor cells per milliliter in the peripheral blood are crucial for the diagnosis of SS. In addition, the detection of an identical TCR clone in the skin and the peripheral blood is a useful criterion.

Despite classic MF and SS representing different lymphomas, the histologic features are very similar between SS and MF patch and plaque stage. SS is histologically characterized in many cases by a dense bandlike monotonous lymphocytic infiltrate of small lymphocytes with nuclear atypia (**Fig. 4**). The infiltrate appears more monotonous than in MF. Eosinophils and plasma cells can be admixed. Epidermotropism with formation of Pautrier microabscesses is found in about 60% of the cases, but can be completely absent. Moreover, a pretreatment with topical steroids or ultraviolet light may result in the absence of epidermotropic T cells. Repeated biopsies are useful to enhance the diagnostic accuracy.[32,33] Phenotypically, the tumor cells express CD3, CD4, and often PD-1.[34] However, as outlined earlier, PD-1 does not allow distinguishing SS from other forms of CTCL. The distinction from other CTCL forms presenting with erythroderma such as erythrodermic MF and adult T-cell lymphoma/leukemia requires a history with patches and plaques in MF and the detection of human T-lymphotropic virus type 1 (HTLV1)-DNA integrated into the host genome or serologic demonstration of HTLV1 infection in ATLL, respectively. The distinction of SS from erythrodermic inflammatory dissases (EID) is based on histology only achieved with certainty in less than 60% of the cases.[35] The clinicopathologic correlation and the absence of more than 1000 atypical circulating T cells in the peripheral blood per microliter are essential to differentiate an SS from an EID such as atopic dermatitis, psoriasis, pityriasis rubra pilaris, and in particular, erythrodermic drug eruption.

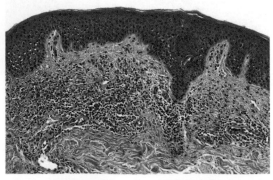

Fig. 4. SS: perivascular monotonous lymphocytic infiltrate in the upper dermis. Note absence of epidermotropism in this biopsy. HE, ×100.

For the distinction of SS and EID, the expression of CD7, PD-1, and TOX may be helpful. PD-1 was expressed by more than 50% of the T cells in 16 of 24 (66%) SS cases, but only in 4 of 30 (13%) EID cases.[34] Although loss of CD7 has been observed in SS as well as in EID, the expression of CD7 by 20% or less of the T cells in skin biopsies was limited to SS. Recent data indicate that the expression of TOX may be an additional marker if more than 50% of the infiltrating T cells show a strong expression of TOX in SS, whereas most cases of EID show only focal and weak expression of this marker.

Primary Cutaneous CD30-Positive Lymphoproliferative Disorders

Primary cutaneous CD30-positive lymphoproliferative disorders represent approximately 20% to 25% of CTCL and comprise a spectrum of lymphoproliferations including LyP and PCALCL as well as so-called borderline lesions.[1,36] The common hallmark of these disorders is the expression of CD30, a tumor necrosis factor superfamily chemokine receptor, by the atypical lymphoid cells.

Lymphomatoid Papulosis

LyP is defined by its characteristic clinical presentation with recurrent papules and small nodules, which undergo spontaneous regression within a few weeks to months. Occasionally, varioliform scars are left behind after regression. The disease has an excellent prognosis without mortality, but patients with LyP are at risk to develop a second lymphoid neoplasm, especially MF, nodal Hodgkin lymphoma, and PCALCL or systemic anaplastic large cell lymphoma (ALCL), before the onset of LyP or during the disease course.

Histology

LyP displays a broad spectrum of histologic manifestations. Five major histologic types can be distinguished (**Table 1**)[37,38]: They differ in regard to the growth pattern (epidermotropic, nodular, angioinvasive), the composition of infiltrate (scattered atypical large CD30+ cells scattered and arranged in small clusters vs cohesive sheets), and the admixture of reactive cells such as neutrophils, eosinophils, and histiocytes. In all histologic types, the atypical lymphocytes express T-cell markers and CD30 except for the histologic type B, characterized by an epidermotropic T-cell infiltrate, which displays variable expression of CD30 (0%–77%) by the small to medium-sized lymphocytes (**Fig. 5**). In addition to these histologic types A to E, a follicular, a granulomatous, and a syringotropic variant of LyP have been described.

Table 1
Lymphomatoid papulosis: histologic types and differential diagnosis

LyP Type	Histology	Differential Diagnosis	Distinguishing Criteria
Type A	Wedge-shaped infiltrate Scattered or in small clusters arranged large CD30+ lymphocytes with nuclear pleomorphism and mitotic activity	• Hodgkin lymphoma (primary or secondary cutaneous)	Staging examination (in nodal HL)
	Background infiltrate of histiocytes, eosinophils, neutrophils	• MF (transformation)	Patches and plaques in MF vs self-regressing papulonodular lesions in LyP
Type B	Epidermotropic infiltrate of small to medium-sized lymphocytes with atypical chromatin-dense nuclei and variable expression of CD30 (0%–77%)	• MF (patch/plaque stage)	Patches and plaques in MF vs self-regressing papulonodular lesions in LyP
		• Cutaneous γ/δ lymphoma (epidermotropic)	Multiple plaques with erosions IHC: Expression of TCR γ
Type C	Nodular cohesive infiltrate of large CD30 + pleomorphic or anaplastic lymphocytes with abundant cytoplasm and mitotic activity	• Anaplastic large-cell lymphoma (primary cutaneous or systemic form)	Clinical presentation with solitary or grouped nodules in PCALCL. Staging examinations in sALCL.
	Admixture of only few eosinophils and neutrophils	• MF (transformation)	Patches and plaques preceding tumors in MF
		• PTCL, NOS (primary cutaneous or nodal)	Lack of CD30 or expression by only a minority of tumor cells, staging examinations
		• Adult T-cell lymphoma/ leukemia	Integration of HTLV-1/2 in tumor cell genome
Type D	Epidermotropism of atypical small to medium-sized pleomorphic lymphocytes with expression of CD8 and CD30	• Pagetoid reticulosis	Unilesional erythematous scaling lesion in pagetoid reticulosis
	Deep dermal or subcutaneous perivascular infiltrates may be present	• Primary cutaneous aggressive epidermotropic CD8+ cytotoxic T-cell lymphoma	Multiple rapidly evolving plaques and nodules with erosions and necrosis Lack of CD30 expression
		• Cutaneous γ/δ lymphoma	Multiple plaques with erosions IHC: Expression of TCR γ
Type E	Angioinvasive (ie, angiocentric and angiodestructive) infiltrates of mostly small to medium-sized pleomorphic CD30+ lymphocytes and expression of CD8+ in 70% of the cases. Admixture of eosinophils.	• Extranodal NK-/T-cell lymphoma, nasal type	Association with EBV, mostly secondary cutaneous involvement (staging)
	Vascular occlusion by atypical lymphocytes or thrombi, hemorrhage, extensive necrosis, and ulceration.	• Cutaneous γ/δ lymphoma	IHC: Expression of TCR γ
		• Anaplastic large-cell lymphoma (primary cutaneous or systemic form) with angiocentric and angiodestructive growth	Clinical presentation with solitary or grouped nodules in PCALCL. Staging examinations in sALCL.

Abbreviations: HL, hodgkin lymphoma; HTLV-1/2, human T-lymphotropic virus type 1/2; IHC, immunohistochemistry; sALCL, systemic anaplastic large-cell lymphoma.

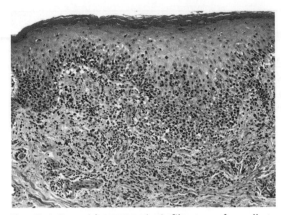

Fig. 5. LyP: epidermotropic infiltrates of small to medium-sized lymphocytes in type B. HE, ×100.

Furthermore, recent genetic studies revealed the presence of IRF4/DUSPP rearrangements on chromosome 6p25.3 in a subset of LyP, which histologically presents with typical histologic findings (ie, an epidermotropic component of atypical small lymphocytes) and, in addition, a dense dermal nodular infiltrate of medium-sized to large atypical CD30+ lymphocytes.[39]

Differential diagnosis

Each of the histologic types of LyP has its differential diagnoses (see **Table 1**). Several infectious and inflammatory skin disorders have been shown to occasionally harbor medium-sized to large CD30+ activated lymphocytes and thus may resemble LyP type A. Detection of clusters of atypical CD30+ cells, the detection of a T-cell clone, and the characteristic clinical presentation allow distinguishing these disorders from LyP type A in most cases.[40,41] LyP type B has to be differentiated from MF, especially because CD30 expression by the epidermotropic lymphocytes can be absent in LyP type B and, on the other hand, MF may show expression of CD30 by epidermotropic lymphocytes even in early disease stage. The clinical presentation, however, allows differentiation between MF (patches, plaques) and LyP (papules and small nodules). A combination of both features within the same lesion has been referred to as persistent agminated LyP. LyP type C resembles the findings in primary cutaneous or systemic ALCL as well as transformed MF. The distinction of those disorders has to rely on clinicopathologic correlation demonstrating patches and plaques in MF and rapidly growing solitary or grouped tumors in ALCL, in contrast to LyP presenting with recurrent papules and small nodules. The distinction of LyP type D from primary cutaneous CD8+ AETCL relies on the clinical presentation with rapidly evolving erosive and ulcerated patches, plaques, and nodules in

the latter (**Table 2**).[42] Moreover, expression of CD30 has not been observed in CD8+ AETCL. The distinction of LyP type D from pityriasis lichenoides et variolaformis acuta (PLEVA) with expression of CD8 and CD30 by the intraepidermal cells may be very challenging in individual cases, especially because clinicopathologic correlation does not allow distinguishing the 2 disorders in all patients. LyP type E needs to be distinguished from the angioinvasive form of ALCL as well as from aggressive T-cell lymphomas with angiodestructive and angioinvasive growth, such as extranodal NK T-cell lymphoma and nasal type, by the presence of Epstein-Barr virus (EBV) in the latter and cutaneous γ/δ T-cell lymphoma by the clinical presentation as well as the expression of TCR γ or δ[43] (**Table 3**).

Table 2 CD8-positive epidermotropic infiltrates	
MF, CD8+ phenotype	Hypopigmented and hyperpigmented patches/plaques, lining-up, and exocytosis of small lymphocytes with nuclear atypia; CD45R0, CD30+/−, T-cell clone[1]
CD8+ AETCL	Rapidly evolving erosive or ulcerated patches, plaques, and nodules. Epidermotropism of small to medium-sized atypical lymphocytes, apoptotic keratinocytes; CD45RA+, CD30−
LyP type D	Recurrent papules and small nodules with spontaneous regression. Epidermotropism of small to medium-sized atypical lymphocytes; CD8+ (100%), CD30+ (90%).
Drug eruption	Maculopapular rash, activated lymphocytes with subtle nuclear atypia; CD8+, CD30−
Pityriasis lichenoides	Papular rash with collerette-like desquamation, vacuolization in the junctional zone, exocytosis of small lymphocytes, apoptotic keratinocytes, focal hyperparakeratosis with inclusion of neutrophils; CD4+ or CD8+, CD30−/+

Note: Clonal T cells may also be detected in pityriasis lichenoides (up to 60%) and drug eruption. Thus, detection of a clonal T-cell population is not a useful marker to differentiate between the listed disorders.

Primary Cutaneous Anaplastic Large T-Cell Lymphoma

In most patients, PCALCL presents with rapidly growing solitary or grouped and often ulcerated tumors (**Fig. 6**). Histologically, in the vast majority of the cases, a dense nodular cohesive infiltrate of large pleomorphic, anaplastic, or immunoblastic T cells is found (**Fig. 7**). Morphologic variants include neutrophil-rich, histiocyte-rich, and sarcomatoid and angioinvasive forms (**Fig. 8**).[44–46] Neutrophil-rich PCALCL is more commonly seen in immunocompromised patients. By definition, more than 75% of the cells express CD30. Remarkably, often a weak expression of CD3 or the absence of CD3 expression can be seen. Various phenotypes have been identified with CD4+ T-helper phenotype being the most common one. The phenotype does not have a prognostic impact. In contrast to nodal or systemic ALCL, almost all cases of PCALCL are negative for ALK1 and the underlying translocation t(2;5).[47] Nevertheless, rare cases of ALK-positive PCALCL have been documented.[48] Recently, genetic analysis revealed the presence of IRF4/DUSP22 rearrangements on chromosome 6p25.3 in approximately a third of PCALCL, but not in systemic ALCL. The detection of this translocation by fluorescence in situ hybridization (FISH) represents a useful method in the diagnostic workup of ALCL.[49] It must, however, be emphasized that certain cases of LyP may carry the same rearrangement, and thus, IRF4/DUSP22 rearrangement is not specific for PCALCL. Differential diagnosis includes LyP type C, which can be only distinguished with certainty by clinicopathologic correlation and tumor stage of MF, which occasionally shows expression of CD30 by most tumor cells. The clinicopathologic correlation with patches and plaques in MF patients allows distinction from PCALCL.

Table 3
Angiocentric and angiodestructive (angioinvasive) lymphocytic infiltrates

Extranodal NK-/T-cell lymphoma, nasal type	Ulcerated plaques and nodules Dermal and subcutaneous infiltrates of medium-sized atypical lymphocytes; $CD3\varepsilon^+$ $CD56^+$, $CD30^{-/+}$, $EBER^+$
Cutaneous γ/δ T-cell lymphoma	Erosive or ulcerated plaques and nodules. Dermal and subcutaneous, occasionally epidermotropic infiltrates of atypical lymphocytes with variable size; $CD3^+$ $CD56^+$, $CD30^{-/+}$, $EBER^-$
PTCL, unspecified	Plaques or nodules Dermal and occasionally subcutaneous infiltrates of variably sized atypical lymphocytes $CD3^-$, $EBER^-$
LyP type E (angioinvasive type)	Recurrent papules and small nodules evolving to ulcers (1–4 cm) with spontaneous regression Dermal and occasionally subcutaneous infiltrates of medium-sized lymphocytes $CD3^+$, $CD8^+$ (70%), $CD30^+$ (100%)
Primary cutaneous anaplastic large-cell lymphoma, angioinvasive type	Solitary or grouped tumors with ulceration. Histology and phenotype identical to LyP type E.

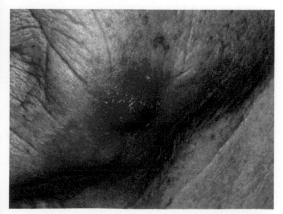

Fig. 6. PCALCL: ulcerated tumor on the left cheek.

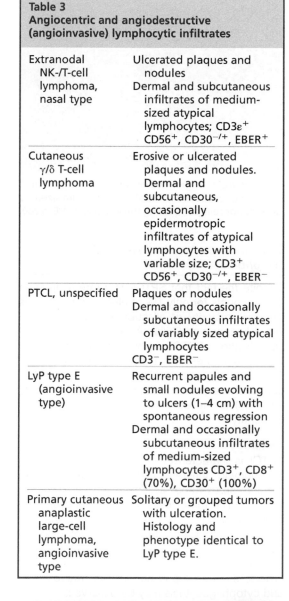

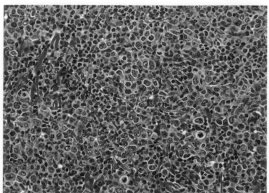

Fig. 7. PCALCL: dense cohesive sheets of anaplastic lymphoid cells. Note mitotic activity. HE, ×200.

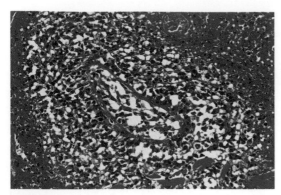

Fig. 8. PCALCL: angioinvasive form with angiocentric and angiodestructive infiltrates of medium-sized to large tumor cells permeating the vessel wall. HE, ×200.

Subcutaneous Panniculitis-Like T-Cell Lymphoma

Despite the fact that SPTCL is a rare lymphoma and accounts for only 1% of all CLs, it represents the vast majority of all subcutaneous forms of T-cell lymphomas (75%). According to the WHO classification, SPTCL is by definition restricted to cases expressing a TCR α/β phenotype.[1,3] Therefore, the immunohistochemical demonstration of the expression of TCR α/β (ie, positivity for β-F1) is the essential diagnostic marker for this entity.

Histology

SPTCL is characterized by a predominantly lobular lymphocytic infiltrate composed of small to medium-sized tumor cells with nuclear pleomorphism.[50] The tumor cells surround lipocytes (so-called rimming). One has to be aware that the rimming of lipocytes, however, is not disease-specific and can be observed in other forms of subcutaneous lymphomas and inflammatory disorders, such as lupus panniculitis. Karyorrhexis and cytophagocytosis may be observed.

Immunophenotype and clonality

Tumor cells in SPTCL express CD3+, CD4−, CD8+, CD56−, TIA 1+, granzyme B+, and as the most important marker, β-F1+. There is no association with epstein-barr virus (EBV) infection. Clonal T cells are found in up to 80% of the cases.

Differential diagnosis

Immunophenotyping is essential to differentiate SPTCL from a subcutaneous form of γ/δ T-cell lymphoma, which expresses the γ/δ chain of TCR. The latter can be demonstrated on archival tissue by immunohistochemical detection of TCR γ or on frozen tissue by immunohistochemical detection of TCR δ. In addition, subcutaneous

γ/δ lymphoma expresses CD56. In contrast to extranodal T-/NK-cell lymphoma, which may also present with subcutaneous involvement, subcutaneous γ/δ T-cell lymphoma is not associated with EBV. In extranodal T-/NK-cell lymphoma, however, EBV-encoded small RNAs (EBER) can be demonstrated by in situ hybridization. Among nonlymphomatous infiltrates, lupus panniculitis is the major differential diagnosis of SPTCL. Both entities show overlapping histologic features with predominantly lobular lymphocytic infiltrates. In both entities, plasma cells can be observed.[51,52] Useful histopathological criteria for distinguishing lupus panniculitis from SPLTCL include epidermal changes, lymphoid follicles with reactive germinal centers, clusters of B cells, and mixed cell infiltrate with prominent plasma cells in lupus panniculitis.[53] In addition, clusters of CD123+ plasmacytoid dendritic cells are found in lupus panniculitis. Nevertheless, the distinction can be impossible in individual cases. Some authors have suggested that both entities may belong to a spectrum of disease, because lupus panniculitis and SPTCL may occur in the same individual. Furthermore, borreliosis manifesting with lobular panniculitis represents a diagnostic pitfall, because the high number of CD8+ lymphocytes mimics SPTCL, and the plasma cells as well as mucin deposition and clusters of CD123+ plasmacytoid dendritic cells are similar to that seen in lupus panniculitis.[54]

Cutaneous Peripheral T-Cell Lymphoma

PTCL comprise a group of rare subtypes including primary cutaneous CD4+ small/medium-sized lymphoma, primary cutaneous CD8+ aggressive epidermotropic T-cell lymphoma, as well as cutaneous γ/δ T-cell lymphoma. For those cases that do not fit into one of these rare subtypes or any other well-defined CTCL entity, the term cutaneous PTCL unspecified (PTCL NOS) can be applied or used.[1,55]

Cutaneous CD4+- Small/Medium-Sized T-Cell Lymphoma

This lymphoproliferative process is listed as a provisional entity in the current WHO classification. Originally considered to be a rare lymphoma form, this lymphoproliferation is nowadays more commonly diagnosed. In most patients, the disease presents clinically with a solitary nodule on the head or neck (**Fig. 9**).

Histologically, a dense nodular infiltrate composed of small to medium-sized lymphocytes with chromatin dense nuclei and a slight nuclear pleomorphism with admixture of eosinophils,

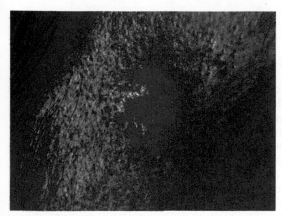

Fig. 9. Cutaneous CD4-positive SMTL: nonulcerated solitary nodule on the right temple.

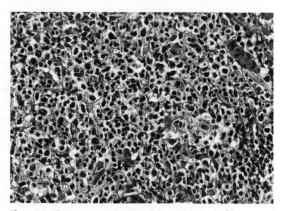

Fig. 11. Cutaneous CD4-positive SMTL: infiltrate of small to medium-sized lymphocytes with slight nuclear pleomorphism. HE, ×200.

plasma cells, and other B cells as well as histiocytes are found (**Fig. 10**). The small to medium-sized lymphocytes express CD4 and a subset of the CD4$^+$ cells also express PD-1 (**Fig. 11**).[56] The expression of PD-1, however, is not restricted to CD4$^+$SMTL, but can be found in various stages of MF, SS, as well as other CTCLs. Therefore, PD-1 cannot be considered a diagnostic marker specific for CD4$^+$SMTL, and additional markers, such as bcl-6, ICOS, CXCL-13, or CD10, need to be expressed by the tumor cells to prove a follicular helper T phenotype. The proliferation rate usually does not extend more than 30%.[34,57] In about 60% of the cases, a clonal T-cell population can be detected.[57] Because of this relatively low detection rate, the value of clonality studies in CD4$^+$ SMTL is limited.

Differential diagnosis includes tumor stage of MF, which can be distinguished by the presence of patches and plaques preceding the development

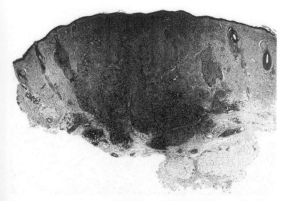

Fig. 10. Cutaneous CD4-positive SMTL: nodular dermal lymphocytic infiltrate without epidermotropism. HE, ×2.5.

of nodular lesions (**Table 4**). Secondary cutaneous involvement by angioimmunoblastic T-cell lymphoma is based on the results of staging examinations and additional laboratory findings. Infiltrates of cutaneous marginal zone (MZL) B-cell lymphoma have to be considered particularly if there are monotypic plasma cells present. The most challenging differential diagnosis is nodular T-cell pseudolymphoma due to overlapping histologic and phenotypic findings. In 5% of the patients, the development of nodular T-cell pseudolymphoma is linked to drug intake, particularly of antiepileptics.

The prognosis of CD4$^+$ SMTL in its solitary or localized form is excellent with a 5-year survival rate greater than 95%. Patients with multiple lesions, however, and a higher proliferation rate of tumor cells as well as a lower number of infiltrating CD8$^+$ cells carry an impaired prognosis and should be treated more aggressively.[58] In regard to the overlapping features, some authors consider CD4$^+$ SMTL and nodular T-cell pseudolymphoma to represent one disease and therefore refer to the process as primary cutaneous CD4$^+$ small/medium-sized lymphoproliferative disorder to underline its indolent course. Considering the impaired prognosis of CD4$^+$ SMTL presenting with multifocal lesions, this constellation should rather be referred to as PTCL NOS.

Primary Cutaneous CD8$^+$ Aggressive Epidermotropic Cytotoxic T-Cell Lymphoma

This lymphoma is a very rare, but highly aggressive form of CTCL characterized by widespread erosive patches, plaques, papules, and nodules with necrosis and ulceration.[59,60] Men are more commonly affected. Usually the patients are in their fifth to seventh decade at diagnosis. Diagnostic criteria for CD8$^+$ AECTCL include short

Table 4
Nodular infiltrates of small/medium-sized atypical T cells

CD4+ SMTL	Mostly solitary nodules on the head and neck; admixture of B cells. Expression of follicular helper T-cell markers (eg, PD-1, bcl-6, ICOS). Admixture of B cells (in clusters) and plasma cells.
Transformed MF	Patches and plaques Often admixture of large pleomorphic lymphocytes; variable expression of CD30 and PD-1.
Angioimmunoblastic T-cell lymphoma	Often multiple lesions. Admixture of Bcells and plasma cells. Expression of follicular helper T-cell markers. Association with EBV (in 50% of the skin infiltrates).
Nodular T-cell pseudolymphoma	Identical clinical and histologic as well as phenotypic findings as in CD4+ SMTL.

history, widespread lesions, epidermotropism of pleomorphic T cells, a CD8+/CD4− phenotype, and an aggressive course as essential diagnostic elements.[61] Histologically, this lymphoma entity is characterized by an epidermotropic infiltrate of small to medium-sized to even large atypical lymphocytes with pleomorphic chromatin dense nuclei (**Fig. 12**). Commonly, apoptotic keratinocytes, spongiosis, intraepidermal vesicles, and blister formation as well as epidermal necrosis can be seen. In addition to the epidermotropic component, a deeper component involving the dermis and subcutis and presenting occasionally with angioinvasive growth can be observed. Phenotyping is crucial for the diagnosis of this lymphoma entity because the tumor cells express a characteristic phenotype (CD3+e, CD4+, CD8+, CD30−, CD45RA+, CD45RO−, TIA1+, and β F1+) (**Fig. 13**). There is no association with EBV.

The differential diagnosis of CD8+ AECTCL is broad and includes primarily CD8+ MF (See Table 2). The latter, however, presents with nonulcerated and nonerosive patches and plaques and shows an indolent course in contrast to CD8+ AECTCL. In addition, usually there is no significant number of apoptotic keratinocytes. In addition, LyP type D must be considered, which differs from CD8+ AECTCL by the expression of CD30 (in 90% of the cases) and the lack of expression of CD45RA. Moreover and most importantly, LyP type D shows recurrent papulonodular lesions with spontaneous regression and exhibits an indolent course. As a differential diagnosis among the inflammatory disorders, CD8+, CD30+ PLEVA can be distinguished by the lack of nuclear atypia as is seen in CD8+ AECTCL. Moreover, the clinical presentation differs significantly from CD8+ AECTCL.

Cutaneous γ/δ T-Cell Lymphoma

This rare and aggressive lymphoma is characterized by a clonal proliferation of mature and

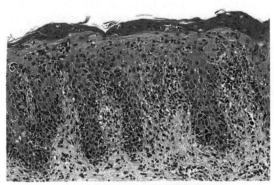

Fig. 12. Cutaneous CD8-positive AETCL: epidermotropic infiltrates of atypical lymphocytes. Note apoptotic keratinocytes. HE, ×200.

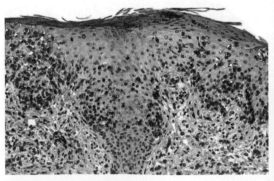

Fig. 13. Cutaneous CD8-positive AETCL: expression of CD8 by the epidermotropic atypical lymphocytes. Immunohistochemistry, ×200

activated γ/δ T cells. Histologically, epidermotropic (pagetoid), dermal diffuse, or nodular or subcutaneous infiltrates or a combination of these patterns can be found.[50,62] In particular, the subcutaneous form of γ/δ T-cell lymphoma is often accompanied by a dermal and an epidermotropic component. In the subcutaneous form, a lobular infiltrate of medium-sized to large cells with chromatin-dense atypical nuclei is present. Angiocentric and angiodestructive infiltrates are common features.[63] The tumor cells exhibit a CD2$^+$, CD3$^+$, CD56$^+$ phenotype being often CD4/CD8-double-negative. In addition, cytotoxic molecules (TIA1, granzyme B, and perforin) are typically expressed. By definition, the tumor cells lack expression of TCR α/β (β F1), but express TCR γ/δ, which can be demonstrated by the expression of TCR γ on formalin-fixed, paraffin-embedded sections or by TCR δ on fresh frozen tissue. Clonality studies reveal a clonal rearrangement of TCR γ/δ. The vast majority of cutaneous γ/δ lymphoma is not associated with EBV, but rare cases of EBV$^+$ primary cutaneous gamma/delta T-cell lymphoma (PCGD-TCL) have been reported. Cutaneous γ/δ T-cell lymphoma can be accompanied by a hemophagocytic syndrome defined by fever, splenomegaly, cytopenia, hypertriglyceridemia, or hypofibrinogenemia, elevated serum ferritin, CD25$^+$ cells, and the evidence of hemophagocytic histiocytosis in bone marrow, spleen, or lymph nodes.

Differential diagnosis includes the epidermotropic form of PCGD-TCL MF (plaque stage). Because classic MF cases with expression of TCR γ/δ have been documented in the literature, the definite distinction between MF and PCGD-TCL requires, however, careful clinicopathologic correlation and should not only be based on the phenotype of the tumor cells.[64] In the presence of predominantly dermal infiltrates in PCGD-TCL with angiocentric features, other aggressive forms of T-cell lymphomas with angiocentric/angiodestructive infiltrates need to be considered. In this context, one has to be aware that distinction from extranodal NK-/T-cell lymphoma, nasal type may be very challenging, because this lymphoma and PCGD-TCL show overlapping histologic as well phenotypic features. The presence of EBV highlighted by in situ hybridization rather argues for extranodal NK-/T-cell lymphoma, nasal type.

Cutaneous Peripheral T-Cell Lymphoma, Unspecified

PTCL NOS is a very rare form of CTCL that is in most cases associated with an aggressive course. Patients usually present with rapidly growing large solitary ulcerated tumors or disseminated nodular lesions without preceding patches and plaques. Histologically, in most cases diffuse or nodular dense infiltrates of mostly medium to large-sized lymphocytic tumor cells with significant nuclear pleomorphism are found.[65,66] Epidermotropism is found in a subset of cases. An angiocentric component can be present. Eosinophils of variable numbers and plasma cells are admixed. Variable T-cell phenotypes (CD4$^+$ or CD8$^+$ or CD4/CD8-double-negative and -double-positive) with or without expression of cytotoxic proteins are found.[66-68] By definition, most tumor cells do not express CD30.[1] An aberrant expression of CD20, but not additional B-cell markers, can be observed in a subset of cases. Clonal rearrangement can be detected, but is often not required for diagnostic purposes.

The differential diagnosis includes primarily transformed MF, which differs from PCTL NOS by preceding patches and plaques (**Table 5**). Importantly, radiologic staging examinations have to exclude secondary cutaneous involvement by a nodal PTCL NOS. Primary cutaneous or systemic ALCL is distinguished by the expression of CD30 by at least 75% of tumor cells. The differentiation from extranodal NK-/T-cell lymphoma and γ/δ T-cell lymphoma is primarily based on the phenotype (EBV-positivity) in extranodal NK-/T-cell lymphoma and expression of TCR γ/δ in PCGD-TCL. Adult T-cell leukemia/lymphoma shows an association with HTLV1, which is not present in PCTL NOS.

Extranodal Natural Killer-/T-Cell Lymphoma, Nasal Type

This rare, but aggressive form of lymphoma is characterized phenotypically by a phenotype resembling NK/T cells and NK cells. Hydroa vacciniformia-like lymphoma represents a variant of EBV$^+$ NK-/T-cell lymphoma occurring mostly in Central and South America in young adults and children.[69,70] Facial or periorbital edema is typically found. Skin lesions further include blister formation and ulcerations, particularly on sun-exposed areas.

The histology shows predominantly angiocentric and angiodestructive infiltrates of tumor cells of variable size with nuclear pleomorphism and mitotic activity. Usually numerous eosinophils, plasma cells, and histiocytes can be observed. Phenotypically, the tumor cells lack expression of surface CD3, but express CD3ε, CD56, and cytotoxic markers.[71,72] Most importantly, EBV can be demonstrated by in situ hybridization or immunohistochemistry.

Table 5
Large T-cell lymphoid infiltrates: differential diagnoses

Cutaneous anaplastic large cell lymphoma	Solitary or grouped ulcerated nodule or nodules. Expression of CD30 by more than 75% of the tumor cells.
LyP (type C)	Recurrent papules and nodules. Expression of CD30 by the large atypical lymphocytes.
MF, transformation	Patches, plaques (and tumors). Presence of more than 25% of large pleomorphic cells with variable expression of CD30. Variable loss of T-cell markers. Admixture of B cells possible.
Primary cutaneous peripheral T-cell lymphoma, unspecified	Solitary or multiple nodules/tumors. Variable phenotype (cytotoxic vs noncytotoxic, CD4 vs CD8 or double-negative); expression of CD30 by <30% of the cells.
Extranodal NK-/T-cell lymphoma, nasal type	Ulcerated tumors. Angiocentric and angiodestructive growth. Expression of $CD3\varepsilon^+$, $CD56^+$, $EBER^+$.
Cutaneous γ/δ-T-cell lymphoma	Erosive or ulcerated plaques and tumors. Expression of $CD3^+$ $CD8^+$ $TCR\gamma^+$ $EBER^-$.

CUTANEOUS B-CELL LYMPHOMAS

Cutaneous B-cell lymphomas are the second most common group of CLs, accounting for about 25% to 35% of all CLs.[73]

Primary Cutaneous Marginal Zone Lymphoma

In the WHO classification, primary cutaneous marginal zone lymphoma (PCMZL) belongs to the group of extranodal MZL of mucosa-associated lymphoid tissue (MALT-lymphoma).[74,75] Recent data indicate that PCMZL differs from other MALT-lymphoma with regard to the expression of class-switched immunoglobulins, chemokine receptors, translocations, and associated infections.[76,77] In the WHO-EORTC (European Organization For Research and Treatment of Cancer) classification and WHO classification, cutaneous immunocytoma, and primary cutaneous plasmocytoma are considered to represent variants of PCMZL.[1,78] These variants are characterized by a dense dermal infiltrate, which is almost entirely composed of plasma cells with monotypic expression of Ig light chains.[1,78] A systemic manifestation has to be excluded by staging procedures. An overview of the diagnostic characteristics is given in **Table 6**.

Histology

PCMZL is characterized by a nodular dermal lymphocytic infiltrate, separated from the uninvolved epidermis by a grenz zone and sometimes extending into the subcutaneous fat (**Fig. 14**). The infiltrate consists of small lymphocytes, lymphoplasmacytoid cells, and plasma cells, which are commonly located in the edge of the infiltrates and next to the epidermis (**Fig. 15**). Reactive germinal centers can be seen. The infiltrate is typically accompanied by abundant admixed T lymphocytes.

Morphologic variants of PCMZL are reported with (i) marked plasmacytoid differentiation,[79] (ii) a high number of admixed T lymphocytes,[79] (iii) a predominance of monocytoid B cells instead of lymphoplasmocytoid cells. A blastic transformation is a rare event in PCMZL and has been linked to an aggressive clinical course. Because of a reported CD5 and CD23 expression,[80] these lesions have to be differentiated from B-cell chronic lymphocytic leukemia (B-CLL) with large cell transformation (so-called Richter transformation).[81]

Two subtypes of PCMZL have been described based on different expression profiles of immunoglobulins[76,77]: (i) the more common class-switch form, which predominantly consists of a nodular and perivascular infiltrate with numerous admixed T cells. The plasma cells express IgG, IgA, or IgE. An IgD expression is found in reactive lymph follicles. The B cells lack CXCR3; (ii) the rare nonclass-switch form, which presents with larger nodular dermal infiltrates predominantly composed of B cells. The number of admixed T cells is only moderate. The plasma cells express IgM. The CXCR3 expression is strong in T and

Table 6
Cutaneous B-cell lymphomas

	Cutaneous Marginal Zone Lymphoma	Cutaneous Follicle Center Lymphoma	Diffuse Large B-Cell Lymphoma, Leg Type	Diffuse Large B-Cell Lymphoma, Other
Pattern	Nodular, geographic	Nodular, diffuse	Diffuse	Diffuse
Infiltrate composition	Small lymphocytes, lymphoplasmocytoid cells, plasma cells	Predominantly centrocytes	Predominantly centroblasts and immunoblasts	Predominantly centroblasts and immunoblasts
Follicular structures	Reactive GC (bcl6+, bcl2−)	In follicular growth pattern: neoplastic follicles (bcl6+, bcl2−/+)	No germinal centers	No germinal centers
Phenoytpe	CD20/CD79a/PAX5+ bcl2+, bcl6− κ, λ	CD20/CD79a/PAX5+ bcl2−, bcl6+, MUM-1−, IgM−, irregular networks of FDC (CD21+/CD35+)	CD20/CD79a/PAX5+ bcl2++, bcl6−/+, MUM-1+, IgM+, lack of FDC networks (CD21/CD35)	CD20/CD79a/PAX5+ bcl2−, bcl6+, MUM-1+/−, IgM−, FOX-P1 +/− lack of FDC networks (CD21/CD35)
Genetics	t(14;18)(q32;q21)IGH/BCL2 and t(14;18) (q32,q21) IGH/MALT translocation is an indicator for transformation toward higher-grade B-cell lymphoma.	t(14;18) translocation was found in up to 50%. This translocation was not linked to differences in clinical presentation and prognosis. Deletion of chromosome 14q32.33 has been reported.	Translocations involving MYC, BCL6, IGH genes. High levels of DNA amplifications of 18q21.31-q21.33, including BCL2 and MALT genes. Loss of 9p21 is a negative prognostic marker. Chromosomal imbalances with gains in 18q and 7p and loss of 6q.	

Abbreviation: GC, germinal centers.

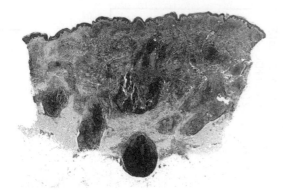

Fig. 14. Cutaneous MZL: dermal and superficial subcutaneous nodular and confluent lymphohcytic infiltrate. Note the grenz zone beneath the epidermis. HE, ×2.5.

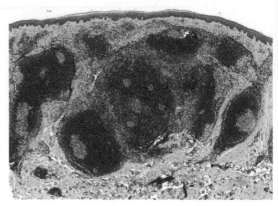

Fig. 16. Cutaneous MZL: expression of bcl-2 by tumor cells. Note the spared reactive germinal centers. HE, ×5.

mild in B cells. In the non-class-switched form, extracutaneous involvement is more often observed.

In contrast to noncutaneous MZL, IgG4 expression is found in approximately 40% of PCMZL and may represent a marker for PCMZL.[82]

Immunophenotype and clonality
The tumor cells express CD20, CD79a, and bcl-2 and are negative for bcl-6, CD5, CD10, and CD43 (**Fig. 16**).[1,83] Plasma cells could be highlighted by CD138. To detect monotypic plasma cells, immunohistochemistry or in situ hybridization must be performed. Most experts consider monoclonal a ratio of 5:1 or 10:1. Monotypic plasma cells can be found in 85% of the cases[84]: in two-thirds of cases, kappa is predominant,[84] and a heavy chain rearrangement is detected in about 60% to 70% of the cases.[84]

Genetics
t(14;18) (q32;q21) IGH/BCL2 and t(14;18) (q32;q21) IGH/MALT-1 were seen in cases of

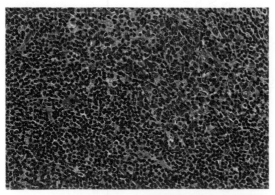

Fig. 15. Cutaneous MZL: proliferation of small lymphocytes in the interfollicular component and reactive germinal centers. HE, ×200.

PCMZL with transformation toward higher-grade B-cell lymphoma.[85]

Differential diagnosis
Distinction of PCMZL from cutaneous B-cell pseudolymphoma (B-PSL), which shows similar features as PCMZL with small B cells, plasma cells, and reactive germinal centers, is based also on clinical presentation (mostly solitary lesion in B-PSL, characteristic predilection sites of ears, scrotum, and nipples in Borrelia-associated B-PSL [Synonym Borrelia-associated lymphocytoma cutis] and a polytypic expression of Ig light chains in B-PSL). In primary cutaneous follicle center cell lymphoma (PCFCL), the tumor cells show a centrocyte-like differentiation. Plasma cells are usually sparse or absent in PCFCL. Cutaneous involvement by B-cell chronic lymphocytic leukemia (B-CLL) may sometimes simulate PCMZL and could be differentiated by their immunohistochemical profiles. In contrast to PCMZL, the tumor cells in B-CLL express CD5, CD23, and CD43.[83,86] Another diagnostic pitfall is a secondary cutaneous infiltrate of extracutaneous MALT lymphoma, which must be excluded by staging procedures. It remains a matter of debate whether PCMZL represents a de novo neoplastic process or whether B-PSL and PCMZL represent different evolutionary steps of the same disease. Therefore, a clear differentiation between both entities could be difficult or impossible in individual cases. Monotypic plasma cells or a monoclonal IgH rearrangement (same clone in repeated assays) argues for a PCMZL. In certain areas of Europe, PCMZL is rarely associated with *Borrelia burgdorferi* infection, but this link has not been found in PCMZL from Asia and the United States.[87–89]

In plasma cell predominate variants (primary cutaneous plasmocytoma, immunocytoma), other differential diagnoses have to be considered.

Secondary cutaneous plasmocytoma could be excluded by staging procedures. Rare, but important differential diagnoses are vegetating herpes virus infections in HIV patients,[90] lymphoplasmacytoid plaque,[91,92] and cutaneous plasmocytosis.[93] These entities can show a plasma cell–rich infiltrate, but the plasma cells are polyclonal in contrast to most cases of PCMZL.

Primary Cutaneous Follicle Center Lymphoma

PCFCL is listed as a separate entity in the WHO classification.[74] It is characterized by a tumor of neoplastic follicle centers and is predominantly composed of centrocyte-like cells. It occurs typically on the scalp, large tumors of PCFCL on the back that had been originally referred to as reticulohistiocytoma dorsi (Crosti lymphoma). Miliary and agminated types of PCFCL can be challenging, histologically and clinically.[94] The diagnostic criteria are given in **Table 6**.

Histology
Three growth patterns can be discerned, but in all of them, a proliferation of tumor cells with centrocyte-like differentiation predominates (**Fig. 17**):

i. The follicular growth pattern is characterized by predominantly large neoplastic follicles, which are composed of centrocyte-like cells. Tingible body macrophages are only rarely found (less than 10%).
ii. The diffuse growth pattern is defined by diffuse aggregates of medium and large centrocytes with admixed small lymphocytes. Follicular structures cannot be detected.
iii. In the mixed growth pattern, areas with diffuse arrangement of centrocyte-like cells, next to areas with follicular structures, can be observed.

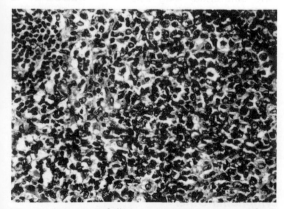

Fig. 17. Cutaneous follicle center lymphoma: proliferation of tumor cells with centrocyte-like differentiation. HE, ×200.

As a morphologic variant of PCFCL, a spindle cell differentiation has been described.[95]

Cases with coexpression of CD30 or with blastic transformation can cause diagnostic difficulties.[96,97]

Immunophenotype and clonality
The tumor cells in PCFCL express CD20, CD79a, PAX-5, and bcl-6. They are predominantly negative for bcl-2 (90%), in contrast to nodal follicular lymphoma.[98] The presence of bcl-2 expression or t(14; 18) translocation in PCFCL is not linked to differences in clinical presentation or prognosis.[1] Proliferating cells (Ki-67+ or MIB-1+) are scattered throughout the entire infiltrate. CD21 highlights large irregular networks of follicular dendritic cells (FDC). FOX-P1 expression is an indicator for a worse prognosis.[99] A heavy chain rearrangement could be detected in about 90% of the cases (BIOMED-2 protocol).[100]

Genetics
In nodal follicular lymphoma, t(14;18) translocation is presented in approximately 90% of cases. In PCFCL t(14;18), translocation was found in up to 50%, but was not linked to differences in clinical presentation and prognosis.[1,98] Deletion of chromosome 14q32.33 has been reported.

Differential diagnosis
Some B-PSLs show features accounting for a significant overlap with PCFCL.[101,102] In those cases, coalescing lymphoid follicles with nonpolarized germinal centers lacking mantle zones and smudged infiltrate of lymphoid cells spreading into collagen (often as single cell files), smooth muscle, vessel walls, and peripheral nerve sheets may result in diagnostic challenge and mimic PCFCL. In cases with germinal centers, in B-PSL the proliferative activity (Ki-67+ or MIB-1+) and bcl-6 expression are more restricted to the germinal centers. Tingible body macrophages are more often found in B-PSL.[103] The networks of CD21-positive FDCs are more sharply restricted to the germinal centers.

Comparing CBCL, recent publications have demonstrated that PD-1 expression is significantly higher in PCMZL and PCFCL in contrast to primary cutaneous diffuse large B-cell lymphoma-leg type (PCDLBCL-LT) and showed PD-1-positive cells forming so-called pseudorosettes or clusters. The tumor cells themselves were negative for PD-1.[34,104] Moreover, clusters of CD123-positive plasmocytoid dendritic cells have been described, which are found in only a minority of PCFCL and are absent in PCDLBCL-LT.[105]

Distinction of PC-FCL from secondary cutaneous infiltrates of nodal follicular lymphoma, which often show expression of bcl-2, requires staging. Secondary cutaneous involvement of mantle cell lymphoma has to be considered in the differential diagnosis. The diffuse infiltrates are composed of blasts and centrocyte-like tumor cells. The tumor cells are positive for CD5 and cyclin D1, but negative for CD23.[106]

Primary Cutaneous Diffuse Large B-Cell Lymphoma-Leg Type

PCDLBCL is characterized by dense nodular or diffuse infiltrates predominated by centroblast-like and immunoblast-like tumor cells with noncleaved, round nuclei.[1] The PCDLBCL-LT represents the most common type of diffuse large B-cell lympoma (DLBCL) and is listed as a distinct subtype of DLBCL in the current WHO classification.[3] The diagnostic criteria are outlined in **Table 6**.

Histology
There is a diffuse dermal infiltrate of centroblast-like and immunoblast-like cells with mitotic activity and only a few admixed reactive lymphocytes (**Fig. 18**). Epidermal involvement is uncommon and rarely described. Usually a subepidermal grenz zone can be found. An infiltration in the subcutis can be observed. An uncommon histologic presentation includes a spindle cell and an anaplastic variant.[107] Moreover, an angiocentric infiltrate[108] and expression of CD30 have been described.[109,110]

Immunophenotype and clonality
The tumor cells are positive for CD20, CD79a, and PAX-5 and show a strong expression for bcl-2 and

multiple myeloma oncogene-1 (MUM-1). In most cases, they are negative for bcl-6 and CD10 or show only a weak expression.[111] IgM expression was identified as an additional adjunctive diagnostic marker, which is found in all cases of DLBCL-LT but only rarely in PCFCL (9%).[112] Networks of CD21-positive FDC are not found. FOX-P1 expression was linked to a worse prognosis.[99]

A diagnostic pitfall may result from CD30 expression in large B-cell lymphoma mimicking ALCL, but expression of CD20 and absence of T-cell markers led to the diagnosis.[109,110] PD-1 expression is significantly lower in PCDLBCL-LT than in PCMZL and PCFCL.[34,104] The tumor cells are predominantly negative for PD-1, but in some cases an expression of PD-1 in the tumor cells can be observed.[34,104] There may be detection of heavy chain rearrangement by PCR.

Genetics
Genetic analysis has revealed chromosomal loss of 9p21, which encodes p16 as a negative prognostic marker in PCDLCBL-LT.[113] Loss of p16 assessed by immunohistochemistry, however, does not correlate with these findings, indicating the necessity for genetic analysis by reverse transcription–PCR or FISH analysis. Recurrent deletions in 9p21 (p14 [ARF]/p16 [INK4a/CDKN2A]) have been found to be a constant finding in PCDLBCL-LT, whereas PCFCL does not exhibit this change.[114] Chromosomal imbalances have been identified in up to 85% of PCDLCBL-LT, with gains in 18q and 7p and loss of 6q as the most common findings.[115,116] A high prevalence of MYD88L265P mutation shows an association with a shorter survival.[117]

Differential diagnosis
Secondary cutaneous involvement has to be excluded by staging procedures. The most important differential diagnosis of PCDLBCL-LT is PCFCL with a diffuse growth pattern. The tumor cells of PCFCL are predominantly negative for bcl-2 and positive for bcl-6 and CD10. Networks of FDCs cannot be found in the vast majority of PCDLBCL-LT. IgM expression has been identified as an additional adjunctive diagnostic marker, which is found in all cases of PCDLBCL-LT but only rarely in PCFCL (9%).[112] In sharp contrast to PCDLBCL-LT, the tumor cells of PCDLBCL-other express bcl-6 in all cases and are negative for bcl-2.

Primary Cutaneous Diffuse Large B-Cell Lymphoma-Other

The term PCDLBCL-other refers to cases of large B-cell lymphomas not belonging to PCDLBCL-

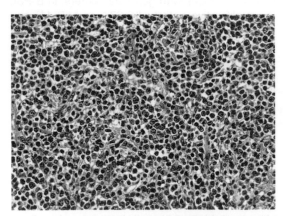

Fig. 18. Cutaneous diffuse large B-cell lymphoma, leg type: cohesive sheets of blasts resembling centroblasts and immunoblasts. HE, ×200.

LT.[1] PCDLBCL-other is a very rare and still poorly characterized form of DLBCL that shares cytologic features with PCDLBCL-LT. Histologically, PCDLBCL-other presents with a diffuse infiltrate of centroblast-like and immunoblast-like cells with mitotic activity. Occasionally, numerous small lymphocytes in addition to the large centroblast-like and immunoblast-like tumor cells may be present. Anaplastic, plasmablastic, and T-cell/histiocyte-rich variants have been described.[1] The tumor cells express bcl-6 in all cases and are negative for bcl-2. Expression of MUM-1 is found in 67%. FOX-P1 is positive in 50% of the cases.[99] In sharp contrast to PCDLBCL-LT, the tumor cells of PCDLBCL-other express bcl-6 in all cases and are negative for bcl-2.[99] Secondary cutaneous involvement by nodal DLBCL has to be excluded by staging procedures.

Intravascular Large B-Cell Lymphoma

Intravascular large B-cell lymphoma is a rare form of extranodal large B-cell lymphoma. As the designation implies, intravascular large B-cell lymphoma is characterized by the intravascular growth of large B cells, especially in small vessels, particularly capillaries and venules (**Fig. 19**).[118] A defect in homing receptors on tumor cells (CD29 = β1 Integrin; CD54 = ICAM1) is considered to be responsible for the unique intravascular growth pattern.[119] Any organ can be involved, although lymph nodes are usually spared. A systemic form and a cutaneous form are distinguished. Histology of skin lesions shows small dermal and subcutaneous vessels filled with large B cells with pleomorphic, moderately chromatin dense nuclei and abundant cytoplasm. Occasionally, tumor cells colonize in hemangiomas.[120,121]

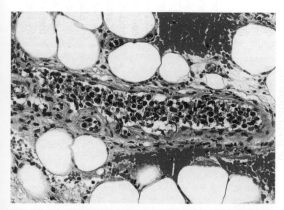

Fig. 19. Intravascular large B-cell lymphoma: accumulation of blasts within small vessels in the subcutis. HE, ×200.

The tumor cells express CD20 and bcl-2 and may be positive for CD5 or CD10.

Differential diagnosis includes other forms of intravascular lymphomas and reactive intralymphatic accumulations of lymphocytes. A rare T-cell and NK cell variant of intravascular lymphomas has been described and is associated in some cases with EBV.[122] Iacobelli and colleagues[123] reported a case of intravascular ALCL restricted to the skin. The T-cell and NK-cell variant is not included as a distinct entity or subtype in the current WHO classification. Differential diagnosis includes intralymphatic histiocytosis as it can be seen after orthopedic metal implantation.[124] Benign intravascular CD30+ T-cell proliferation occurring after trauma or as a consequence of inflammatory skin diseases has to be differentiated from the rare T-cell variant of intravascular lymphoma.[125,126] The distinction could be easily made by immunohistochemistry.

Epstein-Barr Virus–Associated B-Cell Lymphoproliferations

EBV is a γ-herpes virus, which is associated with a range of lymphoproliferative disorders. Among the increasing spectrum of EBV-associated B-cell lymphoproliferations, EBV-positive DLBCL of the elderly, plasmablastic lymphoma, EBV-positive mucocutaneous ulcer, lymphomatoid granulomatosis posttransplant, and methotrexate (MTX)-associated B-cell lymphoproliferative diseases are of particular dermatopathologic interest.[127] An overview of the diagnostic characteristics of EBV-associated lymphoproliferations in the skin is given in **Table 7**.

EBV-positive DLBCL of the elderly is an EBV-positive B-cell lymphoma that occurs in patients older than 50 years of age (with a median age of 71 years) and without any known immunodeficiency or previous lymphoma (see **Table 7**).[128] Nevertheless, the immunologic deterioration or senescence in immunity as part of the aging process is assumed to play a pathogenetic role in the development of this lymphoma, which involves most commonly extranodal sites (70%), especially skin, lung, tonsil, and stomach. The primary cutaneous form is very rare.

Plasmablastic lymphoma is a rare variant of DLBCL that almost exclusively develops in the setting of HIV infection or other immune deficiencies, including posttransplant.[129,130] Risk factors for the development of the lymphoma in the setting of organ transplantation include younger age, higher rejection frequency, and high-dose cyclosporine therapy.

Table 7
Overview of the diagnostic characteristics of Epstein-Barr virus–associated lymphoproliferations in the skin

	EBV-Positive DLBCL of the Elderly	EBV-Positive Mucocutaneous Ulcer	MTX-Associated B-Cell Lymphoproliferative Disease	Posttransplant Lymphoproliferative Disorder	Plasmablastic Lymphoma	Lymphomatoid Granulomatosis
Histology	Diffuse infiltrate of immunoblast-like or plasmablast-like cells. Intermingled tingible body macrophages. Geographic necrosis.	Ulceration. Polymorphous infiltrate, mixture of lymphocytes and immunoblasts. Often Hodgkin-/Reed-Sternberg-like cell morphology. Dispersed apoptotic cells. Abundant small T cells in the background. Scattered plasma cells, histiocytes, and eosinophils. "Cartwheel" nuclear appearance of plasma cells. Angio-invasion with associated thrombosis may be found.	Diffuse infiltrate of centroblasts and immunoblasts. Some polymorphous tumor cells with a Reed-Sternberg-like appearance. Admixed T cells. The EBV-cases were more monomorphous with either centrocytes or immunoblasts.	Dense diffuse or nodular monomorphous infiltrates of centroblastic, immunoblastic, or plasmablastic cells. Often numerous mitotic figures.	Diffuse or multinodular proliferation. Immunoblast-like cells or markedly atypical cells with plasmablastic differentiation. Eccentric nucleus with a "clock-faced" chromatin, a discrete perinuclear hof and abundant cytoplasm. Multinucleated forms can be observed. Numerous/atypical mitotic figures.	Skin involvement found in 40%–50% of the cases. Patchy infiltration of the dermis and subcutis, only little or no epidermal involvement. Angiocentric lymphohistiocytic infiltrate with lymphocytic angiitis and admixed atypical B cells. Multifocal areas of necrosis.

Phenotype	CD20+,CD79a+, PAX-5+, MUM-1/IRF4+, CD10−, bcl-6−, CD30+/−, light chain restriction +/−, Ki-67/MIB-1+++	CD30++, CD20(+/−), CD45+ (56%), CD15+ (43%), PAX-5+, Oct-2+, MUM-1+, CD10−, bcl6+/− (focal)	CD20(+), PAX5+, CD79a(+), MUM-1+ (80%), FOXP1+ (70%), bcl-2+ (70%), bcl-6 (70%), CD30+ (60%). Reduced expression of B-cell markers in EBV+ cases.	CD20+ or CD79a, MUM-1+, Ki-67/ MIB-1+++	CD20−, PAX-5−, CD38+ CD138+, VS38c+, CD10+/−, CD79a+/−, CD30+/−, CD56+/−	Predominating CD3/ CD4+ T-cell infiltrate with scattered atypical CD20+ B cells.
Viruses	In situ hybridization for EBER. Some cases also show expression of latent membrane protein 1 and EBNA-2.	The CD30+ B cells were positive for EBER.	EBER is positive in 50% of the cases.	EBV detection (in situ hybridization or PCR) in 90% of the cases.	EBV has been demostrated in most cases. EBER transcripts often found in virtually all tumor cells. HHV-8 has also been implicated in this lymphoma type.	Association with EBV was found in most cases with EBER transcripts present in B cells.

Abbreviations: EBNA-2, epstein barr virus nuclear antigen-2; HHV-8, human herpesvirus 8.

Lymphomatoid granulomatosis is a rare B-cell proliferation with primarily extranodal involvement, affecting the lungs, skin, central nervous system, and kidneys. The skin is secondarily involved in 20% to 50% of patients with lymphomatoid granulomatosis.[131] Histologically, angiocentric infiltrates with large atypical B cells are found in a background of a dense infiltrate of reactive T cells, histiocytes, and plasma cells.[132,133] Association with EBV is found in most of the cases with EBER transcripts present in B cells.

EBV-positive mucocutaneous ulcer is a recently described B-cell lymphoproliferative disease that manifests with isolated sharply demarcated ulceration most commonly in the oropharynx, skin, and gastrointestinal tract (see **Table 7**).[134] One-third of the affected patients have a drug-related immunosuppression, but age-related immune suppression is also a feature.[134,135] Polymorphous infiltrates of atypical large B-cell blasts, often with Hodgkin or Reed-Sternberg cell-like morphology in the background of abundant small T cells and eosinophils, are found. The large cells express CD20 and CD30 and are positive for EBER.[134]

Posttransplant B-cell lymphoproliferative disorders represent a spectrum of lymphoid tissue disease, ranging from early lesions, such as plasmacytic hyperplasia, to monomorphic neoplasm.[136] They usually manifest years after transplantation, are frequently EBV linked, and are associated with a favorable clinical outcome.[136]

Methotrexate-associated B-cell lymphoproliferative disease presents with ulcerating or generalized skin lesions. Histologically, it shares features with PCDLBCL-LT.[137] In cases with a reduced staining for CD79a and marked tumor cell polymorphism, this diagnosis should be taken into account.

SUMMARY

Considering the overlap in clinical presentation and histologic as well as phenotypic features of CLs, the final diagnosis in cutaneous lymphoproliferative disorders must be based on a multiparameter approach integrating clinicopathologic correlation and detailed phenotypic studies. Molecular studies are indicated in selected cases, but will most probably become more important in the near future to identify prognostic factors and therapeutic targets.

REFERENCES

1. Willemze R, Jaffe ES, Burg G, et al. WHO-EORTC classification for cutaneous lymphomas. Blood 2005;105(10):3768–85.

2. Burg G, Jaffe ES, Kempf W, et al. WHO/EORTC classification of cutaneous lymphomas. In: LeBoit P, Burg G, Weedon D, et al, editors. World Health Organization classification of tumours. Pathology and genetics of skin tumors. Lyon (France): WHO IARC; 2006. p. 166.

3. Swerdlow SH, Campo E, Harris NL, et al. WHO classification of tumours of haematopoietic and lymphoid tissues. 4th edition. Lyon (France): IARC Press; 2008.

4. Harris NL, Jaffe ES, Stein H, et al. A revised European-American classification of lymphoid neoplasms: a proposal from the International Lymphoma Study Group. Blood 1994;84(5):1361–92.

5. Harris NL, Jaffe ES, Vardiman JW, et al. WHO classification of tumours of hematopoietic and lymphoid tissues: introduction. In: Swerdlow SH, Campo E, Harris NL, et al, editors. WHO classification of tumours of haematopoietic and lymphoid tissues. 4th edition. Lyon (France): IARC Press; 2008. p. 12–3.

6. Goeldel AL, Cornillet-Lefebvre P, Durlach A, et al. T-cell receptor gamma gene rearrangement in cutaneous T-cell lymphoma: comparative study of polymerase chain reaction with denaturing gradient gel electrophoresis and GeneScan analysis. Br J Dermatol 2010;162(4):822–9.

7. Massone C, Kodama K, Kerl H, et al. Histopathologic features of early (patch) lesions of mycosis fungoides: a morphologic study on 745 biopsy specimens from 427 patients. Am J Surg Pathol 2005;29(4):550–60.

8. Kazakov DV, Burg G, Kempf W. Clinicopathological spectrum of mycosis fungoides. J Eur Acad Dermatol Venereol 2004;18(4):397–415.

9. Pavlovsky L, Mimouni D, Amitay-Laish I, et al. Hyperpigmented mycosis fungoides: an unusual variant of cutaneous T-cell lymphoma with a frequent CD8+ phenotype. J Am Acad Dermatol 2012;67(1):69–75.

10. Massone C, Crisman G, Kerl H, et al. The prognosis of early mycosis fungoides is not influenced by phenotype and T-cell clonality. Br J Dermatol 2008;159(4):881–6.

11. Edinger JT, Clark BZ, Pucevich BE, et al. CD30 expression and proliferative fraction in nontransformed mycosis fungoides. Am J Surg Pathol 2009;33(12):1860–8.

12. Pimpinelli N, Olsen EA, Santucci M, et al. Defining early mycosis fungoides. J Am Acad Dermatol 2005;53(6):1053–63.

13. Zhang Y, Wang Y, Yu R, et al. Molecular markers of early-stage mycosis fungoides. J Invest Dermatol 2012;132(6):1698–706.

14. Hodak E, David M, Maron L, et al. CD4/CD8 double-negative epidermotropic cutaneous T-cell lymphoma: an immunohistochemical variant of mycosis fungoides. J Am Acad Dermatol 2006; 55(2):276–84.

15. Kempf W, Kazakov DV, Cipolat C, et al. CD4/CD8 double negative mycosis fungoides with PD-1 (CD279) expression—a disease of follicular helper T-cells? Am J Dermatopathol 2012;34(7):757–61.

16. Benner MF, Jansen PM, Vermeer MH, et al. Prognostic factors in transformed mycosis fungoides: a retrospective analysis of 100 cases. Blood 2012;119(7):1643–9.

17. Laharanne E, Chevret E, Idrissi Y, et al. CDKN2A-CDKN2B deletion defines an aggressive subset of cutaneous T-cell lymphoma. Mod Pathol 2010; 23(4):547–58.

18. Lehman JS, Cook-Norris RH, Weed BR, et al. Folliculotropic mycosis fungoides: single-center study and systematic review. Arch Dermatol 2010; 146(6):607–13.

19. Rongioletti F, De Lucchi S, Meyes D, et al. Follicular mucinosis: a clinicopathologic, histochemical, immunohistochemical and molecular study comparing the primary benign form and the mycosis fungoides-associated follicular mucinosis. J Cutan Pathol 2010;37(1):15–9.

20. Camp B, Horwitz S, Pulitzer MP. Adult T-cell leukemia/lymphoma with follicular mucinosis: an unusual histopathological finding and a commentary. J Cutan Pathol 2012;39(9):861–5.

21. Kempf W, Kazakov DV, Baumgartner HP, et al. Follicular lymphomatoid papulosis revisited: a study of 11 cases, with new histopathological findings. J Am Acad Dermatol 2013;68(5):809–16.

22. van Doorn R, Van Haselen CW, van Voorst Vader PC, et al. Mycosis fungoides: disease evolution and prognosis of 309 Dutch patients. Arch Dermatol 2000;136(4):504–10.

23. Flaig MJ, Cerroni L, Schuhmann K, et al. Follicular mycosis fungoides. A histopathologic analysis of nine cases. J Cutan Pathol 2001;28(10):525–30.

24. de Masson A, Battistella M, Vignon-Pennamen MD, et al. Syringotropic mycosis fungoides: clinical and histologic features, response to treatment, and outcome in 19 patients. J Am Acad Dermatol 2014;71(5):926–34.

25. Scarabello A, Leinweber B, Ardigo M, et al. Cutaneous lymphomas with prominent granulomatous reaction: a potential pitfall in the histopathologic diagnosis of cutaneous T- and B-cell lymphomas. Am J Surg Pathol 2002;26(10):1259–68.

26. Kempf W, Ostheeren-Michaelis S, Paulli M, et al. Granulomatous mycosis fungoides and granulomatous slack skin: a multicenter study of the Cutaneous Lymphoma Histopathology Task Force Group of the European Organization For Research and Treatment of Cancer (EORTC). Arch Dermatol 2008;144(12):1609–17.

27. Dabiri S, Morales A, Ma L, et al. The frequency of dual TCR-PCR clonality in granulomatous disorders. J Cutan Pathol 2011;38(9):704–9.

28. Pfaltz K, Kerl K, Palmedo G, et al. Clonality in sarcoidosis, granuloma annulare, and granulomatous mycosis fungoides. Am J Dermatopathol 2011;33(7):659–62.

29. Haghighi B, Smoller BR, LeBoit PE, et al. Pagetoid reticulosis (Woringer-Kolopp disease): an immunophenotypic, molecular, and clinicopathologic study. Mod Pathol 2000;13(5):502–10.

30. Ally MS, Pawade J, Tanaka M, et al. Solitary mycosis fungoides: a distinct clinicopathologic entity with a good prognosis: a series of 15 cases and literature review. J Am Acad Dermatol 2012;67(4): 736–44.

31. Campbell JJ, Clark RA, Watanabe R, et al. Sezary syndrome and mycosis fungoides arise from distinct T-cell subsets: a biologic rationale for their distinct clinical behaviors. Blood 2010;116(5):767–71.

32. Zip C, Murray S, Walsh NM. The specificity of histopathology in erythroderma. J Cutan Pathol 1993; 20(5):393–8.

33. Walsh NM, Prokopetz R, Tron VA, et al. Histopathology in erythroderma: review of a series of cases by multiple observers. J Cutan Pathol 1994;21(5):419–23.

34. Cetinozman F, Jansen PM, Willemze R. Expression of programmed death-1 in primary cutaneous CD4-positive small/medium-sized pleomorphic T-cell lymphoma, cutaneous pseudo-T-cell lymphoma, and other types of cutaneous T-cell lymphoma. Am J Surg Pathol 2012;36(1):109–16.

35. Ram-Wolff C, Martin-Garcia N, Bensussan A, et al. Histopathologic diagnosis of lymphomatous versus inflammatory erythroderma: a morphologic and phenotypic study on 47 skin biopsies. Am J Dermatopathol 2010;32(8):755–63.

36. Kempf W, Kazakov DV, Mitteldorf C. Cutaneous lymphomas: an update. Part 2: B-cell lymphomas and related conditions. Am J Dermatopathol 2014;36(3):197–208 [quiz: 209–10].

37. El Shabrawi-Caelen L, Kerl H, Cerroni L. Lymphomatoid papulosis: reappraisal of clinicopathologic presentation and classification into subtypes A, B, and C. Arch Dermatol 2004;140(4):441–7.

38. Kempf W. Cutaneous CD30-positive lymphoproliferative disorders. Surg Pathol Clin 2014;7: 203–28.

39. Karai LJ, Kadin ME, Hsi ED, et al. Chromosomal rearrangements of 6p25.3 define a new subtype of lymphomatoid papulosis. Am J Surg Pathol 2013; 37(8):1173–81.

40. Kempf W. CD30+ lymphoproliferative disorders: histopathology, differential diagnosis, new variants, and simulators. J Cutan Pathol 2006;33(Suppl 1): 58–70.

41. Werner B, Massone C, Kerl H, et al. Large CD30-positive cells in benign, atypical lymphoid infiltrates of the skin. J Cutan Pathol 2008;35(12):1100–7.

42. Saggini A, Gulia A, Argenyi Z, et al. A variant of lymphomatoid papulosis simulating primary cutaneous aggressive epidermotropic CD8+ cytotoxic T-cell lymphoma. Description of 9 cases. Am J Surg Pathol 2010;34(8):1168–75.

43. Kempf W, Kazakov DV, Scharer L, et al. Angioinvasive lymphomatoid papulosis: a new variant simulating aggressive lymphomas. Am J Surg Pathol 2013;37(1):1–13.

44. Burg G, Kempf W, Kazakov DV, et al. Pyogenic lymphoma of the skin: a peculiar variant of primary cutaneous neutrophil-rich CD30+ anaplastic large-cell lymphoma. Clinicopathological study of four cases and review of the literature. Br J Dermatol 2003;148(3):580–6.

45. Massone C, El-Shabrawi-Caelen L, Kerl H, et al. The morphologic spectrum of primary cutaneous anaplastic large T-cell lymphoma: a histopathologic study on 66 biopsy specimens from 47 patients with report of rare variants. J Cutan Pathol 2008; 35(1):46–53.

46. Kempf W, Kazakov DV, Paredes BE, et al. Primary cutaneous anaplastic large cell lymphoma with angioinvasive features and cytotoxic phenotype: a rare lymphoma variant within the spectrum of CD30+ lymphoproliferative disorders. Dermatology 2013;227(4):346–52.

47. DeCoteau JF, Butmarc JR, Kinney MC, et al. The t(2;5) chromosomal translocation is not a common feature of primary cutaneous CD30+ lymphoproliferative disorders: comparison with anaplastic large-cell lymphoma of nodal origin. Blood 1996; 87(8):3437–41.

48. Kadin ME, Pinkus JL, Pinkus GS, et al. Primary cutaneous ALCL with phosphorylated/activated cytoplasmic ALK and novel phenotype: EMA/MUC1+, cutaneous lymphocyte antigen negative. Am J Surg Pathol 2008;32(9):1421–6.

49. Wada DA, Law ME, Hsi ED, et al. Specificity of IRF4 translocations for primary cutaneous anaplastic large cell lymphoma: a multicenter study of 204 skin biopsies. Mod Pathol 2011;24(4):596–605.

50. Willemze R, Jansen PM, Cerroni L, et al. Subcutaneous panniculitis-like T-cell lymphoma: definition, classification, and prognostic factors: an EORTC Cutaneous Lymphoma Group Study of 83 cases. Blood 2008;111(2):838–45.

51. Magro CM, Crowson AN, Kovatich AJ, et al. Lupus profundus, indeterminate lymphocytic lobular panniculitis and subcutaneous T-cell lymphoma: a spectrum of subcuticular T-cell lymphoid dyscrasia. J Cutan Pathol 2001;28(5):235–47.

52. Pincus LB, LeBoit PE, McCalmont TH, et al. Subcutaneous panniculitis-like T-cell lymphoma with overlapping clinicopathologic features of lupus erythematosus: coexistence of 2 entities? Am J Dermatopathol 2009;31(6):520–6.

53. Massone C, Kodama K, Salmhofer W, et al. Lupus erythematosus panniculitis (lupus profundus): clinical, histopathological, and molecular analysis of nine cases. J Cutan Pathol 2005;32(6):396–404.

54. Kempf W, Kazakov DV, Kutzner H. Lobular panniculitis due to Borrelia burgdorferi infection mimicking subcutaneous panniculitis-like T-cell lymphoma. Am J Dermatopathol 2013;35(2): e30–3.

55. Kempf W, Rozati S, Kerl K, et al. Cutaneous peripheral T-cell lymphomas, unspecified/NOS and rare subtypes: a heterogeneous group of challenging cutaneous lymphomas. G Ital Dermatol Venereol 2012;147(6):553–62.

56. Rodriguez Pinilla SM, Roncador G, Rodriguez-Peralto JL, et al. Primary cutaneous CD4+ small/medium-sized pleomorphic T-cell lymphoma expresses follicular T-cell markers. Am J Surg Pathol 2009;33(1):81–90.

57. Beltraminelli H, Leinweber B, Kerl H, et al. Primary cutaneous CD4+ small-/medium-sized pleomorphic T-cell lymphoma: a cutaneous nodular proliferation of pleomorphic T lymphocytes of undetermined significance? A study of 136 cases. Am J Dermatopathol 2009;31(4):317–22.

58. Garcia-Herrera A, Colomo L, Camos M, et al. Primary cutaneous small/medium CD4+ T-cell lymphomas: a heterogeneous group of tumors with different clinicopathologic features and outcome. J Clin Oncol 2008;26(20):3364–71.

59. Berti E, Tomasini D, Vermeer MH, et al. Primary cutaneous CD8-positive epidermotropic cytotoxic T cell lymphomas. A distinct clinicopathological entity with an aggressive clinical behavior. Am J Pathol 1999;155(2):483–92.

60. Robson A, Assaf C, Bagot M, et al. Aggressive epidermotropic cutaneous CD8+ lymphoma: a cutaneous lymphoma with distinct clinical and pathological features. Report of an EORTC Cutaneous Lymphoma Task Force Workshop. Histopathology 2014, Jan 18, in press.

61. Nofal A, Abdel-Mawla MY, Assaf M, et al. Primary cutaneous aggressive epidermotropic CD8(+) T-cell lymphoma: proposed diagnostic criteria and therapeutic evaluation. J Am Acad Dermatol 2012;67(4):748–59.

62. Berti E, Cerri A, Cavicchini S, et al. Primary cutaneous gamma/delta T-cell lymphoma presenting as disseminated pagetoid reticulosis. J Invest Dermatol 1991;96(5):718–23.

63. Arnulf B, Copie-Bergman C, Delfau-Larue MH, et al. Nonhepatosplenic gamma delta T-cell lymphoma: a subset of cytotoxic lymphomas with mucosal or skin localization. Blood 1998;91(5): 1723–31.

64. Rodriguez-Pinilla SM, Ortiz-Romero PL, Monsalvez V, et al. TCR-gamma expression in

primary cutaneous T-cell lymphomas. Am J Surg Pathol 2013;37(3):375–84.

65. Bekkenk MW, Vermeer MH, Jansen PM, et al. Peripheral T-cell lymphomas unspecified presenting in the skin: analysis of prognostic factors in a group of 82 patients. Blood 2003;102(6):2213–9.

66. Hagiwara M, Takata K, Shimoyama Y, et al. Primary cutaneous T-cell lymphoma of unspecified type with cytotoxic phenotype: clinicopathological analysis of 27 patients. Cancer Sci 2009;100(1):33–41.

67. Reich A, Maj J, Schlue J, et al. Primary cutaneous peripheral T-cell non-Hodgkin lymphoma, not otherwise specified, with cytotoxic features. Int J Dermatol 2010;49(8):967–9.

68. Yamamoto M, Nakada T, Iijima M. Primary cutaneous T-cell lymphoma, unspecified, exhibiting an aggressive clinical course and a cytotoxic phenotype. Int J Dermatol 2008;47(7):720–2.

69. Magana M, Sangueza P, Gil Beristain J, et al. Angiocentric cutaneous T-cell lymphoma of childhood (hydroa-like lymphoma): a distinctive type of cutaneous T-cell lymphoma. J Am Acad Dermatol 1998;38(4):574–9.

70. Barrionuevo C, Anderson VM, Zevallos-Giampietri E, et al. Hydroa-like cutaneous T-cell lymphoma: a clinicopathologic and molecular genetic study of 16 pediatric cases from Peru. Appl Immunohistochem Mol Morphol 2002;10(1):7–14.

71. Chan JKC, Quintanilla-Martinez L, Ferry JA, et al. Extranodal NK/T-cell lymphoma, nasal type. In: Swerdlow SH, Campo E, Harris NL, et al, editors. WHO classification of tumours of haematopietic and lymphoid tissues. Lyon (France): IARC Press; 2008. p. 285–8.

72. Berti E, Recalcati S, Girgenti V, et al. Cutaneous extranodal NK/T-cell lymphoma: a clinicopathologic study of 5 patients with array-based comparative genomic hybridization. Blood 2010;116(2):165–70.

73. Bradford PT, Devesa SS, Anderson WF, et al. Cutaneous lymphoma incidence patterns in the United States: a population-based study of 3884 cases. Blood 2009;113(21):5064–73.

74. Swerdlow SH, Campo E, Harris NL, et al. WHO Classification of tumors of the haematopoietic and lymphoid tissues. Lyon (France): IARC Press; 2008.

75. Isaacson PG, Chott A, Nakamura S, et al. Extranodal marginal zone lymphoma of mucosa-associated lymphoid tissue (MALT lymphoma). In: Swerdlow SH, Campo E, Harris NL, et al, editors. World Health Organization classification of tumours of haematopoietic and lymphoid tissues. 4th edition. Lyon (France): IARC Press; 2008. p. 214–7.

76. van Maldegem F, van Dijk R, Wormhoudt TA, et al. The majority of cutaneous marginal zone B-cell lymphomas expresses class-switched immunoglobulins and develops in a T-helper type 2 inflammatory environment. Blood 2008;112(8):3355–61.

77. Edinger JT, Kant JA, Swerdlow SH. Cutaneous marginal zone lymphomas have distinctive features and include 2 subsets. Am J Surg Pathol 2010; 34(12):1830–41.

78. Kempf W, Ralfkiaer E, Duncan LM, et al. Cutaneous marginal zone B-cell lymphoma. In: LeBoit P, Burg G, Weedon D, et al, editors. World Health Organization classification of tumours. Pathology and genetics of skin tumors. Lyon (France): WHO IARC; 2006. p. 194–5.

79. Geyer JT, Ferry JA, Longtine JA, et al. Characteristics of cutaneous marginal zone lymphomas with marked plasmacytic differentiation and a T cell-rich background. Am J Clin Pathol 2010;133(1): 59–69.

80. Magro CM, Yang A, Fraga G. Blastic marginal zone lymphoma: a clinical and pathological study of 8 cases and review of the literature. Am J Dermatopathol 2013;35(3):319–26.

81. Yamazaki ML, Lum CA, Izumi AK. Primary cutaneous Richter syndrome: prognostic implications and review of the literature. J Am Acad Dermatol 2009;60(1):157–61.

82. Brenner I, Roth S, Puppe B, et al. Primary cutaneous marginal zone lymphomas with plasmacytic differentiation show frequent IgG4 expression. Mod Pathol 2013;26(12):1568–76.

83. Levin C, Mirzamani N, Zwerner J, et al. A comparative analysis of cutaneous marginal zone lymphoma and cutaneous chronic lymphocytic leukemia. Am J Dermatopathol 2012;34(1): 18–23.

84. Servitje O, Estrach T, Pujol RM, et al. Primary cutaneous marginal zone B-cell lymphoma: a clinical, histopathological, immunophenotypic and molecular genetic study of 22 cases. Br J Dermatol 2002; 147(6):1147–58.

85. Palmedo G, Hantschke M, Rutten A, et al. Primary cutaneous marginal zone B-cell lymphoma may exhibit both the t(14;18)(q32;q21) IGH/BCL2 and the t(14;18)(q32;q21) IGH/MALT1 translocation: an indicator for clonal transformation towards higher-grade B-cell lymphoma? Am J Dermatopathol 2007;29(3):231–6.

86. Kash N, Fink-Puches R, Cerroni L. Cutaneous manifestations of B-cell chronic lymphocytic leukemia associated with Borrelia burgdorferi infection showing a marginal zone B-cell lymphoma-like infiltrate. Am J Dermatopathol 2011;33(7):712–5.

87. Aberer E, Fingerle V, Wutte N, et al. Within European margins. Lancet 2011;377(9760):178.

88. Ponzoni M, Ferreri AJ, Mappa S, et al. Prevalence of Borrelia burgdorferi infection in a series of 98 primary cutaneous lymphomas. Oncologist 2011; 16(11):1582–8.

89. Li C, Inagaki H, Kuo TT, et al. Primary cutaneous marginal zone B-cell lymphoma: a molecular and

clinicopathologic study of 24 asian cases. Am J Surg Pathol 2003;27(8):1061–9.

90. Gubinelli E, Cocuroccia B, Lazzarotto T, et al. Nodular perianal herpes simplex with prominent plasma cell infiltration. Sex Transm Dis 2003; 30(2):157–9.

91. Moulonguet I, Hadj-Rabia S, Gounod N, et al. Tibial lymphoplasmacytic plaque: a new, illustrative case of a recently and poorly recognized benign lesion in children. Dermatology 2012;225(1):27–30.

92. Kempf W, Kazakov DV, Scheidegger PE, et al. Two cases of primary cutaneous lymphoma with a gamma/delta+ phenotype and an indolent course: further evidence of heterogeneity of cutaneous gamma/delta+ T-cell lymphomas. Am J Dermatopathol 2014;36(7):570–7.

93. Leonard AL, Meehan SA, Ramsey D, et al. Cutaneous and systemic plasmacytosis. J Am Acad Dermatol 2007;56(2 Suppl):S38–40.

94. Massone C, Fink-Puches R, Laimer M, et al. Miliary and agminated-type primary cutaneous follicle center lymphoma: report of 18 cases. J Am Acad Dermatol 2011;65(4):749–55.

95. Rozati S, Kerl K, Kempf W, et al. Spindle-cell variant of primary cutaneous follicle center lymphoma spreading to the hepatobiliary tree, mimicking Klatskin tumor. J Cutan Pathol 2013;40(1):56–60.

96. Kempf W, Kazakov DV, Rutten A, et al. Primary cutaneous follicle center lymphoma with diffuse CD30 expression: a report of 4 cases of a rare variant. J Am Acad Dermatol 2014;71(3):548–54.

97. Plaza JA, Kacerovska D, Sangueza M, et al. Can cutaneous low-grade B-cell lymphoma transform into primary cutaneous diffuse large B-cell lymphoma? An immunohistochemical study of 82 cases. Am J Dermatopathol 2014;36(6):478–82.

98. Child FJ, Russell Jones R, Woolford AJ, et al. Absence of the t(14;18) chromosomal translocation in primary cutaneous B-cell lymphoma. Br J Dermatol 2001;144(4):735–44.

99. Kodama K, Massone C, Chott A, et al. Primary cutaneous large B-cell lymphomas: clinicopathologic features, classification, and prognostic factors in a large series of patients. Blood 2005; 106(7):2491–7.

100. Morales AV, Arber DA, Seo K, et al. Evaluation of B-cell clonality using the BIOMED-2 PCR method effectively distinguishes cutaneous B-cell lymphoma from benign lymphoid infiltrates. Am J Dermatopathol 2008;30(5):425–30.

101. Boudova L, Kazakov DV, Sima R, et al. Cutaneous lymphoid hyperplasia and other lymphoid infiltrates of the breast nipple: a retrospective clinicopathologic study of fifty-six patients. Am J Dermatopathol 2005;27(5):375–86.

102. Belousova IE, Nemcova J, Kacerovska D, et al. Atypical histopathological features in cutaneous lymphoid hyperplasia of the scrotum. Am J Dermatopathol 2008;30(4):407–8.

103. Leinweber B, Colli C, Chott A, et al. Differential diagnosis of cutaneous infiltrates of B lymphocytes with follicular growth pattern. Am J Dermatopathol 2004;26(1):4–13.

104. Mitteldorf C, Bieri M, Wey N, et al. Expression of PD-1 (CD279) in cutaneous B-cell lymphomas with correlation to lymphoma entities and biologic behaviour. Br J Dermatol 2013;169(6):1212–8.

105. Kutzner H, Kerl H, Pfaltz MC, et al. CD123-positive plasmacytoid dendritic cells in primary cutaneous marginal zone B-cell lymphoma: diagnostic and pathogenetic implications. Am J Surg Pathol 2009;33(9):1307–13.

106. Sen F, Medeiros LJ, Lu D, et al. Mantle cell lymphoma involving skin: cutaneous lesions may be the first manifestation of disease and tumors often have blastoid cytologic features. Am J Surg Pathol 2002;26(10):1312–8.

107. Plaza JA, Comfere NI, Gibson LE, et al. Unusual cutaneous manifestations of B-cell chronic lymphocytic leukemia. J Am Acad Dermatol 2009;60(5):772–80.

108. Plaza JA, Kacerovska D, Stockman DL, et al. The histomorphologic spectrum of primary cutaneous diffuse large B-cell lymphoma: a study of 79 cases. Am J Dermatopathol 2011;33(7):649–55.

109. Herrera E, Gallardo M, Bosch R, et al. Primary cutaneous CD30 (Ki-1)-positive non-anaplastic B-cell lymphoma. J Cutan Pathol 2002;29(3):181–4.

110. Magro CM, Nash JW, Werling RW, et al. Primary cutaneous CD30+ large cell B-cell lymphoma: a series of 10 cases. Appl Immunohistochem Mol Morphol 2006;14(1):7–11.

111. Grange F, Beylot-Barry M, Courville P, et al. Primary cutaneous diffuse large B-cell lymphoma, leg type: clinicopathologic features and prognostic analysis in 60 cases. Arch Dermatol 2007;143(9):1144–50.

112. Koens L, Vermeer MH, Willemze R, et al. IgM expression on paraffin sections distinguishes primary cutaneous large B-cell lymphoma, leg type from primary cutaneous follicle center lymphoma. Am J Surg Pathol 2010;34(7):1043–8.

113. Senff NJ, Zoutman WH, Vermeer MH, et al. Fine-mapping chromosomal loss at 9p21: correlation with prognosis in primary cutaneous diffuse large B-cell lymphoma, leg type. J Invest Dermatol 2009;129(5):1149–55.

114. Belaud-Rotureau MA, Marietta V, Vergier B, et al. Inactivation of p16INK4a/CDKN2A gene may be a diagnostic feature of large B cell lymphoma leg type among cutaneous B cell lymphomas. Virchows Arch 2008;452(6):607–20.

115. Hallermann C, Kaune KM, Siebert R, et al. Chromosomal aberration patterns differ in subtypes of primary cutaneous B cell lymphomas. J Invest Dermatol 2004;122(6):1495–502.

116. Mao X, Lillington D, Child F, et al. Comparative genomic hybridization analysis of primary cutaneous B-cell lymphomas: identification of common genomic alterations in disease pathogenesis. Genes Chromosomes Cancer 2002;35(2):144–55.

117. Pham-Ledard A, Beylot-Barry M, Barbe C, et al. High frequency and clinical prognostic value of MYD88 L265P mutation in primary cutaneous diffuse large B-cell lymphoma, leg-type. JAMA Dermatol 2014;150(11):1173–9.

118. Ferreri AJ, Campo E, Seymour JF, et al. Intravascular lymphoma: clinical presentation, natural history, management and prognostic factors in a series of 38 cases, with special emphasis on the 'cutaneous variant'. Br J Haematol 2004;127(2):173–83.

119. Ponzoni M, Arrigoni G, Gould VE, et al. Lack of CD 29 (beta1 integrin) and CD 54 (ICAM-1) adhesion molecules in intravascular lymphomatosis. Hum Pathol 2000;31(2):220–6.

120. Krokowski M, Sellmann L, Feller AC. Intravascular large B-cell lymphoma within a subcutaneous cavernous haemangioma. Br J Haematol 2010; 151(1):2.

121. Ishida M, Hodohara K, Yoshida T, et al. Intravascular large B-cell lymphoma colonizing in senile hemangioma: a case report and proposal of possible diagnostic strategy for intravascular lymphoma. Pathol Int 2010;61(9):555–7.

122. Cerroni L, Massone C, Kutzner H, et al. Intravascular large T-cell or NK-cell lymphoma: a rare variant of intravascular large cell lymphoma with frequent cytotoxic phenotype and association with Epstein-Barr virus infection. Am J Surg Pathol 2008;32(6):891–8.

123. Iacobelli J, Spagnolo DV, Tesfai Y, et al. Cutaneous intravascular anaplastic large T-cell lymphoma: a case report and review of the literature. Am J Dermatopathol 2012;34(8):e133–8.

124. Requena L, El-Shabrawi-Caelen L, Walsh SN, et al. Intralymphatic histiocytosis. A clinicopathologic study of 16 cases. Am J Dermatopathol 2009; 31(2):140–51.

125. Baum CL, Stone MS, Liu V. Atypical intravascular CD30+ T-cell proliferation following trauma in a healthy 17-year-old male: first reported case of a potential diagnostic pitfall and literature review. J Cutan Pathol 2009;36(3):350–4.

126. Riveiro-Falkenbach E, Fernandez-Figueras MT, Rodriguez-Peralto JL. Benign atypical intravascular CD30(+) T-cell proliferation: a reactive condition mimicking intravascular lymphoma. Am J Dermatopathol 2013;35(2):143–50.

127. Eminger LA, Hall LD, Hesterman KS, et al. Epstein-Barr virus: dermatologic associations and implications: part II. Associated lymphoproliferative disorders and solid tumors. J Am Acad Dermatol 2015;72(1): 21–34 [quiz: 35–6].

128. Nakamura S, Jaffe ES, Swerdlow SH. EBV-positive diffuse large B-cell lymphoma of the elderly. In: Swerdlow SH, Campo E, Harris NL, et al, editors. WHO classification of tumours of haematopoietic and lymphoid tissues. Lyon (France): WHO IARC Press; 2008. p. 243–4.

129. Flaitz CM, Nichols CM, Walling DM, et al. Plasmablastic lymphoma: an HIV-associated entity with primary oral manifestations. Oral Oncol 2002; 38(1):96–102.

130. Black CL, Foster-Smith E, Lewis ID, et al. Post-transplant plasmablastic lymphoma of the skin. Australas J Dermatol 2013;54(4):277–82.

131. Rysgaard CD, Stone MS. Lymphomatoid granulomatosis presenting with cutaneous involvement: a case report and review of the literature. J Cutan Pathol 2014;42(3):188–93.

132. McNiff JM, Cooper D, Howe G, et al. Lymphomatoid granulomatosis of the skin and lung. An angiocentric T-cell-rich B-cell lymphoproliferative disorder. Arch Dermatol 1996;132(12):1464–70.

133. Beaty MW, Toro J, Sorbara L, et al. Cutaneous lymphomatoid granulomatosis: correlation of clinical and biologic features. Am J Surg Pathol 2001; 25(9):1111–20.

134. Dojcinov SD, Venkataraman G, Raffeld M, et al. EBV positive mucocutaneous ulcer—a study of 26 cases associated with various sources of immunosuppression. Am J Surg Pathol 2010;34(3):405–17.

135. McGinness JL, Spicknall KE, Mutasim DF. Azathioprine-induced EBV-positive mucocutaneous ulcer. J Cutan Pathol 2012;39(3):377–81.

136. Wang E, Stoecker M. Primary cutaneous giant cell plasmacytoma in an organ transplant recipient: a rare presentation of a posttransplant lymphoproliferative disorder. Am J Dermatopathol 2010;32(5): 479–85.

137. Koens L, Senff NJ, Vermeer MH, et al. Methotrexate-associated B-cell lymphoproliferative disorders presenting in the skin: a clinicopathologic and immunophenotypical study of 10 cases. Am J Surg Pathol 2014;38(7):999–1006.

Skin-Directed Therapies in Cutaneous T-Cell Lymphoma

Cuong V. Nguyen, MD, Kimberly A. Bohjanen, MD*

KEYWORDS

- Skin-directed therapy • T cell • Lymphoma • Cancer • Mycosis fungoides

KEY POINTS

- Not all patients with early stage cutaneous T-cell lymphoma (CTCL) require treatment.
- Topical therapies are effective in treatment and management of early stage CTCL and as adjuvant treatment with systemic therapy for more aggressive disease.
- Topical therapies have been most extensively studied for use in mycosis fungoides. Further studies are needed to evaluate their efficacy in other forms of CTCL.

INTRODUCTION

Cutaneous T-cell lymphomas (CTCLs) are an uncommon group of cutaneous lymphoproliferative disorders, characterized by skin infiltration with malignant mature T cells. Mycosis fungoides (MF) and its leukemic variant, Sézary syndrome (SS), are the most common types of CTCL. Given their prevalence, most topical therapies for CTCL are primarily those used, and whose clinical efficacy has been studied, in MF/SS. These therapeutic options are numerous and varied, with treatment often based on physician experience, patient preference, and/or prognostic factors (ie, staging, histology).[1] The National Comprehensive Cancer Network (NCCN) guidelines on MF/SS provide an overall framework for treatment, but, with so many treatment alternatives, determination of regimen efficacy and timing of regimen transitions can be difficult. In 2011, the International Society for Cutaneous Lymphomas, the United States Cutaneous Lymphoma Consortium, and the European Organization for Research and Treatment of Cancer Cutaneous Lymphoma Taskforce released a consensus statement detailing the end points and response criteria of therapy for MF/SS.[2,3] The goal of this statement was to provide a standardized method to evaluate treatment efficacy and allow more consistent research protocols. This article provides a uniform resource for choosing topical therapies for MF/SS. It summarizes the currently available skin-directed therapies for MF/SS and reviews the response rates using the Cutaneous Lymphoma Taskforce consensus statement.

TOPICAL THERAPIES

At present, there is no widely acknowledged cure for MF/SS, with death from disease ranging from 10% to 15%,[4] to up to 43%.[1] However, these adverse survival outcomes primarily apply to those patients with MF with more advanced disease. Most patients with early stage MF (stages IA, IB, and IIA) generally have favorable outcomes. Research studies in stage IA patients showed no difference in survival in those undergoing treatment compared with age-matched and sex-matched controls,[4,5] whereas patients with stage IB and IIA had an increased relative risk of 2.2.[1,6] The overall goal of therapy for MF/SS is to improve quality of life (ie, symptomatic relief, improve appearance) and delay or prevent disease progression. In early stage MF, there are no current data to show that more aggressive systemic

Department of Dermatology, University of Minnesota, 516 Delaware Street S.E., Mail Code 98, Phillips-Wangensteen Building, Suite 4-240, Minneapolis, MN 55455, USA
* Corresponding author.
E-mail address: Bohja003@umn.edu

Dermatol Clin 33 (2015) 683–696
http://dx.doi.org/10.1016/j.det.2015.05.004
0733-8635/15/$ – see front matter © 2015 Elsevier Inc. All rights reserved.

derm.theclinics.com

regimens, including chemotherapy, modify overall survival, and they may be associated with greater morbidity and complications.[7] Thus, treatment of early stage MF tends to focus first on skin-directed therapy (SDT).

Emollients

Emollients have long been studied in the repair of compromised skin barrier.[8] Inflammatory skin conditions, like MF/SS, lead to disruption of the skin barrier, and often result in dry, scaly skin secondary to transepidermal water loss (TEWL). Emollients, or moisturizers, contain occlusive properties that prevent TEWL, and/or humectants that help to absorb water from the surrounding environment, increasing the water-holding capacity of the stratum corneum.[8,9] The most common of these humectants is glycerin, which has been shown to decrease corneocyte loss from the superficial epidermis, and alter the lipid barrier to decrease TEWL.[10,11]

To control symptoms of pruritus or scale, the use of simple emollients can be helpful.

At our site, we recommend application of emollients twice daily in the form of a cream. Although ointments are more occlusive and better moisturizers, patient compliance is often an issue given the greasy quality. In addition, the first and only randomized, placebo-controlled trial of topical emollient therapy for MF only evaluated the use of a cream emollient. This study showed that 24% of 46 patients with patch-stage or plaque-stage MF receiving a placebo of simple emollient cream achieved a partial response (PR).[12] Regardless, this high placebo response suggests an important adjunctive role for simple emollients in the treatment of MF.

Corticosteroids

Topical corticosteroids function through the binding and activation of intracytoplasmic glucocorticoid receptors. In a broad sense, they act through both antiinflammatory and antiproliferative mechanisms. They seem to affect nearly every stage of the inflammatory response. By stabilizing the cell and lysosomal membranes, they inhibit phagocytosis, and decrease monocytic and lymphocytic activity. They decrease chemical mediators such as interleukin (IL)-1, IL-2, interferon-gamma, tumor necrosis factor, and granulocyte-monocyte colony–stimulating factor.[13] Topical corticosteroids further lead to a reduction in mitotic activity and cause apoptosis of malignant cells.[14] They also reduce epidermal thickness, dermal water content, and collagen and elastic fiber production, which explains their common cutaneous side effects (further discussed later).[13]

The pharmacokinetics of topical corticosteroids are complex and depend on several factors, including structure and concentration of the drug, the vehicle, and the condition of the skin on which it is being applied. In addition, the skin can act as a reservoir for the applied drug, allowing for storage for 2 to 14 days in nonoccluded and occluded skin, respectively.[14,15] With so many disparate variables, it is often difficult to assess the pharmacokinetics and pharmacodynamics of topical corticosteroids, and their efficacy is instead assessed by means of their potency as measured through the Stoughton vasoconstriction assay.[13]

Although topical corticosteroids have been used since the 1960s for treatment of MF,[16,17] evidence for their use is still scarce. The largest prospective study to date on topical corticosteroid use in MF is that of Zackheim and colleagues.[18] Seventy-nine patients with skin stage T1 and T2 MF were treated (all of the T1 patients and 68% of the T2 patients) with class 1 topical steroids. Of the 79 patients, 94% of T1 and 82% of T2 patients showed at least a PR to treatment. A complete response (CR) was seen in 63% of T1 and 25% of T2 patients. Once therapy was stopped, only 37% of T1 and 18% of T2 patients retained complete remission. In a 2003 follow-up report, Zackheim[19] noted continued rates of PR to CR in more than 200 cases ranging from 80% to 90% in T1 and T2 patients, respectively. Lower strength topical steroids, such as low-strength to midstrength concentrations of fluocinolone acetonide 0.025% to 0.1% creams, have also been helpful, with response rates of 67% to 89%,[16,17] and can provide symptomatic relief of scale and pruritus.[20] However, for scale and pruritus, patients were treated either under occlusion with saran wrap or with wet wraps: these can be time consuming and burdensome processes for patients when used long term.

Common cutaneous side effects of topical corticosteroids include atrophy, striae, purpura, hypopigmentation, telangiectasias, acne or folliculitis, and perioral dermatitis.[13,21] Other than striae, which are permanent, most of these side effects, tend to resolve over 1 to 4 weeks with cessation of the drug.[13] In addition, allergic contact dermatitis may occur and Cushing syndrome, hyperglycemia, and unmasking of latent diabetes mellitus have been reported from systemic absorption of topical corticosteroids. After 2 weeks of continued use, almost 20% of patients using topical clobetasol for psoriasis had hypothalamus-pituitary-adrenal (HPA) axis suppression as defined by a serum cortisol level of 18 μg/dL or less 30 minutes after cosyntropin stimulation.[22] Recovery of HPA axis function is generally prompt and complete on discontinuation of topical corticosteroids. It has therefore been suggested by the US Food and Drug Administration (FDA) that, when using topical clobetasol, no more than 50 g/wk for 2 consecutive weeks should be used given the concern for adrenal suppression. However, despite twice-daily application of topical clobetasol for months, sometimes under occlusion, none of the more than 200 patients with CTCL treated by Zackheim showed clinical symptoms of adrenal insufficiency,[19,23] and there have been few documented cases of adrenal insufficiency.[24,25] Given that formal HPA axis suppression testing is rarely performed, further studies need to be conducted to evaluate the efficacy and safety of various potencies of topical corticosteroids as currently used in treating MF/SS.

Frequency and choice of topical corticosteroid application for treatment of MF/SS are not standardized. Although research has shown that once-daily application may be just as effective as twice-daily application of topical steroids,[26] current data on MF treatment are based on twice-daily application.[16–18] Alternative or additional therapies should be considered if appropriate response is not obtained by 3 months.

We recommend lesional application of clobetasol 0.05% cream twice daily as the initial treatment of patients with early stage MF to all involved lesions, including those on the face, axillae, and groin. Although clobetasol ointment can also be considered if cream formulation is not adequate, we recommend initiation with a cream-based vehicle, because this is generally more tolerable to the patient. We base our recommendation for topical clobetasol cream use on the 1998 study by Zackheim.[19] Other practitioners frequently incorporate 1-week breaks in the long-term treatment with potent topical steroids in an attempt to reduce the potential for side effects, and may use lower-potency steroids on the face, axillae, or groin. Whether the outcome and side effects are significantly different with a class I versus class II to IV topical corticosteroid in MF, stratified by patch or plaque type lesions, is yet to be determined.

TOPICAL CHEMOTHERAPEUTICS
Mechlorethamine

More colloquially known as nitrogen mustard, mechlorethamine (Mustargen) functions in vitro as an alkylating agent. Its high reactivity to DNA results in alkyl group donation to DNA leading to cell function disruption and, subsequently, through an unclear mechanism, apoptosis.[27] Despite being the most studied of the topical therapies for MF

and in use for MF since as early as 1946,[28] nitrogen mustard's mechanism of action in cutaneous application is unknown, especially because it does not seem to have any significant systemic absorption.[27,29,30] It is has been suggested that it may also interact through an immune-mediated response via the epidermal–Langerhans cell–T-cell axis.[29,31]

Various vehicles for delivery of topical mechlorethamine have been used in treating MF, compounded into formulations of aqueous, ointment, and more recently, an FDA-approved gel formulation.[30,32] Mechlorethamine breaks down quickly in water, making preparations of topical formulations difficult, because the only vehicle completely void of water is an ointment.

Clinical response to aqueous and ointment preparations of mechlorethamine have varied in retrospective studies in the literature (**Table 1**). Most of these studies evaluated efficacy of aqueous preparations of nitrogen mustard in MF.[33–35] In 1982, Hamminga and colleagues[33] reported on a retrospective study of 42 patients with MF, including 10 patients with tumor-stage MF, who were treated with either total-body aqueous mechlorethamine or total-body (skin) electron beam irradiation (TSEB) (2800–3000 rad). Of the patients with early stage MF treated with TSEB, 100% had an initial CR compared with the 82% treated with aqueous mechlorethamine. Ten of 18 patients (including tumor-stage MF) who had CR to TSEB radiation developed a relapse within 4 to 16 months. In comparison, all patients treated with topical mechlorethamine remained in remission, with maintenance mechlorethamine at a frequency of once weekly over a median follow-up period of 41 months. Further retrospective studies have revealed CR rates of 76.6% to 80% in T1 or 51.6% to 68% in T2 patients treated with aqueous preparations, but did not document how soon before initiation of aqueous mechlorethamine patients had discontinued other therapies or whether they had even received other therapies, including emollients, before or concurrently.[34,35] Another retrospective study completed in 2013 is also not included in **Table 1**, because more than 98% of patients treated with aqueous mechlorethamine also received various adjunctive therapies, making interpretation of the clinical response to mechlorethamine difficult.[36]

There has been 1 large report of clinical response in MF to ointment preparation of nitrogen mustard.[31] Two articles related to this subject are not included in **Table 1** because these patients were included in the 2003 retrospective report by Kim and colleagues.[31,37,38] In 2003, Kim and colleagues evaluated a total of 195 patients with stage T1 or T2

Table 1
Clinical response to topical mechlorethamine as initial therapy

Study, Year	Vehicle and Concentration (mg/mL)	T1					T2					Additional Notes, Including Stage of Patients and Initial Therapy
		N	CR	PR	OR	NR	N	CR	PR	OR	NR	
Hamminga et al,[33] 1982	A, 0.25	8	100	0	100	0	9	66.7	33.3	100	0	Unclear what percentage had NM as initial therapy
Ramsay et al,[34] 1988	A, 0.17	40	67.3	—	—	—	67	40.3	—	—	—	Percentage achieving CR after 1 y of therapy. This percentage may be underestimated because these numbers do not exclude T3 patients
Vonderheid et al,[35] 1989	A, 0.17–0.50	89	80	—	—	—	66	68	—	—	—	Stage IIA also evaluated but not separated by T stage. Unclear what percentage had NM as initial therapy
Kim et al,[31] 2003	O/A, 0.1–0.2	107	65	28	93	7	88	34	38	72	28	Results not separated by vehicle
Lessin et al,[30] 2013	—	No Delineation Between Staging										—
	O, 0.20	95	14.7	44.2	58.9	41.1						In the efficacy-evaluable population as measured by CAILS, patients were either stage IA or IB
	G, 0.20	90	18.9	57.8	76.7	23.3						

T1 tumor stage has less than 10% body surface area involvement; T2 has greater than or equal to 10% body surface area involvement. PR represents greater than or equal to 50% improvement.

Abbreviations: A, aqueous; BSA, body surface area; CAILS, Composite Assessment of Index Lesion Severity; Conc, concentration in mg/mL; G, gel; N, number; NM, nitrogen mustard; NR, no response or <50% improvement; O, ointment; OR, objective response.

disease; 158 of these patients applied topical nitrogen mustard ointment and 28 applied an aqueous preparation of topical nitrogen mustard. Patients either received total-body application if disease was extensive or lesional application if disease was limited as their initial and only treatment of MF. By using only mechlorethamine, the investigators were able to show the true effect of nitrogen mustard on disease management without influence from other therapies. There was no statically significant difference in efficacy or survival in patients treated with ointment versus aqueous preparation. The total response rate was 93% and 72% in stage T1 and T2 disease, respectively. Of these, 65% of T1 and 34% of T2 had a CR. Included in Kim and colleagues' 2003 retrospective analysis was Price and colleagues'[38] 1983 study (excluded from table), in which 13 patients with stage IA/IB MF were treated with nitrogen mustard ointment as initial therapy; 6 patients with stage 1A/1B MF as adjuvant to TSEB (30–40 Gy) within 4 to 8 weeks of completion of radiation[39]; and 12 patients with MF (stage unspecified) in the setting of recurrent disease after clearance on alternate therapies, who had never been exposed to nitrogen mustard. Of 13 patients treated with topical nitrogen mustard as initial therapy, 69% had a CR and 23% had a PR. When used as adjuvant therapy after TSEB, of 6 patients, 100% had CR. However, 1 patient developed recurrence, but later had partial clearing with continued nitrogen mustard ointment therapy. Of the 12 patients with recurrent disease who had never been exposed previously to nitrogen mustard, 5 patients (42%) had initial CR, although 1 developed recurrence during the evaluation period, and another 42% had a PR. Price and colleagues'[38] data show that nitrogen mustard ointment may be beneficial in patients in multiple settings, including as both adjuvant therapy and with recurrent disease in patients who have not previously been exposed to nitrogen mustard.

In 2013, the FDA approved the first mechlorethamine preparation for CTCL treatment in the form of Valchlor,[32] a topical gel based on the only randomized controlled trial to date in MF of a topical medication. The study evaluated the efficacy of 0.02% topical mechlorethamine gel compared with 0.02% topical compounded mechlorethamine ointment in stage IA and IB patients.[30] This phase II, multicenter, randomized, observer-blinded, noninferiority study found ORR rates of 58.5% and 47.7% by the Composite Assessment of Index Lesion Severity (CAILS) where target lesion responses were assessed, and 46.9% and 46.2% by the Modified Severity Weighted Assessment Tool for gel compared with ointment, respectively. CRs between the gel and ointment intent-to-treat groups were not significantly different (18.9% vs

14.7% respectively by CAILS in the efficacy-evaluable population). In contrast, the average time needed to achieve PR ($\geq$50% improvement) was significantly shorter (*P*<.01) with the gel (26 weeks) compared with ointment (42 weeks). However, the duration of clinical response was not significantly different in the two treatment groups. Patients enrolled in the study were not initiated on therapy until they went through a 4-week washout period of therapies directed toward the disease. Patients were excluded from the study if they had ever received topical carmustine, if they had received topical nitrogen mustard in the last 2 years, or if they had received irradiation in the last year. Ninety-eight of the 260 patients in the initial 0.02% topical nitrogen mustard trials participated in a phase II, open-label extension study for an additional 6 months of 0.04% mechlorethamine gel.[40] Twenty-six of 98 (26.5%) patients achieved at least a 50% reduction of their CAILS score compared with that at the beginning of this extension study with 6.1% CRs and 20.4% PRs, indicating the possible benefit of additional use of 0.04% mechlorethamine gel in patients who fail to clear with 0.02% mechlorethamine gel.

There have been many local adverse reactions associated with topical mechlorethamine. Mild irritant dermatitis, including pruritus, dysesthesias, and eczematous reactions, are the most common.[30,41] Hyperpigmentation has also been reported in a large number of patients and is reversible after drug cessation.[30,42] One rare case report documented anaphylaxis after application.[43] The most common cause of therapy cessation is a delayed allergic contact dermatitis that can range from mild erythema to bullae formation.[29,34–36,38,41] Irritant and allergic contact dermatitis have been reported in up to 80% of patients treated with the aqueous formulation, 29% with ointment, and 40% with the gel.[30,37] However, therapy discontinuation can usually be prevented by application of topical steroids, prior desensitization in the case of an allergic contact dermatitis, or decreasing the concentration of the medication or frequency of application in cases of irritant dermatitis.[31,42,44]

A 2005 French study of 64 stage T1 and T2 patients with MF, revealed that combination treatment with topical nitrogen mustard and topical steroids could reduce adverse cutaneous reactions and still be effective.[41] Patients were treated with twice-weekly 0.02% mechlorethamine aqueous solution to the entire skin surface, excluding the head. Within 10 minutes of application of nitrogen mustard, up to 15 g of betamethasone cream was applied. Only 33% of patients developed an adverse cutaneous reaction but efficacy was comparable to that found in prior studies (see **Table 1**), with a CR of 58% in both the stage T1 and T2 groups.

In patients in whom local application of topical steroids is not enough to control contact reactions, desensitization may be required. Price's[44] study showed that patients treated with electron beam radiation as adjuvant therapy to aqueous nitrogen mustard displayed a much lower rate of hypersensitivity reactions (8% of 43 patients). In a follow-up study, only 3 of 9 (33%) patients with prior hypersensitivity to nitrogen mustard developed hypersensitivity after receiving adjuvant electron beam radiation with nitrogen mustard ointment therapy.[38] None of the 16 patients without prior history of hypersensitivity treated in the same manner had an adverse cutaneous reaction. It was hypothesized that electron beam radiation depresses the immunologic response, thus leading to a lower incidence of cutaneous reactions. Thus, in patients with concern for hypersensitivity reaction, the use of adjuvant electron beam radiation may be useful in suppressing hypersensitivity reactions.

In addition to electron beam radiation adjuvant therapy, systemic mechlorethamine may also be useful for desensitizing patients who are hypersensitive to topical nitrogen mustard.[45] Vonderheid and colleagues[45] used desensitization with once-weekly intravenous injections of 200 μg of mechlorethamine over 4 to 5 weeks. However, 7 of 31 patients (22.5%) treated with systemic desensitization developed linear dermatitis at the site of administration. This adverse reaction and the need for hospitalization to perform the desensitization led to Vonderheid and colleagues[45] favoring topical immunotherapy to systemic desensitization. Topical immunotherapy for desensitization was performed with either aqueous mechlorethamine at 10, 1, or 0.1 μg in 0.1 mL of water or aqueous dinitrochlorobenzene at 250, 25, or 2.5 μg dissolved in equal parts acetone and water, which was then applied to 15 cm^2 of normal skin. Applications were observed at 48 hours and repeated until a 2+ reaction (erythema and vesiculation) was observed. In some patients, application to involved skin was performed to achieve a 3+ reaction (bullae formation and denudation). In 8 of 19 patients (42%), intentional induction of a delayed hypersensitivity reaction led to CR, with another 42% showing PR in the degree of infiltration of lesions. However, several patients developed excessive pruritus, secondary skin infections, or decreased sensitivity to topical mechlorethamine. Given these side effects and the concern for decreased response following immunotherapy, it is recommended that further studies be performed to evaluate methods of decreasing hypersensitivity reactions to topical nitrogen mustard.

The long-term side effects of topical mechlorethamine are controversial. There have been reports of 1% to 5% increased risk of nonmelanoma skin cancers.[31,35,36,46–48] The largest of these studies, by Vonderheid and colleagues,[35] evaluated 331 patients treated with aqueous nitrogen mustard and 31 cases of squamous cell carcinoma (relative risk, 7.8) and 27 cases of basal cell carcinoma (relative risk, 1.8) were observed. However, a 30-year population-based cohort study revealed no significantly increased risk of secondary cutaneous malignancy in 110 patients treated with topical mechlorethamine for an average of 2.7 years (range, 2 days to 14.6 years), compared with 193 patients not treated with mechlorethamine (hazard ratio, 0.84; 95% confidence interval, 0.46–1.56).[49] The study also did not find an increased risk of comorbidities, including pulmonary disease, in contrast with previous reports of an increased risk of pulmonary cancer development after inhalation of topical nitrogen mustard.[50,51]

Studies suggest that topical application of nitrogen mustard does not lead to systemic absorption. In 203 patients treated with nitrogen mustard ointment over a median of 5 years, Kim and colleagues'[31] study found no abnormalities in complete blood count or chemistries obtained every 2 to 3 months. Reinforcing this, Lessin and colleagues'[30] 2013 study, which led to FDA approval of Valchlor, also revealed no hematologic or chemistry abnormalities in the 260 patients studied with laboratory tests obtained at baseline, 4, 8, and 12 months. In addition, of 16 patients evaluated with liquid chromatography at 0, 1, 3, and 6 hours after application on day 1 and at week 4, there was no detectable blood level of nitrogen mustard. This finding suggests the relative safety of topical nitrogen mustard use. However, use in pregnancy should be pursued only after extensive conversation with the patient about Mustargen's documented mutagenicity as a systemic agent and the topical gel formulation classification as pregnancy class D.[52] The pregnancy classification is based on rat data using 33-fold to 25-fold higher doses than are used as standard for chemotherapy and that were administered in the first weeks of gestation.[53] In a 1976 study, Cytostasan (a nitrogen mustard derivative) at high doses of 20 to 100 mg/kg was injected intraperitoneally into pregnant rats at days 4, 7, 9, 11, and 13 postcoitum, which led to many birth defects (kinked tail, omphalocele, hydronephrosis, hydrocephaly). In contrast, a case report of 2 pregnant women with Hodgkin lymphoma treated with systemic nitrogen mustard at a much lower dose of 0.4 to 0.6 mg/kg in the second trimester revealed no birth defects,[54] although 1 of the infants was born prematurely at 7 months, resulting in jaundice, hepatomegaly, and anemia. Further studies are needed to evaluate the exact mechanism of topical mechlorethamine and to determine its efficacy and safety profile, especially when used in combination with other therapies.

Ideally, treatment with topical nitrogen mustard should start with once-daily application to lesional skin in stage IA and total body surface in stage IB. Patients should continue treatment for at least 3 to 6 months to assess response.[40] For aqueous preparations, 10-mg vials of mechlorethamine should be mixed in 60 mL of water and immediately painted on the skin. Lower concentrations should be used when patients show an allergic or irritant reaction.[31,33-36] Ointment preparations are made by mixing 10 mg of Mustargen first with 95% alcohol to remove the powder in the vial and then in 100 g of Aquaphor (a nonpolar and anhydrous vehicle with a low incidence of sensitization) to a final concentration of 0.2 mg/mL, which can be applied once daily to the whole body in generalized disease or to lesional skin in localized disease.[31,37,38] It is recommended that application of the medication should occur on dry skin 4 hours before or 30 minutes after showering. Patients should also wash their hands completely with soap and water after application.[52] Treatment with Valchlor has not been evaluated in stage IIA patients but, based on earlier studies with the extemporaneous compounded nitrogen mustard preparations, is likely to be effective.[31,33-35] In general, although the mechanism of action of topical nitrogen mustard is unclear, it represents an efficacious option for early stage MF with its use mainly limited by delayed contact hypersensitivity.

Carmustine

Also known as bichlorethylnitrosourea (BCNU), carmustine is an alkylating agent that undergoes spontaneous degradation with the production of electrophiles. Subsequently, DNA is alklyated and cross-links.[27]

Similar to nitrogen mustard, BCNU can be compounded in an aqueous or ointment formulation: to date, there is no FDA-approved formulation. Data on topical BCNU largely come from the experience of Zackheim[55] at the University of California, San Francisco. In 1972, Zackheim[55] first described the use of topical carmustine in MF. In 1990, he published a retrospective study on 87 patients treated with aqueous carmustine.[56] A stock solution was made by dissolving 100 mg of carmustine into 50 mL of 95% ethanol to yield 2 mg/mL. Patients applied 20 to 30 mL to deliver 40 to 60 mg per day for 2 to 3 weeks. If patients developed bone marrow suppression, defined as white blood cell count less than 4000 cells/mL, the dose was decreased to 10 mg/d. To apply 10 mg/d, 10 mg (or 5 mL of stock solution) were dissolved in 60 mL of warm water, producing a concentration of 0.17 mg/mL. If treated with this lower dose of 10 mg/d, patients were treated for up to 17 weeks, median 7 to 14 weeks. In patients who continued to have residual lesions after total-body treatment, individual lesions were treated with the higher-alcohol stock solutions of 2 to 4 mg/mL, limiting use to 70 mg/wk.[56] Patients who had an inadequate response to 10 mg/d were given a 6-week rest period and then retreated with 20 mg/d for 4 to 8 weeks. The study showed a total response rate of 98% (CR, 86%; PR, 12%) in stage T1 and 84% (CR, 47%; PR, 37%) in stage T2 patients.[56] Compared with the 1987 study by the Stanford group,[37] which evaluated the use of topical mechlorethamine in 123 patients, the patients treated with topical carmustine had a much shorter period to CR. Mean time to CR in the Stanford study was 12.9 months, with a median of 7.9 months. In contrast, the mean time to CR in Zackheim and colleagues'[56] 1990 study was 4.6 months with a median of 2.9 months. In comparison, mechlorethamine gel takes average 6.5 months to achieve partial remission,[30] suggesting that perhaps topical carmustine is overlooked as a potential first-line effective treatment of MF. However, there are very few studies evaluating the efficacy of topical carmustine and further randomized controlled trials comparing topical carmustine and topical nitrogen mustard are needed to further assess this.

Myelosuppression represents the most concerning adverse effect of topical carmustine, with percutaneous absorption occurring up to 28% of patients.[57-60] Leukopenia as low as 2700 cells/mm can be seen in 3.7% to 5.0% of patients treated with BCNU 10 to 25 mg/daily for 3 to 17 weeks, although it typically appears after cumulative BCNU dosing of 600 mg. Despite this, there are no case reports of patients developing opportunistic infections while being treating with topical BCNU. More commonly, patients show cutaneous reactions, including erythema, telangiectasias, and hyperpigmentation.[56,59-61] Biopsies of hyperpigmented skin reveal enlarged melanocytes, but not an increased number of melanocytes.[61] Telangiectasias can resolve with discontinuation of topical carmustine, although they typically are permanent.[57] Irritant and contact dermatitis also may occur with topical BCNU, but less frequently (<10%) than with topical nitrogen mustard.[57,61] There have been no reported cases of secondary or nonmelanoma skin cancer associated with topical BCNU.[27,62]

These potentially concerning side effects from use of topical carmustine and its need to be compounded limit its use. Studies have shown that malignancies can circumvent the toxic effects of BCNU through a DNA repair enzyme, O6-alkylguanine DNA alkyltransferase (AGT).[63,64] As such, a 2012 open-label, dose-escalation, phase I clinical trial attempted to use a drug, O6-benzylguanine, to inhibit this DNA repair enzyme. O6-benzylguanine is a guanine analogue that inactivates AGT and prevents DNA repair.[65] In doing so, it may potentiate the effects of topical BCNU in damaging DNA. By potentiating the effects of topical BCNU, O6-benzylguanine may enable a reduction of frequency of topical BCNU application. The study treated 21 patients with early stage MF with topical aqueous BCNU following intravenous administration of O6-benzylguanine. Patients were treated less frequently with topical BCNU at doses of 10 to 40 mg/d from a concentrate of 3.33 mg/mL applied once every 2 weeks for up to 70 weeks compared with previously described daily dosing. The study found an ORR of 76% among all patients. Although this is lower than reported in the previous study published by Zackheim,[57] the investigators noted that their patients may have been examples of more treatment-refractory cases: the median time to treatment following diagnosis of MF for their patients was 78 months compared with the 4 months in Zackheim's[57] study. The investigators reported a lower rate of cutaneous reactions with application of topical BCNU once every 2 weeks compared with daily application (52% vs 100%) and 7.4% of their patients developed leukopenia. In addition, 2 patients had mildly increased aspartate aminotransferase levels.

Although the limited retrospective studies of topical BCNU use in the treatment of MF have shown a good response, given the adverse effects described earlier, its usage remains limited to second-line and third-line treatment.[62] Further studies are needed to evaluate its efficacy and systemic safety in MF.

In clinical practice, the aqueous compound is prepared by dissolving 100 mg of BCNU in 50 mL of 95% ethanol to a stock concentration of 2 mg/mL or 0.2%. This compound is stable in the refrigerator for up to 3 months. Before topical application, 5 mL (10 mg) of the stock solution are then dissolved in 60 mL water to a concentration of 0.17 mg/mL. Patients paint a thin layer onto the involved lesional skin once daily while wearing a pair of plastic gloves.[56,66] Zackheim[57] describes preparation of BCNU ointment in his 2003 article, but its use has never been described in any studies. The ointment is made by taking 50 mL of the 2 mg BCNU/mL ethanol stock solution and mixing it with 100 g of petrolatum. This ointment is applied in the same way as the aqueous solution.[56,57]

We recommend using the aqueous compound, at 10 mg/60 mL to the total-body surface area daily for a maximum of 17 weeks.[57] Typical dose duration should be limited to 6 to 8 weeks (cumulative dose, 420–560 mg) to prevent adverse reactions. Leukopenia is not usually seen at total doses less than 600 mg and cutaneous side effects are not usually seen until after 4 weeks of therapy at 10 mg/60 mL.[66] If response is inadequate after the first course, following a 6-week rest period, a second course using 20 mg/60 mL can be applied daily for up to 30 days. At the end of a total-body course, localized lesions can be treated with the 2 mg/mL stock solution, limited to 70 mg/wk. Zackheim and colleagues[66] recommended monitoring a complete blood count every 2 to 4 weeks during treatment and for 6 weeks after treatment. Before and after complete metabolic panel (CMP) are also advisable.

RETINOIDS

Retinoids are a group of vitamin A–derived compounds that are important in several biological processes, most importantly, in the case of CTCL, cellular differentiation, proliferation, and apoptosis.[67,68] These effects are mediated through 2 families of intracellular receptors: retinoic acid receptors (RAR) and retinoid X receptors (RXR). Each of these intracellular receptors has 3 major subtypes (alpha, beta, gamma), each with multiple different isoforms.[69] Varying receptor subtypes govern the biological effects of different retinoids, whether given systemically or topically. For example, the effect of keratinocyte differentiation by topical retinoids is controlled by RAR-α/RAR-γ heterodimers.[70] The role of topical retinoids in MF may be secondary to their ability to restore normal cellular differentiation across the entire epithelia, thus arresting carcinogenesis.[71] The apoptotic effect of retinoids may require both RAR and RXR activity, with high concentrations (>1 μM) of the FDA-approved RXR-specific retinoid (or rexinoid) bexarotene displaying some cross-reactivation of RAR receptors and, subsequently, cellular apoptosis.[72,73] This function may be secondary to bexarotene's effect on decreasing levels of the protein survivin, an inhibitor of apoptosis that has been found to be at increased levels in CTCL.[74]

Table 2
Other topical therapies for CTCL

	Mechanism of Action	Evidence for Use	Dosing	Adverse Events	Additional Notes
Methotrexate-laurocapram	Prevents DNA synthesis through competitive inhibition of dihydrofolate reductase Laurocapram is a lipophilic compound	One published retrospective study of 10 stage Ia/Ib patients with MF[86] Nine patients completed study Three of 9 (33%) had PR. No patients had CR	12.5–25 g/m² every other day for 24 wk with solution/oil	Pruritus, dryness, erythema	Serum levels of methotrexate undetectable[86] Has been shown to be effective in psoriasis[87]
Calcineurin inhibitors	Binding of calcineurin inhibits dephosphorylation of nuclear factor of activated T cells, leading to decreased T-cell activation, cytokine release, and downregulation of IgE receptors	No studies One case report of a 29-y-old man with patch-stage MF that responded to 0.1% tacrolimus ointment[88]	Twice daily for 1 mo with tacrolimus 0.1% ointment	None discussed	Systemic use has been associated with increased incidence of CTCL in immunosuppressed patients, although never documented with topical application[88,89]
Imiquimod	Acts through TLR7 and through unknown mechanism leads to cellular apoptosis	One open-label study of 6 patients with stage Ia–IIb MF, PR 50%[90] Case report of 4 patients with stage Ia–IIb MF with CR (1 also on IFNα-2a)[91] Isolated case reports (total 7 patients with stage Ia–IIb MF) with CR[92–98]	No standardized method, although in pilot study 3 times per week for 12 wk with 5% cream	Cutaneous reactions of erythema, pruritus, dysesthesias and rarely ulceration, bleeding, crusting	Pilot study did not show clinical CR, but did have histologic clearing in 50%[90] When used in inguinal region for genital warts can have up to 1% systemic absorption[99] MF-like histology after treating actinic keratoses with imiquimod[100]

Abbreviations: IFNα, interferon alfa; IgE, immunoglobulin E; TLR7, Toll-like receptor 7.

However, the exact mechanism of topical retinoid action in CTCL is unclear, especially because systemic absorption of topical retinoids is minimal. Two studies showed that application of topical bexarotene 1% gel up to 4 times daily still resulted in serum concentrations of less than 5 ng/mL in 80% to 95% of the 1074 specimens analyzed.[75,76] In comparison, an oral dose of bexarotene 300 mg/m^2/d results in a serum drug concentration of 1130 ± 269 ng/mL.[75]

Bexarotene

One-percent bexarotene gel (Targretin) was approved for the treatment of refractory early CTCL in 2000.[77,78] Patients are generally instructed to apply the 1% bexarotene gel to lesional skin every other day. Frequency of dosing should then increase to daily, twice daily, 3 times daily, and 4 times daily in 1-week intervals, as the patient is able to tolerate.[75,79]

There have been 2 main studies evaluating the efficacy of bexarotene 1% gel in MF. In a multicenter, phase I/II study of 67 patients, an ORR of 63% was seen (CR, 21%; PR, 42%) with a median onset to response of 12 to 20 weeks and time to CR of 25 weeks.[75] Remissions ranged from 12 to 21 weeks, but up to 5 years with maintenance therapy. Most of these patients had previously received other therapies for their MF. The 12 patients treated in this study, in which bexarotene was the initial therapy for MF, had a slightly higher ORR of 76%. To further evaluate the response rate of refractory disease, a multicenter, phase III trial of 50 patients showed an ORR of only 44% (CR, 8%).[74] Refractory disease was defined in this study as having failed (intolerant to or reached a ≥6-month plateau) of 2 different treatment options. There have also been case reports of the efficacy of topical bexarotene in lymphomatoid papulosis and folliculotropic MF.[79,80]

Tazarotene

In contrast with bexarotene, tazarotene binds with high affinity to RARs, most predominantly RAR-γ in the epidermis. Its use as a topical agent in MF has been assessed in a single pilot study of 20 patients with treatment-refractory MF.[81] Patients applied 0.1% tazarotene gel once daily to lesional skin, with 58% of patients experiencing greater than a 50% improvement in index lesions but no patients showing a CR. These patients were allowed to use topical steroids concomitantly with their treatment to reduce cutaneous irritation. Thus, analysis of the clinical significance of this is difficult.

Alitretinoin

Alitretinoin is the only topical retinoid with both RAR and RXR activity. It has been approved since 1999 for the treatment of Kaposi sarcoma, but has not been evaluated in any complete study for the treatment of MF.[82–84] In the 1990s, 2 phase I/II trials were performed to evaluate the effect of topical bexarotene and topical alitretinoin in MF. The study found that 7 patients had some response to topical alitretinoin 0.1% gel with twice-daily applications. However, the study was terminated and continued evaluation of alitretinoin gel was stopped in favor of topical bexarotene given a lower adverse reaction profile and similar efficacy rate.[84] One case report in 2002 did show complete resolution of tumor stage MF with 0.1% alitretinoin gel, applied daily for an unclear duration.[84]

Adverse cutaneous reactions of all the topical retinoids are similar, with the most frequent symptoms being local dryness, burning, erythema, and desquamation.[75,76,82–84] Vesiculobullous eruptions have also occurred with topical bexarotene use.[85] Rarely, allergic contact dermatitis occurs with topical retinoids.[82,83] The topical retinoids also carry a theoretic risk of teratogenicity. However, 2 cases of women who conceived while on topical tazarotene did not involve any birth complications.[85] Regardless, contraceptives are recommended for women of childbearing age using topical retinoids and the use of topical retinoids should be avoided in pregnancy.

EMERGING TOPICAL THERAPIES

The remaining topical therapies mentioned in this article for treatment in MF have not been extensively studied (**Table 2**), only having been evaluated in MF treatment over the last decade. Imiquimod is noted for local use by the NCCN guidelines. Most instances of their use have been reported in case reports and further studies are needed to validate their efficacy.

SUMMARY

Early stage MF represents the most common clinical presentation of cutaneous lymphoma, with skin-directed therapies long established in its treatment. These therapies continue to change as new treatment regimens emerge. Other skin-directed therapies, such as light and radiation therapy, are discussed by kelsey and Colleagues elsewhere in this issue. Therapies with higher levels of evidence and less systemic toxicity are usually preferred as first-line treatment. However, even these established therapies, like topical corticosteroids and carmustine, lack randomized clinical trials to establish their efficacy. Research is also needed to further define the role of combination topical therapies and how skin-directed therapies can be used as adjuvants to systemic medications.

REFERENCES

1. Kim YH, Liu HL, Mraz-Gernhard S, et al. Long-term outcome of 525 patients with mycosis fungoides and Sezary syndrome: clinical prognostic factors and risk for disease progression. Arch Dermatol 2003;139:857–66.

2. National Comprehensive Cancer Network. Non-Hodgkin's lymphoma (Version 4.2014). Available at: http://www.nccn.org/professionals/physician_gls/pdf/nhl.pdf. Accessed October 18, 2014.

3. Olsen EA, Whittaker S, Kim YH, et al. Clinical end points and response criteria in mycosis fungoides and Sézary syndrome: a consensus statement of the International Society for Cutaneous Lymphomas, the United States Cutaneous Lymphoma Consortium, and the Cutaneous Lymphoma Task Force of the European Organisation for Research and Treatment of Cancer. J Clin Oncol 2011;29:2598–607.

4. Zackheim HS, Amin S, Kashani-Sabet M, et al. Prognosis in cutaneous T-cell lymphoma by skin stage: long-term survival in 489 patients. J Am Acad Dermatol 1999;40:418–25.

5. Kim YH, Jensen RA, Watanabe GL, et al. Clinical stage IA (limited patch and plaque) mycosis fungoides. Arch Dermatol 1996;132:1309.

6. Kim YH, Chow S, Varghese A, et al. Clinical characteristics and long-term outcome of patients with generalized patch and/or plaque (T2) mycosis fungoides. Arch Dermatol 1999;135:1309.

7. Kaye FJ, Bunn PA, Steinberg SM, et al. A randomized trial comparing combination electron-beam radiation and chemotherapy with topical therapy in the initial treatment of mycosis fungoides. N Eng J Med 1989;321:1784–90.

8. Proksch E, Brandner JM, Jensen JM. The skin: an indispensable barrier. Exp Dermatol 2008;17:1063–72.

9. Lodén M, Andersson AC, Andersson C, et al. Instrumental and dermatologist evaluation of the effect of glycerine and urea on dry skin in atopic dermatitis. Skin Res Technol 2001;7:209–13.

10. Froebe CL, Simion A, Ohlmeyer H, et al. Prevention of stratum corneum lipid phase transitions in vitro by glycerol – an alternative mechanism for skin moisturization. J Soc Cosmet Chem 1990;41:51–65.

11. Rawlings A, Harding C, Watkinson A, et al. The effect of glycerol and humidity on desmosome degradation in stratum corneum. Arch Dermatol Res 1995;287:457–64.

12. Duvic M, Olsen EA, Omura GA, et al. A phase III, randomized, double-blind, placebo-controlled study of peldesine (BCX-34) cream as topical therapy for cutaneous T-cell lymphoma. J Am Acad Dermatol 2001;44:940–7.

13. Wolverton S. Topical corticosteroids. In: Wolverton S, editor. Comprehensive dermatologic drug therapy. Philadelphia: Elsevier Inc; 2013. p. 487–504.

14. Schwartzman RA, Cidlowski JA. Glucocorticoid-induced apoptosis of lymphoid cells. Int Arch Allergy Immunol 1994;105:347–54.

15. Vickers CF. Existence of reservoir in the stratum corneum: Experimental proof. Arch Dermatol 1963;88:20–3.

16. Farber EM, Cox AJ, Steinberg J, et al. Therapy of mycosis fungoides with topically applied fluocinolone acetonide under occlusive dressing. Cancer 1966;19:237–45.

17. Farber EM, Zackheim HS, McClintock RP, et al. Treatment of mycosis fungoides with various strengths of fluocinolone acetonide cream. Arch Dermatol 1968;97:165–72.

18. Zackheim HS, Kashani-Sabet M, Amin S. Topical corticosteroids for mycosis fungoides. Experience in 79 patients. Arch Dermatol 1998;134:949–54.

19. Zackheim HS. Treatment of patch-stage mycosis fungoides with topical corticosteroids. Dermatol Ther 2003;16:283–7.

20. Harrison A, Duvic M. Diagnosis and treatment of Sézary syndrome. Int J Dermatol 2004;2.

21. Prawer SE, Katz HI. Guidelines for using superpotent topical steroids. Am Fam Physician 1990;41:1531–8.

22. Katz HI, Hien NT, Prawer SE, et al. Superpotent topical steroid treatment of psoriasis vulgaris: clinical efficacy and adrenal function. J Am Acad Dermatol 1987;16:804–11.

23. Nathan AW, Rose GL. Fatal iatrogenic Cushing's syndrome. Lancet 1979;1:207.

24. Bromberg JS. Adrenal insufficiency. N Engl J Med 1997;336:1105 [author reply: 1106–7].

25. Walsh P, Aeling JL, Huff L, et al. Hypothalamus-pituitary-adrenal axis suppression by superpotent topical steroids. J Am Acad Dermatol 1993;29:501–3.

26. Lagos BR, Maibach HI. Frequency of application of topical corticosteroids: an overview. Br J Dermatol 1998;139:763–6.

27. Wolverton S. Topical and intralesional chemotherapeutic agents. In: Wolverton S, editor. Comprehensive dermatologic drug therapy. Philadelphia: Elsevier Inc; 2013. p. 518–26.

28. Goodman LS, Wintrobe MM. Nitrogen mustard therapy; use of methyl-bis (beta-chloroethyl) amine hydrochloride and tris (beta-chloroethyl) amine hydrochloride for Hodgkin's disease, lymphosarcoma, leukemia and certain allied and

miscellaneous disorders. J Am Med Assoc 1946;132:126–32.

29. Kim YH. Management with topical nitrogen mustard in mycosis fungoides. Dermatol Ther 2003;16:288–98.

30. Lessin SR, Duvic M, Guitart J, et al. Topical chemotherapy in cutaneous T-cell lymphoma: positive results of a randomized, controlled, multicenter trial testing the efficacy and safety of a novel mechlorethamine, 0.02%, gel in mycosis fungoides. JAMA Dermatol 2013;149:25–32.

31. Kim YH, Martinez G, Varghese A, et al. Topical nitrogen mustard in the management of mycosis fungoides. Arch Dermatol 2003;139(2):165–73.

32. Federal Drug Administration. Valchlor (mechlorethamine) gel, for topical use. Available at: http://www.accessdata.fda.gov/drugsatfda_docs/label/2013/202317lbl.pdf. Accessed October 24, 2014.

33. Hamminga B, Noordijk EM, van Vloten WA. Treatment of mycosis fungoides total-skin electron-beam irradiation vs topical mechlorethamine therapy. Arch Dermatol 1982;118:150.

34. Ramsay DL, Halperin PS, Zeleniuch-Jacquotte A. Topical mechlorethamine therapy for early stage mycosis fungoides. J Am Acad Dermatol 1988;19:684–91.

35. Vonderheid EC, Tan ET, Kantor AF, et al. Long-term efficacy, curative potential, and carcinogenicity of topical mechlorethamine chemotherapy in cutaneous T cell lymphoma. J Am Acad Dermatol 1989;20:416–28.

36. Lindahl LM, Fenger-Gron M, Iversen L. Topical nitrogen mustard therapy in patients with mycosis fungoides or parapsoriasis. J Eur Acad Dermatol Venereol 2013;27:163–8.

37. Hoppe RT, Abel EA, Deneau DG, et al. Mycosis fungoides: management with topical nitrogen mustard. J Clin Oncol 1987;5:1796–803.

38. Price NM, Hoppe RT, Deneau DG. Ointment-based mechlorethamine treatment for mycosis fungoides. Cancer 1983;52:2214–9.

39. Navi DRN, Levin YS, Sullivan NC, et al. The Stanford University experience with conventional-dose, total skin electron-beam therapy in the treatment of generalized patch or plaque (T2) and tumor (T3) mycosis fungoides. JAMA Dermatol 2001;147:561–7.

40. Kim YH, Duvic M, Guitart J. Tolerability and efficacy of mechlorethamine 0.04% gel in CTCL (mycosis fungoides) after initial treatment with topical mechlorethamine 0.02% gel. The T-cell Lymphoma Forum. San Francisco, January 23-25, 2014.

41. de Quatrebarbes J, Estève E, Bagot M, et al. Treatment of early-stage mycosis fungoides with twice-weekly applications of mechlorethamine and topical corticosteroids: a prospective study. Arch Dermatol 2005;141:1117–20.

42. Constantine VS. Mechlorethamine desensitization in therapy for mycosis fungoides. Arch Dermatol 1975;111:484.

43. Sánchez Yus E, Surárez Martín E. Contact urticaria and anaphylactic reactions induced by topical application of nitrogen mustard. Actas Dermosifiliogr 1977;68:39–44 [in Spanish].

44. Price N. Topical mechlorethamine. Cutaneous changes in patients with mycosis fungoides after its administration. Arch Dermatol 1977;113:1387–9.

45. Vonderheid EC, Van Scott EJ, Johnson WC, et al. Topical chemotherapy and immunotherapy of mycosis fungoides: intermediate-term results. Arch Dermatol 1977;113:454–62.

46. Abel EA, Sendagorta E, Hoppe RT. Cutaneous malignancies and metastatic squamous cell carcinoma following topical therapies for mycosis fungoides. J Am Acad Dermatol 1986;14:1029–38.

47. Lee LA, Fritz KA, Golitz L, et al. Second cutaneous malignancies in patients with mycosis fungoides treated with topical nitrogen mustard. J Am Acad Dermatol 1982;7:590–8.

48. Du VA, Vonderheid EC, Van Scott EJ, et al. Mycosis fungoides, nitrogen mustard and skin cancer. Br J Dermatol 1978;99:61–3.

49. Lindahl LM, Fenger-Grøn M, Iversen L. Secondary cancers, comorbidities and mortality associated with nitrogen mustard therapy in patients with mycosis fungoides: a 30-year population-based cohort study. Br J Dermatol 2014;170:699–704.

50. Wada S, Miyanishi M, Nishimoto Y, et al. Mustard gas as a cause of respiratory neoplasia in man. Lancet 1968;1:1161–3.

51. Yamada A. On the late injuries following occupational inhalation of mustard gas, with special references to carcinoma of the respiratory tract. Acta Pathol Jpn 1963;13:131–55.

52. Valchlor [package insert]. San Francisco, CA: Actelion Pharmaceuticals, inc; 2013.

53. Wendler D, Pabst R, Bertolini R. The influence of the N-mustard derivative "cytostasan" on pregnancy and fetal development in the rat. Anat Anzr 1976;139:100–14.

54. Deuschle KW, Wiggins WS. The use of nitrogen mustard in the management of two pregnant lymphoma patients. Blood 1953;8:576–9.

55. Zackheim HS. Treatment of mycosis fungoides with topical nitrosourea compounds. Arch Dermatol 1972;106:177–82.

56. Zackheim HS, Epstein EH, Crain WR. Topical carmustine (BCNU) for cutaneous T cell lymphoma: a 15-year experience in 143 patients. J Am Acad Dermatol 1990;22:802–10.

57. Zackheim HS. Topical carmustine (BCNU) in the treatment of mycosis fungoides. Dermatol Ther 2003;16:299–302.

58. Zackheim HS, Feldmann RJ, Lindsay C, et al. Percutaneous absorption of 1,3-bis (2-chlorethyl)-1-nitrosourea (BCNU, carmustine) in mycosis fungoides. Br J Dermatol 1977;97:65–7.

59. Ramsay DL, Meller JA, Zackheim HS. Topical treatment of early cutaneous T-cell lymphoma. Hematol Oncol Clin North Am 1995;9:1031–56.

60. Zackheim HS, Epstein EH Jr, Crain WR, et al. Topical carmustine therapy for lymphomatoid papulosis. Arch Dermatol 1985;121:1410–4.

61. Frost P, DeVita VT. Pigmentation due to a new antitumor agent: effects of topical application of BCNU [1,3-Bis(2-Chloretyhl)-1-Nitrosourea]. Arch Dermatol 1996;94:265–8.

62. Berthelot C, Rivera A, Duvic M. Skin directed therapy for mycosis fungoides: a review. J Drugs Dermatol 2008;7:655–66.

63. Aida T, Cheitlin RA, Bodell WJ. Inhibition of O6-alkylguanine-DNA-alkyltransferase activity potentiates cytotoxicity and induction of SCEs in human glioma cells resistant to 1,3-bis(2-chloroethyl)-1-nitrosourea. Carcinogenesis 1987;8:1219–23.

64. Gudas LJ, Sporn MB, Roberts AB. Cellular biology and biochemistry of retinoids. In: Sporn MB, Roberts AB, Goodman DS, editors. The retinoids. New York: Raven Press; 1994. p. 210–86.

65. Apisarnthanarax N, Wood GS, Stevens SR, et al. Phase I clinical trial of O6-benzylguanine and topical carmustine in the treatment of cutaneous T-cell lymphoma, mycosis fungoides type. Arch Dermatol 2012;148:613–20.

66. Zackheim HS, Epstein EH Jr, McNutt S, et al. Topical carmustine (BCNU) for mycosis fungoides and related disorders: a 10-year experience. J Am Acad Dermatol 1983;9:363–74.

67. Wolverton S. Topical retinoids in comprehensive dermatologic drug therapy. In: Wolverton S, editor. Comprehensive dermatologic drug therapy. Philadelphia: Elsevier Saunders Inc; 2013.

68. Chambon P. A decade of molecular biology of retinoic acid receptors. FASEB J 1996;10:940–54.

69. Zhang C, Duvic M. Retinoids: therapeutic applications and mechanisms of action in cutaneous T-cell lymphoma. Dermatol Ther 2003;16:322–30.

70. Sporn MB, Roberts AB. Role of retinoids in differentiation and carcinogenesis. J Natl Cancer 1984;73. p. 3034–40.

71. Lippman SM, Kavanagh JJ, Paredes-Espinoza M, et al. 13-cis-retinoic acid plus interferon-2a: highly active systemic therapy for squamous cell carcinoma of the cervix. J Natl Cancer Inst 1992;84:241–5.

72. Boehm MF, Zhang L, Zhi L, et al. Design and synthesis of potent retinoid X receptor selective ligands that induce apoptosis in leukemia cells. J Med Chem 1995;38:3146–55.

73. Zhang C, Hazarika P, Ni X, et al. Induction of apoptosis by bexarotene in cutaneous T-cell lymphoma cells: relevance to mechanism of therapeutic action. Clin Cancer Res 2002;8:1234–40.

74. Heald P, Mehlmauer M, Martin AG, et al. Topical bexarotene therapy for patients with refractory or persistent early-stage cutaneous T-cell lymphoma: results of the phase III clinical trial. J Am Acad Dermatol 2003;49:801–15.

75. Breneman D, Duvic M, Kuzel T, et al. Phase 1 and 2 trial of bexarotene gel for skin-directed treatment of patients with cutaneous T-cell lymphoma. Arch Dermatol 2002;138:325–32.

76. Hurst RE. Bexarotene ligand pharmaceuticals. Curr Opin Investig Drugs 2000;1:514–23.

77. Liu HL, Kim YH. Bexarotene gel: a Food and Drug Administration-approved skin-directed therapy for early-stage cutaneous T-cell lymphoma. Arch Dermatol 2002;138:398–9.

78. Targretin® (bexarotene) gel 1% [package insert]. Available at: http://www.drugbank.ca/system/fda_labels/DB00307.pdf?1265922814. Accessed October 27, 2014.

79. Krathen RA, Ward S, Duvic M. Bexarotene is a new treatment option for lymphomatoid papulosis. Dermatol 2003;206:142–7.

80. Walling HW, Swick BL, Gerami P, et al. Folliculotropic mycosis fungoides responding to bexarotene gel. J Drugs Dermatol 2008;7:169–71.

81. Apisarnthanarax N, Talpur R, Ward S, et al. Tazarotene 0.1% gel for refractory mycosis fungoides lesions: an open-label pilot study. J Am Acad Dermatol 2004;50:600–7.

82. Duvic M, Friedman-Kien AE, Looney DJ, et al. Topical treatment of cutaneous lesions of acquired immunodeficiency syndrome–related Kaposi sarcoma using alitretinoin gel. Arch Dermatol 2000;136(12):1461–9.

83. Bodsworth NJ, Bloch M, Bower M, et al. Phase III vehicle-controlled, multi-centered study of topical alitretinoin gel 0.1% in cutaneous AIDS-related Kaposi's sarcoma. Am J Clin Dermatol 2001;2:77–87.

84. Bassiri-Tehrani S, Cohen DE. Treatment of cutaneous T-cell lymphoma with alitretinoin gel. Int J Dermatol 2002;41:104–6.

85. Weinstein G. Tazarotene gel: efficacy and safety in plaque psoriasis. J Am Acad Dermatol 1997;37:S33–8.

86. Demierre MF, Vachon L, Ho V, et al. Phase 1/2 pilot study of methotrexate-laurocapram topical gel for the treatment of patients with early-stage mycosis fungoides. Arch Dermatol 2003;139:624–8.

87. Syed TA, Hadi SM, Qureshi ZA, et al. Management of psoriasis vulgaris with methotrexate 0.25% in a hydrophilic gel: a placebo-controlled, double-blind study. J Cutan Med Surg 2001;5:299–302.

88. Rallis E, Economidi A, Verros C, et al. Successful treatment of patch type mycosis fungoides with

tacrolimus ointment 0.1%. J Drugs Dermatol 2006; 5:906–7.

89. Pomerantz RG, Campbell LS, Jukic DM, et al. Post-transplant cutaneous T-cell lymphoma: case reports and review of the association of calcineurin inhibitor use with posttransplant lymphoproliferative disease risk. Arch Dermatol 2010;146:513–6.

90. Deeths MJ, Chapman JT, Dellavalle RP, et al. Treatment of patch and plaque stage mycosis fungoides with imiquimod 5% cream. J Am Acad Dermatol 2005;52:275–80.

91. Martínez-González MC, Verea-Hernando MM, Yebra-Pimentel MT, et al. Imiquimod in mycosis fungoides. Eur J Dermatol 2008;18:148–52.

92. Suchin KR, Junkins-Hopkins JM, Rook AH. Treatment of stage IA cutaneous T-cell lymphoma with topical application of the immune response modifier imiquimod. Arch Dermatol 2002;138:1137–9.

93. Dummer R, Urosevic M, Kempf W, et al. Imiquimod induces complete clearance of a PUVA-resistant plaque in mycosis fungoides. Dermatol 2003;207:116–8.

94. Ariffin N, Khorshid M. Treatment of mycosis fungoides with imiquimod 5% cream. Clin Exp Dermatol 2006;31:822–3.

95. Onsun N, Ufacik H, Kural Y, et al. Efficacy of imiquimod in solitary plaques of mycosis fungoides. Int J Tissue React 2005;27:167–72.

96. Soler-Machin J, Gilaberte-Calzada Y, Vera-Alvarez J, et al. Imiquimod in treatment of palpebral mycosis fungoides. Arch Soc Esp Oftalmol 2006;81:221–3 [in Spanish].

97. Chiam LY, Chan YC. Solitary plaque mycosis fungoides of the penis responding to topical imiquimod therapy. Br J Dermatol 2007;156: 560–2.

98. Ardigò M, Cota C, Berardesca E. Unilesional mycosis fungoides successfully treated with topical imiquimod. Eur J Dermatol 2006;16:446.

99. Owens ML, Bridson WE, Smith SL, et al. Percutaneous penetration of Aldara cream, 5% during the topical treatment of genital and perianal warts. Prim Care Update Ob Gyns 1998;5:151.

100. Altamura D, Simonacci F, Hirbod T, et al. Histologic features mimicking mycosis fungoides induced by imiquimod, 5%: a potential pitfall for dermatopathologists. JAMA Dermatol 2014; 150(11):1–2.

Phototherapy of Mycosis Fungoides

Emmilia Hodak, MD*, Lev Pavlovsky, MD, PhD

KEYWORDS

- Mycosis fungoides • Phototherapy • Ultraviolet light B • Narrow-band ultraviolet light B
- Ultraviolet A • Psoralen plus ultraviolet A

KEY POINTS

- Phototherapy, specifically ultraviolet light B (UVB) phototherapy and psoralen plus ultraviolet A (PUVA) photochemotherapy, is still the first-line treatment of early stage mycosis fungoides (MF).
- The main goal is to induce complete response. Whether prolonged maintenance treatment results in longer sustained remissions and better prognosis is still unclear. The benefit of long maintenance treatment in a given patient should be weighed against the cost and potential adverse effects of extended periods of ultraviolet light exposure.
- Patients with early stage MF refractory to phototherapy, or patients with advanced MF may benefit from combination treatment with systemic treatment.

INTRODUCTION

Phototherapy, specifically, ultraviolet B (UVB) phototherapy, and psoralen plus ultraviolet A (PUVA) photochemotherapy, has been a mainstay of treatment of mycosis fungoides (MF) for the last several decades. Initially, both types of phototherapy were used as monotherapy for early stage MF, but in recent years, the use has been expanded to include combinations of ultraviolet light (UVL) with systemic treatments in cases of treatment refractory early stage MF, and in patients with advanced MF. Although broadband (BB) UVB therapy was widely used in the past, currently most phototherapy delivered around the world is in the form of narrowband (NB) UVB. This article reviews the efficacy and safety profile of the most commonly used forms of phototherapy for MF.

ULTRAVIOLET B PHOTOTHERAPY IN MYCOSIS FUNGOIDES
Background

The clinically relevant electromagnetic radiation emitted by the sun consists of UVB, 290 to 320 nm and UVA, 320 to 400 nm.[1,2] BB-UVB units available in clinical practice emit broadly between 270 to 390 nm with a peak at 313 nm. NB-UVB refers to a radiation source with a sharp emission peak between 311 and 312 nm.[1]

For a given dose, UVB at 300 nm is approximately 1000-fold more erythemogenic compared with UVA at 360 nm,[2,3] but because of its shorter

Potential Conflict of Interest: None.
Department of Dermatology, Rabin Medical Center, Beilinson Hospital, Sackler Faculty Medicine, Tel Aviv University, Derech Ze'ev Jabotinsky 39, Petah Tikva 49100, Israel
* Corresponding author. Department of Dermatology, Rabin Medical Center, Beilinson Hospital, Derech Ze'ev Jabotinsky 39, Petah Tikva 49100, Israel.
E-mail address: hodake@post.tau.ac.il

Dermatol Clin 33 (2015) 697–702
http://dx.doi.org/10.1016/j.det.2015.05.005
0733-8635/15/$ – see front matter

wavelength, UVB has less depth of penetration than UVA.

Treatment Schedule

Most centers recommend phototherapy 2 or 3 times a week; for practical convenience, twice-weekly phototherapy will clear the skin involvement, albeit it at a slower pace than 3 times a week. It is best to have the treatments given at least 48 hours apart. Phototherapy directions are usually those recommended for psoriasis.[4,5] The starting dose can be determined from minimal erythema dose (MED) or skin type; MED is usually utilized only in the face of a history of sun sensitivity. Increments in the light dose are best determined by a percentage of the previous dose based on the skin type and any unexpected or undesired erythema. Different phototherapy centers target a different endpoint and different maintenance schedule after clearing, which makes it difficult to determine overall efficacy and duration of response. Patients on NB-UVB may not be able to tolerate less frequent treatments than every 10 days due to burning. The United States Cutaneous Lymphoma Consortium (USCLC) has developed guidelines for MF that will hopefully alleviate this issue.[6]

Efficacy

In a review of the published literature for both BB-UVB and NB-UVB, a complete response (CR) was defined as at least 90% clearance. The CR rates have been shown not unexpectedly to be greater for patch (>80%) than plaque disease (≤50%), but the majority of patients relapsed after discontinuing therapy.[7–10] BB-UVB has largely now been replaced by NB-UVB.

The published reported CR rates for NB-UVB have ranged from 54% to 90% in patients with Stage IA–IIA disease.[10–26] As with BB-UVB, patients with patch-only disease did better than those with plaques, but patients with one B (IB) disease did much better with NB-UVB versus BB-UVB in 1 study (78% vs 44% respectively).[10] The relapse rate without maintenance therapy (defined as continued treatment post near clearing) varied from approximately 30 to 100%[11,15,18] versus 4% to 83% in those with maintenance.[16,21]

The literature describing the use of NB-UVB in combination with other treatment modalities in MF is sparse, and comparative studies of mono versus combination therapy are lacking. Case reports of NB-UVB combined with bexarotene suggest efficacy in MF.[27,28]

PSORALEN PLUS ULTRAVIOLET A THERAPY IN MYCOSIS FUNGOIDES
Background

Psoralen, taken orally or applied topically, conjugates and forms covalent bonds directly with DNA following exposure to UVA, resulting in the formation of DNA-psoralen cross-links with inhibition of DNA replication.[29]

Treatment Schedule

An optimized form of methoxalen, or 8-MOP, called Oxsoralen-Ultra, is the current oral formulation available in the United States. This should be dosed at 0.5 mg/kg 1 to 1.5 hours before exposure to UVA. There is also a 1% topical formulation available for localized treatment. PUVA treatments are given 2 to 3 times a week in the United States, potentially more frequently elsewhere in the world. As with NBUVB, less frequent treatments take longer to achieve remission. The starting dose and incremental doses are based primarily on skin type as with psoriasis.[4,5] Maintenance treatment is generally done as for NB-UVB, although it is possible for patients on PUVA to tolerate treatments even given as infrequently as once a month; there may be no need to reduce amount of UVL at a given treatment when decreasing the frequency.

Efficacy

Complete clearance rates in MF being 85% for stage IA, 65% for stage IB, and 85% for stage IIA disease.[19,30–32] Based on the experience of experts, patches and thin plaques are known to respond better to PUVA than thick plaques. Most physicians treating patients with MF do use some sort of tapering frequency when the patient has achieved a maximum response. Although expert opinion reflects that most MF experts do use some kind of maintenance PUVA because of the feeling that it prolongs remission, the literature is not as clear-cut. Querfeld and colleagues[33] reported the long-term outcome of 66 patients with early stage MF (IA-IIA) who achieved a CR, most (94%) patients were then put on continuous maintenance therapy. Although 50% of the patients experienced relapse, the time to relapse was 39 months (range 2–127 months), and the other 50% of the patients had a sustained remission of a median duration of 84 months (7 years) (range 5–238 months, ie, 0.5–20 years). There was another study that compared the follow-up data between a group of patients with and without maintenance treatment after initial clearing phase of PUVA; there was no significant difference in the relapse rate or in the time to relapse between the group of 25 early MF patients who stopped PUVA after clearing phase, and the group of 9 patients who received maintenance treatment for a further 15 treatments (range 0.3–10.5 months).[34] The results of this study suggest that relatively short-term PUVA maintenance treatment may not necessarily slow disease recurrence.

PUVA is ineffective as a monotherapy for tumor-stage disease.[15,32,35,36] Patients with erythroderma generally require a greater number of treatments to clear compared with patients with plaque-stage disease, but this may be because the dose of UVA utilized is much lower due to extreme photosensitivity. Blood involvement has been shown to be affected by PUVA therapy.[37]

Combination therapy, primarily with retinoic acid receptor (RAR) retinoids,[38] or bexarotene,[39,40] a retinoid X receptor (RXR) retinoid, or alpha interferon,[41–43] has been used in early disease to improve efficacy, possibly prolong remissions, or to treat those patients in whom lower response rates with PUVA alone are expected. Despite the fact that a combination of skin-directed and systemic treatment is usually considered more effective than either alone in MF, there are few studies to support this. A combination of PUVA with systemic therapy, however, may decrease the total UVA exposure and thus reduce long-term adverse effects. Although multimodality therapy including PUVA is frequently used in clinical practice, there are few published reports.[44]

HAND/FOOT PSORALEN PLUS ULTRAVIOLET A

This is an important adjunct that can be used to treat the top and soles of feet that are otherwise excluded from UVA exposure while standing in the phototherapy box. This can be done at the end of the whole-body treatment with systemic psoralen on board or this can be done at an alternate time with prior application of topical psoralen.

SAFETY OF PHOTOTHERAPY

There are many common adverse effects shared by all forms of phototherapy, but there are some striking differences between NB-UVB compared with PUVA.

The most common acute adverse effects of all forms of phototherapy are erythema, maximum at 12 to 24 hours in NB-UVB with resolution at 48 hours and maximum at 48 to 96 hours in PUVA with resolution over the week following treatment.[45,46] Other cutaneous adverse effects that are not uncommon to all forms of phototherapy include pruritus and stinging pain in circumscribed areas. These adverse effects can be managed by altering the dosage of light and holding therapy when clinically indicated. Photosensitivity to concurrent medications is usually caused by UVA and not UVB, but it can occur with either. Retinoids used in conjunction with phototherapy for MF have the greatest chance of increasing photosensitivity. Precipitation of polymorphous light eruption can occur with PUVA but is not usually seen with UVB. In some patients, phototherapy will unmask underlying MF lesions that are not apparent. Subungual hemorrhage, photoonycholysis, and melanonychia are common to PUVA[29] but not UVB. Acute pigmentary changes other than tanning are much more common with PUVA than UVB. PUVA induces immediate pigment darkening and persistent pigment darkening due to oxidation of preexisting melanin.[47] Nausea may be seen with the intake of psoralen, and fatigue and headache have been reported with PUVA.

Many studies have been published regarding the adverse effects of long-term phototherapy. The most common are pigmentary changes. With PUVA, patients may develop PUVA lentigos, which are usually persistent after treatment. Mottled guttate hypopigmentation can occur with either NBUVB or PUVA.

Photoaging is another known adverse effect of long-term treatment with PUVA,[48] but xerosis can be seen with either form of phototherapy.

Damage to the eye can occur with either form of phototherapy if protection is not given in the light box with UVL protective goggles. The risk with UVB is conjunctivitis or keratitis,[49] and the risk with PUVA is cataracts. The risk of ocular damage with PUVA persists for 24 hours after taking psoralen until the medication is eliminated from the body. During that time, patients must wear UVA-protective wrap around sunglasses upon exposure to sunlight or if sitting by window glass that permits UVA to come through. A 25-year prospective study of patients treated with PUVA from a large US cohort study did not demonstrate an increased risk of either visual impairment or cataract formation with increasing exposure to PUVA,[50] most likely because of the regular adherence to this recommendation for eye protection.

The main concern with both forms of phototherapy is an increased risk of skin cancer. Although there is no question that exposure to sunlight and sunburn can be associated with skin cancer, 2 publications summarizing more than 7000 patients with primarily psoriasis treated with either BB-UVB or NB-UVB did not show an increased risk other than those given both UVB and PUVA.[51,52] In contrast, high cumulative exposure (>200 treatments or >2000 J/cm^2) to oral PUVA is associated with a dose-related increase in the risk of nonmelanoma skin cancer (NMSC), particularly squamous cell carcinoma (SCC).[53–55] Although some US studies do not show an increased risk of melanoma in patients with psoriasis treated with PUVA,[56] one 15-year follow-up US study has shown a higher risk of melanoma after a latency period of at least 15 years and/or high level of exposure (more than 250 PUVA treatments used as benchmark), with a relative risk of 3.1 if both were present.[57] It should be noted that the duration of treatment in MF with PUVA is often greater than in psoriasis.

SUMMARY: PRACTICAL PEARLS FOR PHOTOTHERAPY

For patients with early stage MF

- Patches can be treated well with NB-UVB alone.
- Thick plaques or folliculotropic involvement are better served by PUVA than NB-UVB.
- Patients who have failed to clear on PUVA may benefit from NB-UVB.[58]
- Systemic retinoids (acitretin or isotretinoin) specifically may be of value in patients with sun-damaged skin who are candidates for either NB-UVB or PUVA.[59]
- Patients who have failed to clear with NB-UVB or PUVA alone, or who have associated poor prognostic factors, are best served with combination of phototherapy with a systemic agent.
- Because the goal of treatment is clearing, it is important to continue until reaching this end point and not to stop before it. Notably, it generally takes longer to induce a remission in MF versus psoriasis. Areas not accessible to UVL may be treated with topical steroids or targeted localized chemotherapy
- Although extended periods of remission may be achieved with the use of maintenance treatment for either PUVA or NB-UVB, the decision to have it and the duration of this period is best determined by weighing the risk factors of chronic phototherapy treatment in a given patient including additional adverse effects, cost of therapy, patient time, psychological burden versus the risk of a clinical relapse with the potential need to restart therapy at frequency of 2 to 3 times per week. Guidelines for the specifics of maintenance therapy in MF are needed.
- Most of the patients who respond to the first course of NB-UVB or PUVA therapy will respond to the second course.

For patients with advanced MF

- It is best to combine phototherapy with a systemic agent
- Erythrodermic MF may be helped with either NB-UVB or PUVA alone, but because of the preexisting cutaneous erythema, it may be difficult in these patients to assess any burning from the UVL and hence to safely increase the UVL dose.
- PUVA may have an additional effect on the blood involvement in MF or sezary syndrome (SS) that NB-UVB does not

REFERENCES

1. Kochevar IE, Taylor CR, Krutmann J. Fundamentals of cutaneous photobiology and photoimmunology. In: Goldsmith LA, Katz SI, Gilchrest BA, et al, editors. Fitzpatrick's dermatology in general medicine. 8th edition. New York: McGraw Hill; 2012. p. 1031–48.
2. Runger T. Ultraviolet light. In: Bolognia JL, Jorizzo JL, Schaffer JV, editors. Dermatology. 3rd edition. Philadelphia: Saunders; 2012. p. 1455–86.
3. Anderson RR, Parrish JA. The optics of human skin. J Invest Dermatol 1981;77(1):13–9.
4. Menter A, Korman NJ, Elmets CA, et al. Guidelines of care for the management of psoriasis and psoriatic arthritis: section 5. Guidelines of care for the treatment of psoriasis with phototherapy and photochemotherapy. J Am Acad Dermatol 2010;62(1):114–35.
5. Zanolli MD, Feldman SR. Phototherapy treatment protocols for psoriasis and other phototherapy-responsive dermatoses. 2nd edition. New York: Taylor & Francis; 2004.
6. Olsen EA. Guidelines for phototherapy of mycosis fungoides and sézary syndrome: a consensus statement of the united states cutaneous lymphoma consortium (USCLC). JAAD 2015, in press.
7. Milstein HJ, Vonderheid EC, Van Scott EJ, et al. Home ultraviolet phototherapy of early mycosis fungoides: preliminary observations. J Am Acad Dermatol 1982;6(3):355–62.
8. Resnik KS, Vonderheid EC. Home UV phototherapy of early mycosis fungoides: long-term follow-up observations in thirty-one patients. J Am Acad Dermatol 1993;29(1):73–7.
9. Ramsay DL, Lish KM, Yalowitz CB, et al. Ultraviolet-B phototherapy for early-stage cutaneous T-cell lymphoma. Arch Dermatol 1992;128(7):931–3.
10. Pavlotsky F, Barzilai A, Kasem R, et al. UVB in the management of early stage mycosis fungoides. J Eur Acad Dermatol Venereol 2006;20(5):565–72.
11. Hofer A, Cerroni L, Kerl H, et al. Narrowband (311-nm) UV-B therapy for small plaque parapsoriasis and early-stage mycosis fungoides. Arch Dermatol 1999;135(11):1377–80.

12. Clark C, Dawe RS, Evans AT, et al. Narrowband TL-01 phototherapy for patch-stage mycosis fungoides. Arch Dermatol 2000;136(6):748–52.

13. Xiao T, Xia LX, Yang ZH, et al. Narrow-band ultraviolet B phototherapy for early stage mycosis fungoides. Eur J Dermatol 2008;18(6):660–2.

14. Ponte P, Serrao V, Apetato M. Efficacy of narrowband UVB vs PUVA in patients with early-stage mycosis fungoides. J Eur Acad Dermatol Venereol 2010;24(6):716–21.

15. Ahmad K, Rogers S, McNicholas PD, et al. Narrowband UVB and PUVA in the treatment of mycosis fungoides: a retrospective study. Acta Derm Venereol 2007;87(5):413–7.

16. Boztepe G, Sahin S, Ayhan M, et al. Narrowband ultraviolet B phototherapy to clear and maintain clearance in patients with mycosis fungoides. J Am Acad Dermatol 2005;53(2):242–6.

17. Brazzelli V, Antoninetti M, Palazzini S, et al. Narrow-band ultraviolet therapy in early-stage mycosis fungoides: study on 20 patients. Photodermatol Photoimmunol Photomed 2007;23(6):229–33.

18. Dereure O. The role of electron therapy in the treatment of mycosis fungoides: optimised indications and ease of access. Ann Dermatol Venereol 2009; 136(3):235–7.

19. Diederen PV, van Weelden H, Sanders CJ, et al. Narrowband UVB and psoralen-UVA in the treatment of early-stage mycosis fungoides: a retrospective study. J Am Acad Dermatol 2003;48(2):215–9.

20. El-Mofty M, El-Darouty M, Salonas M, et al. Narrow band UVB (311 nm), psoralen UVB (311 nm) and PUVA therapy in the treatment of early-stage mycosis fungoides: a right-left comparative study. Photodermatol Photoimmunol Photomed 2005;21(6):281–6.

21. Gathers RC, Scherschun L, Malick F, et al. Narrowband UVB phototherapy for early-stage mycosis fungoides. J Am Acad Dermatol 2002; 47(2):191–7.

22. Ghodsi SZ, Hallaji Z, Balighi K, et al. Narrow-band UVB in the treatment of early stage mycosis fungoides: report of 16 patients. Clin Exp Dermatol 2005;30(4):376–8.

23. Gokdemir G, Barutcuoglu B, Sakiz D, et al. Narrowband UVB phototherapy for early-stage mycosis fungoides: evaluation of clinical and histopathological changes. J Eur Acad Dermatol Venereol 2006; 20(7):804–9.

24. Kural Y, Onsun N, Aygin S, et al. Efficacy of narrowband UVB phototherapy in early stage of mycosis fungoides. J Eur Acad Dermatol Venereol 2006; 20(1):104–5.

25. Ohtsuka T. Narrow band UVB phototherapy for early stage mycosis fungoides. Eur J Dermatol 2008;18(4): 464–6.

26. Jang MS, Baek JW, Park JB, et al. Narrowband ultraviolet B phototherapy of early stage mycosis fungoides in korean patients. Ann Dermatol 2011; 23(4):474–80.

27. Lokitz ML, Wong HK. Bexarotene and narrowband ultraviolet B phototherapy combination treatment for mycosis fungoides. Photodermatol Photoimmunol Photomed 2007;23(6):255–7.

28. D'Acunto C, Gurioli C, Neri I. Plaque stage mycosis fungoides treated with bexarotene at low dosage and UVB-NB. J Dermatolog Treat 2010;21(1):45–8.

29. Gupta AK, Anderson TF. Psoralen photochemotherapy. J Am Acad Dermatol 1987;17(5 Pt 1):703–34.

30. Honigsmann H, Brenner W, Rauschmeier W, et al. Photochemotherapy for cutaneous T cell lymphoma. A follow-up study. J Am Acad Dermatol 1984;10(2 Pt 1):238–45.

31. Abel EA, Sendagorta E, Hoppe RT, et al. PUVA treatment of erythrodermic and plaque-type mycosis fungoides. Ten-year follow-up study. Arch Dermatol 1987;123(7):897–901.

32. Herrmann JJ, Roenigk HH Jr, Hurria A, et al. Treatment of mycosis fungoides with photochemotherapy (PUVA): long-term follow-up. J Am Acad Dermatol 1995;33(2 Pt 1):234–42.

33. Querfeld C, Rosen ST, Kuzel TM, et al. Long-term follow-up of patients with early-stage cutaneous T-cell lymphoma who achieved complete remission with psoralen plus UV-A monotherapy. Arch Dermatol 2005;141(3):305–11.

34. Wackernagel A, Hofer A, Legat F, et al. Efficacy of 8-methoxypsoralen vs 5-methoxypsoralen plus ultraviolet A therapy in patients with mycosis fungoides. Br J Dermatol 2006;154(3):519–23.

35. Briffa DV, Warin AP, Harrington CI, et al. Photochemotherapy in mycosis fungoides. A study of 73 patients. Lancet 1980;2(8185):49–53.

36. Molin L, Thomsen K, Volden G, et al. Photochemotherapy (PUVA) in the tumour stage of mycosis fungoides: a report from the scandinavian mycosis fungoides study group. Acta Derm Venereol 1981; 61(1):52–4.

37. Raphael BA, Morrissey KA, Kim EJ, et al. Psoralen plus ultraviolet A light may be associated with clearing of peripheral blood disease in advanced cutaneous T-cell lymphoma. J Am Acad Dermatol 2011;65(1):212–4.

38. Lebwohl M. Acitretin in combination with UVB or PUVA. J Am Acad Dermatol 1999;41(3 Pt 2):S22–4.

39. Singh F, Lebwohl MG. Cutaneous T-cell lymphoma treatment using bexarotene and PUVA: a case series. J Am Acad Dermatol 2004;51(4):570–3.

40. Whittaker S, Ortiz P, Dummer R, et al. Efficacy and safety of bexarotene combined with psoralen-ultraviolet A (PUVA) compared with PUVA treatment alone in stage IB-IIA mycosis fungoides: final results from the EORTC cutaneous lymphoma task force phase III randomized clinical trial (NCT00056056). Br J Dermatol 2012;167(3):678–87.

41. Roenigk HH, Kuzel T, Rosen S. Interferons for cutaneous T-cell lymphoma monotherapy or combination with PUVA. Australas J Dermatol 1993;34(1):13–5.

42. Chiarion-Sileni V, Bononi A, Fornasa CV, et al. Phase II trial of interferon-alpha-2a plus psolaren with ultraviolet light A in patients with cutaneous T-cell lymphoma. Cancer 2002;95(3):569–75.

43. Kuzel TM, Roenigk HH Jr, Samuelson E, et al. Effectiveness of interferon alfa-2a combined with phototherapy for mycosis fungoides and the sezary syndrome. J Clin Oncol 1995;13(1):257–63.

44. Booken N, Weiss C, Utikal J, et al. Combination therapy with extracorporeal photopheresis, interferonalpha, PUVA and topical corticosteroids in the management of sezary syndrome. J Dtsch Dermatol Ges 2010;8(6):428–38.

45. Laube S, George SA. Adverse effects with PUVA and UVB phototherapy. J Dermatolog Treat 2001; 12(2):101–5.

46. Martin JA, Laube S, Edwards C, et al. Rate of acute adverse events for narrow-band UVB and psoralen-UVA phototherapy. Photodermatol Photoimmunol Photomed 2007;23(2–3):68–72.

47. Beitner H, Wennersten G. A qualitative and quantitative transmission electronmicroscopic study of the immediate pigment darkening reaction. Photodermatol 1985;2(5):273–8.

48. Stern RS, Parrish JA, Fitzpatrick TB, et al. Actinic degeneration in association with long-term use of PUVA. J Invest Dermatol 1985;84(2):135–8.

49. Ibbotson SH, Bilsland D, Cox NH, et al. An update and guidance on narrowband ultraviolet B phototherapy: a British photodermatology group workshop report. Br J Dermatol 2004;151(2):283–97.

50. Malanos D, Stern RS. Psoralen plus ultraviolet A does not increase the risk of cataracts: a 25-year prospective study. J Am Acad Dermatol 2007; 57(2):231–7.

51. Lee E, Koo J, Berger T. UVB phototherapy and skin cancer risk: a review of the literature. Int J Dermatol 2005;44(5):355–60.

52. Hearn RM, Kerr AC, Rahim KF, et al. Incidence of skin cancers in 3867 patients treated with narrowband ultraviolet B phototherapy. Br J Dermatol 2008;159(4):931–5.

53. Stern RS, Laird N, Melski J, et al. Cutaneous squamous-cell carcinoma in patients treated with PUVA. N Engl J Med 1984;310(18):1156–61.

54. Nijsten TE, Stern RS. The increased risk of skin cancer is persistent after discontinuation of psoralen+ultraviolet A: a cohort study. J Invest Dermatol 2003;121(2):252–8.

55. Stern RS, Lunder EJ. Risk of squamous cell carcinoma and methoxsalen (psoralen) and UV-A radiation (PUVA). A meta-analysis. Arch Dermatol 1998; 134(12):1582–5.

56. Chuang TY, Heinrich LA, Schultz MD, et al. PUVA and skin cancer. A historical cohort study on 492 patients. J Am Acad Dermatol 1992;26(2 Pt 1):173–7.

57. Stern RS, Nichols KT, Vakeva LH. Malignant melanoma in patients treated for psoriasis with methoxsalen (psoralen) and ultraviolet A radiation (PUVA). The PUVA follow-up study. N Engl J Med 1997; 336(15):1041–5.

58. Khaled A, Fazaa B, Goucha S, et al. PUVA therapy and narrowband UVB therapy in Tunisian patients with mycosis fungoides. Therapie 2009;64:389–94.

59. Bettoli V, Zauli S, Virgili A. Retinoids in the chemoprevention of non-melanoma skin cancers: why, when and how. J Dermatolog Treat 2013;24(3): 235–7.

Radiation Therapy for Cutaneous T-Cell Lymphomas

Daniel J. Tandberg, MD, Oana Craciunescu, PhD,
Chris R. Kelsey, MD*

KEYWORDS

- Mycosis fungoides • Cutaneous T-cell lymphoma • Radiation therapy
- Total skin electron beam therapy • CD30$^+$ lymphoproliferative disorders

KEY POINTS

- Radiation therapy is one of the most effective treatment modalities in cutaneous T-cell lymphomas.
- Local radiation therapy is potentially curative in unilesional mycosis fungoides.
- Local radiation therapy can effectively palliate symptomatic lesions in patients with cutaneous T-cell lymphoma.
- Total skin electron beam therapy should be used in patients with diffuse mycosis fungoides unresponsive to other modalities or when thick plaques or tumors are present.

INTRODUCTION

Cutaneous T-cell lymphomas (CTCLs) are comprised of several histologic subtypes of non-Hodgkin lymphoma characterized by localization of malignant lymphocytes to the skin. Mycosis fungoides (MF) is the most common type of CTCL, accounting for 54% of CTCL diagnoses from 2001 to 2005 in one Surveillance, Epidemiology, and End Results registry review.[1] Other subtypes of CTCL include cutaneous CD30$^+$ T-cell lymphoproliferative disorders and primary cutaneous peripheral T-cell lymphomas.

Radiation therapy (RT) is one of the most effective treatment modalities for CTCL. Lymphocytes are among the most radiosensitive of all cells. Low doses of radiation yield impressive local responses with minimal side effects. For patients with MF, RT has several different clinical applications. For the rare patient with unilesional disease, RT alone is potentially curative. For patients with more advanced cutaneous disease, RT to local lesions or to the entire skin can effectively palliate symptomatic disease and provide local disease control. Finally, symptomatic nodal or visceral disease can also be palliated with RT if necessary. This article reviews basic information regarding the administration of RT and reviews the published literature supporting the use of such for MF and primary cutaneous anaplastic large cell lymphoma (cALCL). Cutaneous peripheral T-cell lymphomas are rare and are not discussed further.

MYCOSIS FUNGOIDES
Local Radiation Therapy

In rare circumstances, MF presents as a solitary lesion, or small number of clustered lesions, that are amenable to a definitive course of therapy where the goal of treatment is long-term disease control. More commonly, patients with MF have more diffuse presentations where symptom palliation

---

No disclosures.
Department of Radiation Oncology, Duke University Medical Center, DUMC BOX 3085, Durham, NC 27710, USA
* Corresponding author.
E-mail address: christopher.kelsey@duke.edu

and local disease control are the fundamental goal of treatment. In circumstances where other modalities are not effective or a rapid response is desired, local RT can be efficacious. These circumstances include cosmetically disfiguring lesions on the face; tumors and thick plaques where radiation can effectively treat to the necessary depth; and lesions that are painful, pruritic, or weeping.

Clinical applications of local radiation therapy

Minimal stage IA disease Patients with patches or plaques covering less than 10% of the body surface area without significant blood, nodal, or visceral involvement have clinical stage IA MF. These patients have a favorable prognosis with survival similar to age-matched control subjects without MF.[2] In a retrospective cohort analysis including 121 patients with clinical stage IA disease, the median survival had not been reached after more than 32 years of follow-up. Three (2%) of 122 patients had died of MF during the study period.

The subgroup of patients with "minimal" stage IA MF (ie, unilesional or up to three close lesions) have an especially favorable prognosis. Patients with this disease may experience long-term remission or ostensibly even "cure" with local RT alone. Several small studies have reported outcomes of local RT in minimal stage IA disease. Results of these studies are summarized in **Table 1**. Wilson and colleagues[3] evaluated 21 patients with minimal disease treated with local RT. Thirteen patients had unilesional MF. The complete response (CR) rate to localized RT was 97%. Disease-free survival (DFS) for the entire group at 5 and 10 years was 75% and 64%, respectively. Improved DFS at 10 years was reported in patients with unilesional disease (85%) and those receiving doses of at least 20 Gy (91%).

Micaily and colleagues[4] reported on the outcomes of 18 patients with unilesional stage IA MF. This represented only 5% (18 of 325) of patients with MF treated at the study institution. Most patients received 30.6 Gy of local RT. The CR rate was 100%. Relapse-free survival (RFS) and overall survival at 10 years was 86%

and 100%, respectively. Two relapses occurred, both confined to the skin at distant sites and subsequently treated with topical nitrogen mustard.

Finally, Piccinno and colleagues[5] evaluated 15 patients with minimal stage MF treated with a median dose of 22 Gy. Complete remission of treated lesions was observed in 95% with the other 5% achieving a partial remission. At 5 and 10 years the overall relapse-free rate was 51%.

In summary, less than 5% of patients present with minimal stage IA MF. This unique subgroup may be managed effectively with local RT alone. Available studies report excellent responses to local RT with 95% to 100% of lesions experiencing a CR. Many patients have a prolonged disease-free interval with the best outcomes seeming to be with RT doses of 20 to 30 Gy.

Palliation of individual lesions Local RT is an effective palliative therapy for patients with all stages of MF with symptomatic cutaneous lesions. Local RT is often used to treat MF lesions refractory to other skin-directed or systemic therapies. Several retrospective studies have demonstrated very high rates of CR (>95%) of individual MF lesions with fractionated courses of RT.[3–6] A dose–response relationship has emerged with higher doses being associated with higher rates of CR and local control. Cotter and colleagues[6] evaluated the impact of radiation dose on local control in 111 MF lesions (53% plaques, 47% tumors). They demonstrated a CR to treatment in all lesions receiving greater than 20 Gy. Local recurrence was inversely associated with dose. The rate of local in-field recurrence was 42% with doses less than or equal to 10 Gy, 32% for doses 10 to 20 Gy, 21% for doses 20 to 30 Gy, and 0% when the dose was greater than 30 Gy. There was no difference in response rates between plaques and tumors. It was suggested that tumor doses equivalent to 30 Gy at 2 Gy per fraction were required for adequate control of MF lesions.

Palliation of individual skin lesions with very short courses of RT has also been reported. Short courses of radiation are more convenient for

Table 1
Outcomes of local radiation therapy in minimal stage IA mycosis fungoides

Study (Ref)	Extent of Disease	No. of Patients	No. of Sites	RT Dose (Median)	CR Rate	Relapse in RT Field	DFS 5 y	DFS 10 y
Wilson et al,[3] 1998	1–3 lesions	21	32	20 Gy	97%	3/31	75%	64%
Micaily et al,[4] 1998	1 lesions	18	18	30.6 Gy	100%	0/18	NR	86%
Piccinno et al,[5] 2009	1–4 lesions	15	22	22 Gy	95%	4/22	51%	51%

Abbreviations: CR, complete response; DFS, disease-free survival.

patients and are potentially more cost effective compared with multiple fractions. Thomas and colleagues[7] reported their experience treating 270 CTCL lesions (primarily MF) with a single fraction of local RT. Of the 58 patients included in the study, 21 (36%) had patch/plaque disease, 34 (59%) had tumor-stage disease, and 3 (5%) had erythroderma only. Most patients (97%) were treated with a single dose of greater than or equal to 7 Gy. A CR was observed in 94% of lesions and the rate of relapse in the radiation field was 1% with a median follow-up of 41.8 months. Large-cell transformation and tumor morphology were associated with a lower CR rate. Neelis and colleagues[8] reported a CR rate of 92% when patients with MF were treated to a total dose of 8 Gy in two fractions. Local relapse occurred in 8% of treated sites. Of note, only 30% of lesions treated with 4 Gy in two fractions achieved a CR. Patients who either did not have a CR or failed locally were retreated with 20 Gy in eight fractions without complication. No significant acute or long-term toxicities were reported in either study.

In summary, local RT is very effective in the palliation of MF skin lesions. Short courses of one to two fractions (7–8 Gy) have yielded favorable results and can be used for patients requiring rapid palliation or who would have a difficult time coming in for a more conventional regimen. Generally, smaller lesions are optimally suited for a single fraction of treatment, whereas larger lesions are often better managed with a more protracted fractionated approach.

Palliation of nodal and visceral disease Most patients with MF never develop symptomatic nodal or visceral disease. However, just as with other malignancies, local RT can be used in this setting for symptom palliation. Patients with advanced-stage MF may experience pain, swelling, or other local symptoms secondary to bulky lymphadenopathy. Visceral metastatic disease can impact the function of an involved organ. RT in these circumstances is typically performed with computed tomography (CT)–based three-dimensional planning with megavoltage photon RT. Typical doses used in our institution range from 20 to 30 Gy using 2- to 3-Gy fractions.

Side effects
Acute and long-term side effects of local RT directed at skin lesions are minimal. Patients may develop erythema and occasionally dry or moist desquamation within the treatment field. Ulcerated lesions sometimes appear worse shortly after starting RT. The skin generally heals rapidly after a course of radiation. Nothing more than topical symptom management is typically necessary during treatment. In the long-term patients may have pigmentation changes and alopecia in the treated areas. There is a theoretic risk of secondary cutaneous malignancies, although reports of this in the literature are rare.[9]

Technique and administration
Local RT is typically delivered by means of a linear accelerator (**Fig. 1**). Most linear accelerators can produce high-energy photon (x-rays) and electron beams. Both photons and electrons can be used depending on the clinical circumstances. Electrons have unique properties that make them particularly suited to treating cutaneous lesions. Electron beam therapy delivers dose close to the skin surface after which the dose falls off extremely rapidly, limiting radiation exposure to deeper tissues. Increasing electron energies can be chosen to treat deeper lesions. The association between the depth dose and electron energy is plotted in **Fig. 2**.

Most electron beam treatments for superficial skin lesions are planned clinically rather than with imaging modalities, such as CT or MRI (**Fig. 3**). The radiation oncologist delineates a margin of 1- to 2-cm around visible and/or palpable disease. A lead cutout is then created conforming to the shape of the target. The lead cutout is inserted into the treatment machine thus focusing the radiation beam to the desired shape. As electrons begin depositing their dose on contact with the skin, there can be some degree of "skin sparing" with electron beam therapy (see **Fig. 2**). To address this phenomenon, material referred to as bolus is placed over skin lesions before treatment. Bolus is a tissue-equivalent material that starts the process of dose deposition allowing the maximum dose to be at the skin surface. The radiation dose is often fractionated, or divided into multiple smaller doses. Patients are treated daily excluding weekends until their course is completed. Each treatment, including time for set-up, lasts approximately 15 minutes.

Photon radiation is often used to treat nodal and visceral disease because the dose penetrates deeper than electrons. Photon beams are occasionally required to treat thick cutaneous tumors. Patients receiving photon radiation must first undergo a radiation planning session termed a simulation. The patient is immobilized and a planning CT is performed. The radiation oncologist then uses the planning CT scan and advanced treatment planning software to plan the radiation treatment. The gross disease is identified and contoured on the planning scan. Margins are created around this volume to account for

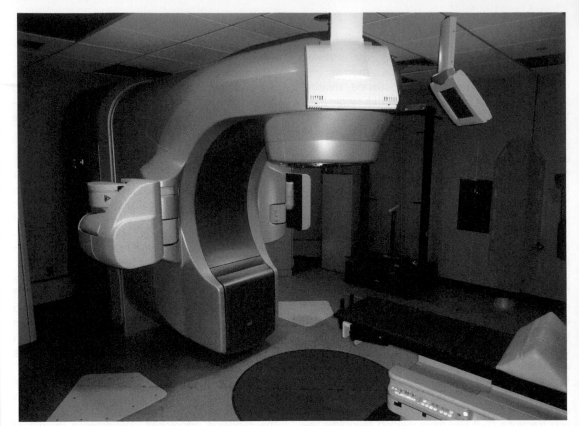

Fig. 1. Medical linear accelerator used to generate and deliver external beam radiation therapy.

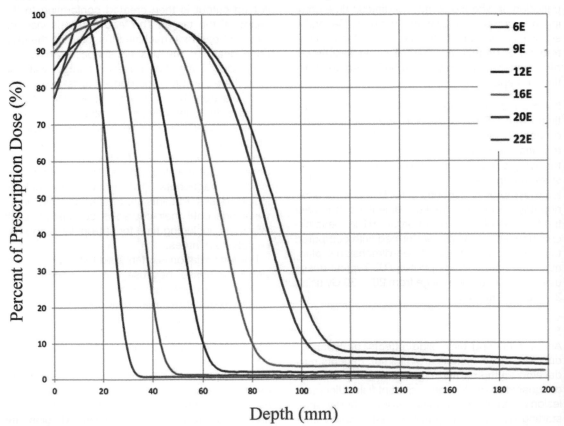

Fig. 2. Plot of percentage of radiation dose (%) versus depth (mm) for various electron beam energies from 6 to 22 MeV.

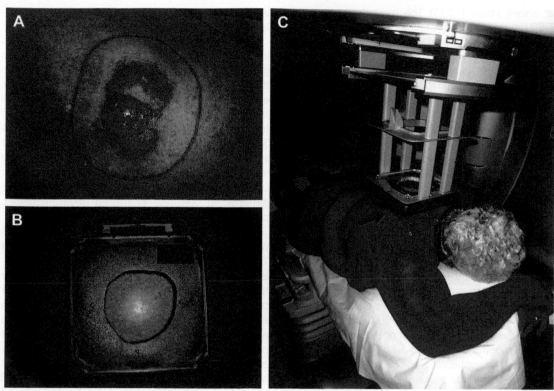

Fig. 3. Method of local electron beam radiation therapy to cutaneous lymphoma lesions. A margin is drawn around visible or palpable disease (*A*). A lead cutout is created conforming to the target volume (*B*). The patient is positioned on the treatment table and the electron beam therapy is delivered by a medical linear accelerator (*C*). Note the bolus material placed over the cutaneous lesion that ensures the maximum dose is delivered to the skin surface (*arrow*).

subclinical disease and variations in daily set-up. The optimal number and configuration of radiation beams to treat the target volume and limit dose to normal sensitive tissues is then determined. Patients are treated daily in the same position as their planning scan. Proper positioning is ensured by alignment to skin markings placed at the time of planning and imaging taken immediately before treatment.

Total Skin Electron Beam Therapy

Many patients with MF present with diffuse cutaneous disease or develop such during the course of their illness. Multiple systemic and skin-directed therapies have been used for diffuse disease, including total skin electron beam therapy (TSEBT). TSEBT is used when RT is recommended and the distribution of disease is such that the entire skin surface requires treatment.

TSEBT is a technically challenging procedure where radiation is delivered to the entire skin surface. It requires special commissioning (ie, configuring) of a linear accelerator and significant support from medical physics. Thus, this treatment is generally only available at larger centers that treat many patients a year. As with local RT, TSEBT is very effective with nearly all patients experiencing significant clinical improvement. Continued research is exploring dose reduction of TSEBT and concurrent and adjuvant therapies.

Clinical indications
Early stage (T1) TSEBT has shown favorable results in early stage MF. Ysebaert and colleagues[10] demonstrated an 88% CR rate in patients T1 MF treated to a mean dose of 30 Gy. Five-year RFS was 75%. Hoppe and colleagues[11] showed complete regression of all skin lesions in 86% of patients with limited plaque disease. Finally, Jones and colleagues[12] reported a CR rate of 95% in patients with stage IA MF treated with 31 to 36 Gy. Progression-free survival (PFS) at 15 years was 35%. However, because there are numerous other effective therapies with less acute side effects, TSEBT is generally not recommended as first-line treatment of patients with limited or localized skin involvement (T1).[13,14]

Advanced stage (T2-T3) The major indication for TSEBT is the palliation of patients with severe skin symptoms or generalized thick plaque or tumor disease (T2-T3).[14] These patients have often had a poor response to previous therapies. Clinical responses are correlated to tumor stage at presentation (T2 vs T3)[15] and the extent of skin involvement.[16] For patients with T2 disease the rate of CR has been reported to be 75% to 85% with 50% RFS at 5 years but only 10% at 10 years.[10,15,17] With T3 disease, CR rates of 43% to 78% have been reported with nearly all patients eventually experiencing recurrent disease.[15,16]

The largest reported series on TSEBT in T2 and T3 MF was published by Navi and colleagues[15] from Stanford. They included 103 patients with T2 MF and 77 patients with T3 MF, all treated with doses greater than 30 Gy. All patients had clinically significant improvement in their disease (>50% improvement in skin involvement). The CR rate was 63%, including 75% in patients with T2 MF and 43% in patients with T3 MF. The median duration of response (in complete responders) was 29 months in patients with T2 disease and 9 months for patients with T3 disease. The 5- and 10-year overall survival rates for the cohort were 59% and 40%, respectively.

Ysebaert and colleagues[10] reported an 85% CR to TSEBT in patients with T2 MF. Five-year RFS was 28%. Quiros and colleagues[16] reported the outcomes of 46 patients with T3 MF treated with TSEBT. A total of 36 of 46 patients (78%) had a cutaneous CR. DFS was 12% at 36 months.

Erythrodermic (T4) disease There is limited experience of TSEBT for patients with erythrodermic (T4) MF. Jones and colleagues[18] reported the outcomes of 45 patients with T4 disease treated with TSEBT without neoadjuvant, concurrent, or adjuvant therapies. The rate of complete cutaneous remission was 60% with 26% remaining disease-free at 5 years. Improved outcomes were seen in patients with stage III disease without blood involvement and in patients treated with a more intensive TSEBT regimen (32–40 Gy). Another retrospective study demonstrated improved PFS and cancer-specific survival with the addition of extracorporeal photophoresis (ECPP) to TSEBT in T4 MF.[19]

Special circumstances with total skin electron beam therapy

Retreatment A second course of TSEBT is feasible and safe in most circumstances. Ideal candidates for such include those who achieved a good response to the first course of TSEBT with reasonable response duration, failure of subsequent treatments, and generalized symptomatic skin involvement.[20]

Several small studies support the tolerability and efficacy of multiple courses of TSEBT in MF. In general, the dose of a second (and sometimes third) course of TSEBT should be reduced. Becker and colleagues[21] described the experience of 15 patients treated with a second course of TSEBT to a mean of 23.4 Gy (mean of first course was 32.6 Gy). A CR to the first course was achieved in 11 of 15. Six patients had a CR and nine achieved a partial response to the second course. Long-term toxicities were mild and consisted of generalized xerosis, scattered telangiectasias, pigmentation changes, and partial alopecia.

Wilson and colleagues[22] reported on 14 patients with recurrent MF treated with multiple courses of TSEBT (two to three courses). The median cumulative dose for the entire cohort was 57 Gy. After the first course, 13 of 14 patients had a CR. After the second course, 12 of 14 had a CR, again showing that a good response can be achieved even when disease relapses after prior RT. The median disease-free interval after the first course of therapy for those with a CR was 20 months and 11.5 months after the second course. Overall the repeat treatments were well tolerated with no severe toxicities.

Adjuvant therapies Patients with advanced MF receiving TSEBT inevitably relapse. Several studies have attempted to lengthen the disease-free interval after TSEBT by using adjuvant therapies, such as topical nitrogen mustard, oral psoralen plus ultraviolet light, oral etretinate, ECPP, interferon, and cytotoxic chemotherapy. Unfortunately, most of these studies are small, retrospective, and from single institutions. Prospective, randomized data are needed to confirm their results.

Chinn and colleagues[23] initially demonstrated a longer freedom from relapse in patients with T2 disease treated with adjuvant topical nitrogen mustard compared with observation after TSEBT. However, a larger more recent series from the same institution showed no clinical advantage to adjuvant topical nitrogen mustard.[15] Quirós and colleagues[24] reported a significant benefit in DFS but no significant overall survival advantage in patients receiving adjuvant psoralen plus ultraviolet A. Roberge and colleagues[25] demonstrated concurrent and adjuvant alpha interferon to be tolerable but there was no significant difference in PFS or overall survival. A more recent study similarly showed no clinical benefit with the addition of interferon to TSEBT.[26] Wilson and colleagues[19,27] have reported on their experience with concurrent/adjuvant ECPP in patients with

T3/T4 disease. In one study they demonstrated a borderline significant improvement in overall survival with ECPP.[27] Another reported improved DFS and cancer-specific survival in patients with T4 disease.[19] Finally, adjuvant systemic chemotherapy (cyclophosphamide/doxorubicin) has been shown to have no benefit for RFS or overall survival in one study[27] but to improve RFS among stage I/II patients in another.[28] In short, the data are mixed whether adjuvant therapies after TSEBT are clinically beneficial.

Total skin electron beam therapy before stem cell transplant Select patients with advanced-stage, refractory MF are deemed appropriate candidates for an autologous or allogeneic stem cell transplant. Patients should, ideally, be in CR before initiating the conditioning regimen for transplant. TSEBT can be used to control cutaneous disease and achieve remission in the skin. Total-body irradiation can also be used in the conditioning regimen.

Duvic and colleagues[29] reported their experience with 19 patients who received TSEBT (36 Gy) immediately before allogeneic transplantation for refractory MF (median of four prior therapies). Three patients had stage IIB disease (all with large cell transformation), six had stage IVA disease, and 10 had stage IVB disease. The rate of CR was 58% after TSEBT and transplant. At 2 years, overall survival was 79% and PFS 53%. The authors also suggested that TSEBT may have helped to reduce the severity of posttransplantation cutaneous graft-versus-host disease.

Technique and administration
The European Organization for Research and Treatment of Cancer (EORTC) has published consensus guidelines regarding the use of TSEBT in MF.[17] The goal of TSEBT is to deliver a relatively uniform dose of radiation to the entire skin while limiting acute and long-term toxicities. Modern TSEBT as delivered by linear accelerator was largely developed at Stanford and today the "Stanford technique" is commonly used.[20,30] Many modifications of this technique now exist.

The patient is positioned standing approximately 3 to 4 m from the linear accelerator. A 6- to 9-MeV electron beam is used. A polycarbonate screen is often placed between the linear accelerator and the patient, which attenuates or scatters the beam to increase the dose to the skin surface.

The patient is treated in six different standing positions including anterior, posterior, right posterior oblique, left posterior oblique, left anterior oblique, and right anterior oblique (**Fig. 4**). All six positions are treated over the course of 2 treatment days, three positions on Day 1 and three positions on Day 2. This cycle is repeated twice per week. Treatment of each position is accomplished with a dual-field technique where the linear accelerator is angled up to treat the superior field and down to treat the inferior field. The use of angled beams helps to fit the patient in the radiation treatment field. The EORTC recommends that the 80% isodose line extend to 4 mm below the skin surface.[17]

Certain areas of the body are more susceptible to side effects from RT and may require shielding during portions of the treatment. Internal or external eye shields are used to protect the eyes during treatment (**Fig. 5**). Internal lead shields placed underneath the eyelids are used when there is disease on the face. External eye shields can be used for portions of the treatment, especially in the absence of disease on the face. At our institution we also commonly use mouth shields covering the lips and oral mucosa to prevent the development of mucositis. Blisters can occasionally develop on the feet, which can cause significant disability and delay patients from completing the treatment as planned. At our institution, the hands and feet are shielded in the TSEBT fields and treated separately with photon fields.

Certain areas of the body may be underdosed or even overdosed during TSEBT because of shadowing, body habitus, or peculiarities inherent in treating with TSEBT. In a study by Weaver and colleagues,[31] thermoluminescent monitors were placed on several body locations to record the dose received during TSEBT. Areas that routinely receive a lower dose include the top of head, perineum, upper inner thighs, and inframammary fold region in women. These areas may be treated with supplemental local electron beam either during or after completion of the TSEBT. For patients with tumors, a supplemental course of local RT can be given at the start of TSEBT to rapidly reduce the thickness of the tumor allowing for better dosimetry through the course of therapy.

Some patients cannot be treated with the modified Stanford technique because of their inability to stand safely or comfortably for extended periods. An alternative technique exists where the patient is treated in three supine and three prone positions (lying-on-the-floor position). This technique has shown comparable radiation quality and uniformity with the modified Stanford technique.[32]

Dose
When RT is delivered to discrete lesions, larger daily doses can be safely administered. In contrast, treating the entire skin surface with

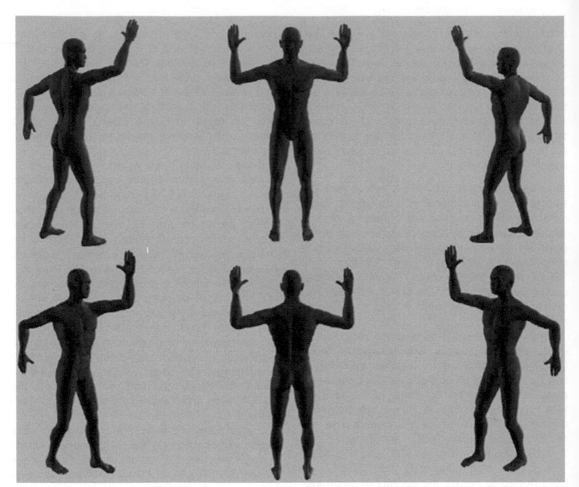

Fig. 4. The six treatment positions used for total skin electron beam therapy. (*From* Smith BD, Wilson LD. Management of mycosis fungoides. Part 2: treatment. Oncology 2003;17(10):1424; with permission.)

TSEBT necessitates a lower dose of radiation per fraction to prevent significant toxicity. This typically consists of 1 to 1.5 Gy each day. When lower daily doses are used, higher total doses are necessary to achieve comparable tumor responses.

Similar to local RT, a dose–response relationship has been observed with TSEBT. Hoppe and colleagues[11] correlated the rate of CR with TSEBT dose. He demonstrated a CR rate of 18% with less than 10 Gy, 55% with 10 to 20 Gy, 66% with 20 to 25 Gy, 75% with 25 to 30 Gy, and 94% with doses from 30 to 36 Gy. These data provide the rationale for the recommendation that the total TSEBT dose ranges from 30 to 36 Gy.[14,17] At our institution, the typical TSEBT prescription is 36 Gy at 1.5 Gy per fraction using 6-MeV electrons. Treatment is delivered over 6 weeks. Daily doses of 1 Gy per fraction are also commonly used with treatments delivered over 9 weeks.

More recent experience has also shown reasonable clinical outcomes with lower doses of TSEBT. Harrison and colleagues[33] reviewed the Stanford experience with low-dose (<30 Gy) TSEBT. Overall response rates (defined as >50% improvement) were 90% in patients receiving 5 to 10 Gy, 98% in patients receiving 10 to 20 Gy, and 97% in patients receiving 20 to 30 Gy. When compared with the standard dose of greater than or equal to 30 Gy, CR rates were reduced in the lower-dose groups. However, PFS was comparable among the low-dose groups and the standard dose. Furthermore, a pooled analysis of three phase II clinical trials including 33 patients treated with 12-Gy TSEBT demonstrated an overall response rate of 88%.[34] The median duration of response was 71 weeks. These data suggest low-dose TSEBT may be a reasonable option for patients desiring palliation of diffuse disease and who may not tolerate the side effects and time commitment of the standard course. Patients who receive the low-dose TSEBT may also benefit from the ability to repeat the regimen multiple times without considerable toxicity.

Close surveillance of patients by a multidisciplinary team is required to manage the acute side effects of TSEBT. Patients receiving TSEBT are seen formally by the radiation oncologist during weekly treatment check visits. Symptomatic treatments include moisturizers, topical and oral analgesics, antibiotics when clinical infections develop, and appropriate wound care. Close collaboration with a wound care specialist is important in promoting wound healing and preventing infection.

Side effects that may develop following completion of TSEBT include alopecia (temporary vs permanent based on dose), dystrophic nails, decreased ability to sweat, chronically dry skin, cataracts, and telangiectasias. TSEBT has also been associated with increased rates of secondary skin cancers.[36–38]

PRIMARY CUTANEOUS ANAPLASTIC LARGE CELL LYMPHOMA

Primary cutaneous CD30+ lymphoproliferative disorders are less common than MF and include lymphomatoid papulosis (LyP) and primary cutaneous anaplastic large cell lymphoma (cALCL). The Dutch Cutaneous Lymphoma Group published a detailed report on a large series of patients with CD30+ lymphoproliferative disorders with long-term follow-up.[39] In addition, a more recent consensus publication by the International Society for Cutaneous Lymphoma, EORTC Cutaneous Lymphoma Task Force, and the United States Cutanous Lymphoma Consortium has addressed treatment of these conditions.[40] Based on their observations and that of the National Comprehensive Cancer Network, there are clinical guidelines for diagnosis and treatment of the CD30+ lymphoproliferative disorders.

LyP is an indolent lymphoproliferative disorder. Clinically this disorder is characterized by multifocal skin lesions that regress spontaneously within 3 to 12 weeks. The prognosis of LyP is excellent with a 5- and 10-year disease-related survival of 100%.[39] Of note, within the Dutch cohort, 19% of patients with LyP had other associated malignant lymphomas before, after, or concurrent with LyP. There is no clear role for RT for LyP.

In contrast to LyP, cALCL typically presents as a solitary lesion or a localized group of lesions. The prognosis of patients with localized disease is excellent. Local RT is the first choice of treatment in patients with a solitary or few localized nodules or tumors (**Fig. 6**).[39] A series from Stanford demonstrated a CR in six of seven patients treated with RT alone.[41] Yu and colleagues[42] reported on

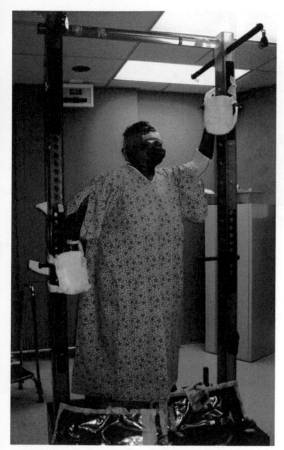

Fig. 5. Patient undergoing total skin electron beam therapy. Both internal eye and mouth shields are used. The hands and feet are shielded and treated separately with photon fields.

Side effects

TSEBT is given over a 6- to 10-week time period, which can be logistically and emotionally challenging for patients. Furthermore, it is also associated with more acute toxicities compared with local RT. However, most patients successfully complete the planned course of therapy without high-grade toxicity and long-term toxicities are generally mild. Some patients might require a 10- to 14-day break after 18 to 30 Gy to recover from the acute toxicities of TSEB. Lloyd and colleagues[35] described the type and grade of acute treatment toxicities in 82 patients receiving TSEB courses from 30 to 36 Gy. The most common toxicities included erythema/desquamation (76%), blisters (52%), hyperpigmentation (50%), and skin pain (48%). In their series, 32% of patients had clinical evidence of a skin infection, which was treated with antibiotics. There were no grade 4 or 5 acute toxicities.

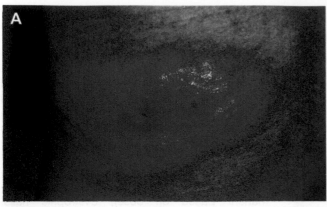
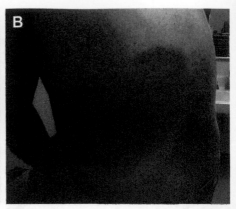

Fig. 6. Localized primary cutaneous anaplastic large cell lymphoma at diagnosis (*A*) and 3 months after radiation therapy (*B*).

eight patients with cALCL treated with 34- to 44-Gy local RT. The CR was 100% and there was no evidence of disease recurrence at a median follow-up of 12 months. Finally, in the Dutch study, 99% of patients had a CR to initial therapy, 48% of which were treated with local RT.[39] Fifty-one percent of patients developed recurrent disease with the skin only being the most common site of relapse (80% of patients with recurrent disease). Relapses are almost always outside the previous radiation field.

REFERENCES

1. Bradford PT, Devesa SS, Anderson WF, et al. Cutaneous lymphoma incidence patterns in the United States: a population-based study of 3884 cases. Blood 2009;113(21):5064–73.
2. Kim YH, Jensen RA, Watanabe GL, et al. Clinical stage IA (limited patch and plaque) mycosis fungoides. A long-term outcome analysis. Arch Dermatol 1996;132(11):1309–13.
3. Wilson LD, Kacinski BM, Jones GW. Local superficial radiotherapy in the management of minimal stage IA cutaneous T-cell lymphoma (mycosis fungoides). Int J Radiat Oncol Biol Phys 1998;40(1):109–15.
4. Micaily B, Miyamoto C, Kantor G, et al. Radiotherapy for unilesional mycosis fungoides. Int J Radiat Oncol Biol Phys 1998;42(2):361–4.
5. Piccinno R, Caccialanza M, Percivalle S. Minimal stage IA mycosis fungoides. Results of radiotherapy in 15 patients. J Dermatolog Treat 2009;20(3):165–8.
6. Cotter GW, Baglan RJ, Wasserman TH, et al. Palliative radiation treatment of cutaneous mycosis fungoides: a dose response. Int J Radiat Oncol Biol Phys 1983;9(10):1477–80.
7. Thomas TO, Agrawal P, Guitart J, et al. Outcome of patients treated with a single-fraction dose of palliative radiation for cutaneous T-cell lymphoma. Int J Radiat Oncol Biol Phys 2013;85(3):747–53.
8. Neelis KJ, Schimmel EC, Vermeer MH, et al. Low-dose palliative radiotherapy for cutaneous B- and T-cell lymphomas. Int J Radiat Oncol Biol Phys 2009;74(1):154–8.
9. Volden G, Larsen TE. Squamous cell carcinoma appearing in X-ray-treated mycosis fungoides. Acta Derm Venereol 1977;57(4):341–3.
10. Ysebaert L, Truc G, Dalac S, et al. Ultimate results of radiation therapy for T1-T2 mycosis fungoides (including reirradiation). Int J Radiat Oncol Biol Phys 2004;58(4):1128–34.
11. Hoppe RT, Fuks Z, Bagshaw MA. The rationale for curative radiotherapy in mycosis fungoides. Int J Radiat Oncol Biol Phys 1977;2(9–10):843–51.
12. Jones G, Wilson LD, Fox-Goguen L. Total skin electron beam radiotherapy for patients who have mycosis fungoides. Hematol Oncol Clin North Am 2003;17(6):1421–34.
13. Trautinger F, Knobler R, Willemze R, et al. EORTC consensus recommendations for the treatment of mycosis fungoides/Sézary syndrome. Eur J Cancer 2006;42(8):1014–30.
14. Zelenetz AD, Wierda WG, Abramson JS, et al. Non-Hodgkin's lymphomas, version 1.2013. J Natl Compr Canc Netw 2013;11(3):257–72 [quiz: 273].
15. Navi D, Riaz N, Levin YS, et al. The Stanford University experience with conventional-dose, total skin electron-beam therapy in the treatment of generalized patch or plaque (T2) and tumor (T3) mycosis fungoides. Arch Dermatol 2011;147(5):561–7.
16. Quiros PA, Kacinski BM, Wilson LD. Extent of skin involvement as a prognostic indicator of disease free and overall survival of patients with T3 cutaneous T-cell lymphoma treated with total skin electron beam radiation therapy. Cancer 1996;77(9):1912–7.
17. Jones GW, Kacinski BM, Wilson LD, et al. Total skin electron radiation in the management of mycosis fungoides: consensus of the European Organization for Research and Treatment of Cancer (EORTC) Cutaneous Lymphoma Project Group. J Am Acad Dermatol 2002;47(3):364–70.

18. Jones GW, Rosenthal D, Wilson LD. Total skin electron radiation for patients with erythrodermic cutaneous T-cell lymphoma (mycosis fungoides and the Sézary syndrome). Cancer 1999;85(9):1985–95.

19. Wilson LD, Jones GW, Kim D, et al. Experience with total skin electron beam therapy in combination with extracorporeal photopheresis in the management of patients with erythrodermic (T4) mycosis fungoides. J Am Acad Dermatol 2000;43(1 Pt 1):54–60.

20. Hoppe RT. Mycosis fungoides: radiation therapy. Dermatol Ther 2003;16(4):347–54.

21. Becker M, Hoppe RT, Knox SJ. Multiple courses of high-dose total skin electron beam therapy in the management of mycosis fungoides. Int J Radiat Oncol Biol Phys 1995;32(5):1445–9.

22. Wilson LD, Quiros PA, Kolenik SA, et al. Additional courses of total skin electron beam therapy in the treatment of patients with recurrent cutaneous T-cell lymphoma. J Am Acad Dermatol 1996;35(1):69–73.

23. Chinn DM, Chow S, Kim YH, et al. Total skin electron beam therapy with or without adjuvant topical nitrogen mustard or nitrogen mustard alone as initial treatment of T2 and T3 mycosis fungoides. Int J Radiat Oncol Biol Phys 1999;43(5):951–8.

24. Quirós PA, Jones GW, Kacinski BM, et al. Total skin electron beam therapy followed by adjuvant psoralen/ultraviolet-A light in the management of patients with T1 and T2 cutaneous T-cell lymphoma (mycosis fungoides). Int J Radiat Oncol Biol Phys 1997;38(5):1027–35.

25. Roberge D, Muanza T, Blake G, et al. Does adjuvant alpha-interferon improve outcome when combined with total skin irradiation for mycosis fungoides? Br J Dermatol 2007;156(1):57–61.

26. Wagner AE, Wada D, Bowen G, et al. Mycosis fungoides: the addition of concurrent and adjuvant interferon to total skin electron beam therapy. Br J Dermatol 2013;169(3):715–8.

27. Wilson LD, Licata AL, Braverman IM, et al. Systemic chemotherapy and extracorporeal photochemotherapy for T3 and T4 cutaneous T-cell lymphoma patients who have achieved a complete response to total skin electron beam therapy. Int J Radiat Oncol Biol Phys 1995;32(4):987–95.

28. Braverman IM, Yager NB, Chen M, et al. Combined total body electron beam irradiation and chemotherapy for mycosis fungoides. J Am Acad Dermatol 1987;16(1 Pt 1):45–60.

29. Duvic M, Donato M, Dabaja B, et al. Total skin electron beam and non-myeloablative allogeneic hematopoietic stem-cell transplantation in advanced mycosis fungoides and Sezary syndrome. J Clin Oncol 2010;28(14):2365–72.

30. Hoppe RT, Fuks Z, Bagshaw MA. Radiation therapy in the management of cutaneous T-cell lymphomas. Cancer Treat Rep 1979;63(4):625–32.

31. Weaver RD, Gerbi BJ, Dusenbery KE. Evaluation of dose variation during total skin electron irradiation using thermoluminescent dosimeters. Int J Radiat Oncol Biol Phys 1995;33(2):475–8.

32. Deufel CL, Antolak JA. Total skin electron therapy in the lying-on-the-floor position using a customized flattening filter to eliminate field junctions. J Appl Clin Med Phys 2013;14(5):115–26.

33. Harrison C, Young J, Navi D, et al. Revisiting low-dose total skin electron beam therapy in mycosis fungoides. Int J Radiat Oncol Biol Phys 2011;81(4):e651–7.

34. Hoppe RT, Harrison C, Tavallaee M, et al. Low-dose total skin electron beam therapy as an effective modality to reduce disease burden in patients with mycosis fungoides: results of a pooled analysis from 3 phase-II clinical trials. J Am Acad Dermatol 2015;72(2):286–92.

35. Lloyd S, Chen Z, Foss FM, et al. Acute toxicity and risk of infection during total skin electron beam therapy for mycosis fungoides. J Am Acad Dermatol 2013;69(4):537–43.

36. Licata AG, Wilson LD, Braverman IM, et al. Malignant melanoma and other second cutaneous malignancies in cutaneous T-cell lymphoma. The influence of additional therapy after total skin electron beam radiation. Arch Dermatol 1995;131(4):432–5.

37. Abel EA, Sendagorta E, Hoppe RT. Cutaneous malignancies and metastatic squamous cell carcinoma following topical therapies for mycosis fungoides. J Am Acad Dermatol 1986;14(6):1029–38.

38. Stein ME, Anacak Y, Zaidan J, et al. Second primary tumors in mycosis fungoides patients: experience at the Northern Israel Oncology Center (1979–2002). J BUON 2006;11(2):175–80.

39. Bekkenk MW, Geelen FA, van Voorst Vader PC, et al. Primary and secondary cutaneous CD30(+) lymphoproliferative disorders: a report from the Dutch Cutaneous Lymphoma Group on the long-term follow-up data of 219 patients and guidelines for diagnosis and treatment. Blood 2000;95(12):3653–61.

40. Kempf W, Pfaltz K, Vermeer MH, et al. EORTC, ISCL, and USCLC consensus recommendations for the treatment of primary cutaneous CD30-positive lymphoproliferative disorders: lymphomatoid papulosis and primary cutaneous anaplastic large-cell lymphoma. Blood 2011;118(15):4024–35.

41. Liu HL, Hoppe RT, Kohler S, et al. CD30$^+$ cutaneous lymphoproliferative disorders: the Stanford experience in lymphomatoid papulosis and primary cutaneous anaplastic large cell lymphoma. J Am Acad Dermatol 2003;49(6):1049–58.

42. Yu JB, McNiff JM, Lund MW, et al. Treatment of primary cutaneous CD30$^+$ anaplastic large-cell lymphoma with radiation therapy. Int J Radiat Oncol Biol Phys 2008;70(5):1542–5.

The Role of Systemic Retinoids in the Treatment of Cutaneous T-Cell Lymphoma

Auris O. Huen, PharmD, MD, Ellen J. Kim, MD*

KEYWORDS

- Retinoids • Rexinoids • Bexarotene • Isotretinoin • Acitretin • Cutaneous T-cell lymphoma
- Mycosis fungoides • Sézary syndrome

KEY POINTS

- Mycosis fungoides and Sézary syndrome subtypes of cutaneous T-cell lymphoma (CTCL) have a variable clinical course, ranging from indolent disease that does not alter life expectancy to aggressive, rapidly progressive disease.
- Goals of treatment, especially in patients with early-stage disease, are to induce remission with agents that have a low toxicity profile. The systemic retinoids are an important component of the treatment options for all stages of this disease because of the ease of administration and relatively low toxicity profile.
- Bexarotene is the only systemic retinoid approved by the Food and Drug Administration specifically for CTCL but does require additional medications to treat the associated hyperlipidemia and hypothyroidism during the duration of bexarotene treatment.
- Combination treatment with retinoids and other agents with activity against mycosis fungoides/Sézary syndrome appear to be well tolerated and associated with high response rates in relapsed or treatment refractory patients in small studies and series.

INTRODUCTION

Retinoids are signaling molecules that are structural and functional derivatives of vitamin A (retinol). The term collectively describes naturally occurring retinol and its metabolites, as well as synthetic analogs. Retinoid receptors are found ubiquitously in virtually all organ systems, and they regulate important functions in the body, including embryonic development, vision, immune and neural function, as well as cell proliferation, differentiation, and apoptosis.[1,2] These compounds exert their effects through control of gene expression. In the treatment of cancer, the retinoids are considered "biologic response modifiers" (BRMs) in that they are dissimilar to traditional cytotoxic chemotherapy, inducing response without immune suppression, and often augmenting the immune response.[3–5] Although there have been a number of clinical studies using retinoids for treatment of breast, ovarian, renal, head and neck, melanoma, and prostate cancers, they are most prominently used in the treatment of hematologic malignancies. In the case of acute promyelocytic leukemia, retinoids in the form of all-*trans* retinoic acid are used as first-line treatment to restore normal myeloid

Department of Dermatology, Perelman School of Medicine, University of Pennsylvania, 3400 Civic Center Boulevard, Suite 330S, Philadelphia, PA 19104, USA
* Corresponding author. Department of Dermatology, Perelman School of Medicine, University of Pennsylvania, 1 Dulles Building, 3400 Spruce Street, Philadelphia, PA 19104.
E-mail address: Ellen.Kim@uphs.upenn.edu

Dermatol Clin 33 (2015) 715–729
http://dx.doi.org/10.1016/j.det.2015.05.007
0733-8635/15/$ – see front matter © 2015 Elsevier Inc. All rights reserved.

differentiation to leukemic cells, inducing the formation of mature granulocytes.[6] In T-cell lymphoma cells, retinoids are thought to induce apoptosis and DNA fragmentation in affected T lymphocytes.[7,8]

Cutaneous T-cell lymphomas (CTCLs) are a heterogeneous group of uncommon primarily mature T-helper lymphoproliferative disorders. The most common form is mycosis fungoides (MF), which accounts for approximately 60% of all cases.[9] It typically displays indolent behavior, although disease progression to higher stages or transformation to large-cell lymphoma can occur. Sézary syndrome (SS) is a related subtype of CTCL presenting as erythroderma, with a significant population of circulating atypical T-lymphocytes and typically has a more aggressive course than MF. Patients with the earliest stages of MF do not have decreased survival due to their disease, and skin-directed therapy, such as phototherapy or topical medications, are the mainstays of treatment.[10] Additionally, treatment with BRMs, such as interferons or retinoids, also are commonly used in these patients, although systemic treatment is generally reserved for patients with MF who have failed local or skin-directed therapy or have more extensive disease.[5,10] The anecdotal use of retinoids for treatment of MF was first reported in the 1980s, both as monotherapy or in combination with chemotherapy.[3,11,12] Currently, topical and systemic retinoids are an integral part of the treatment armamentarium for CTCL. This article focuses primarily on systemic retinoids in MF and SS.

RETINOIDS AND MECHANISM OF ACTION

All retinoids have similar molecular structure, containing a benzene ring, a polyene chain, and a carboxylic end group. In the body, retinol is metabolized to all-*trans* retinoic acid and then further isomerizes to 13-*cis* retinoic acid (isotretinoin) and 9-*cis* retinoic acid in the liver.[2] Subsequently, synthetic retinoids have been derived from retinol, including mono-aromatic second-generation retinoids (eg, etretinate, acitretin) followed by polyaromatic third-generation compounds called arotenoids (eg, bexarotene).[13] More recently, alitretinoin, which is a synthetic analog of 9-*cis* retinoic acid, has been developed with efficacy in atopic dermatitis and a few reports showing effects in MF/SS.

Retinoids bind to 2 distinct families of nuclear receptors regulating gene transcription called retinoic acid receptors (RARs) and retinoic X receptors (RXRs). Each receptor is associated with 3 subtypes, α, β, and, γ, which bind to specific ligands.[1,14] These receptors are part of a larger superfamily of nuclear receptors, including thyroid hormone receptor, vitamin D3 receptor, and glucocorticoid receptor (**Table 1**).[1] Transactivation of some of these other nuclear receptors is believed to be linked to some of the side effects seen with the retinoids.[1]

Despite significant progress in elucidating the mechanism by which retinoids exert their activity, their effect on tumorigenesis and cancer biology remains poorly understood. The RAR receptors

Table 1
Human nuclear receptors and ligands

Receptor	Ligand(s)
Retinoic acid receptor (RAR) α, β, γ	All-*trans* retinoic acid, 9-*cis* retinoic acid, isotretinoin, etretinate, acitretin
Retinoic X receptor (RXR) α, β, γ	9-*cis* retinoic acid, bexarotene
Thyroid hormone receptor (TR)	Thyroid hormone
Vitamin D3 receptor (VDR)	Vitamin D, calcitriol
Peroxisome proliferator-activated receptor (PPAR) α, β, γ	Fatty acids, fibrates, leukotriene B4, thiazolidinediones
Pregnane X receptor	Xenobiotics
Liver X receptor α, β (LXR)	Oxysterols
Estrogen receptor α, β	Estradiol
Progesterone receptor	Progesterone
Glucocorticoid receptor	Cortisol, corticosteroids
Mineralocorticoid receptor	Aldosterone, spironolactone
Androgen receptor	Testosterone

Data from Sokołowska-Wojdyło M, Ługowska-Umer H, Maciejewska-Radomska A. Oral retinoids and rexinoids in cutaneous T-cell lymphomas. Postepy Dermatol Alergol 2013;30:19–29.

bind only to all-*trans* retinoid acid, 9-*cis* retinoic acid or synthetic isotretinoin, etretinate, and acitretin. The RXR receptors exclusively bind to 9-*cis* retinoic acid or synthetic retinoids such as bexarotene (which is often referred to as a rexinoid).[3,15] These receptors can form homodimers or heterodimers with each other or with other nuclear hormone receptors, such as thyroid hormone receptor or liver X receptor. The RXR receptor also can form a tetramer in its resting state. Once bound to a ligand, the receptor induces a conformation change forming a ligand-receptor complex. These complexes bind directly to specific DNA sequences called hormone response elements that affect transcription of specific genes and production of specific peptides downstream, which can induce and maintain terminal differentiation of malignant cells.[1,16] **Fig. 1** is a diagram demonstrating possible combinations of receptor dimers formed by rexinoid receptors.

Retinoids also have been shown to inhibit ornithine decarboxylase activity, an enzyme that is upregulated in the presence of tumor-promoting substances.[17] It is believed that retinoids also

1. 1. RXR homodimer

2. RXR permissive heterodimer

3. RXR non-permissive heterodimer

*= ligand

Fig. 1. Retinoid receptor responses. (1) RXR forms homodimers with itself, and with ligand binding, leads to activation of transcription. (2) RXR also forms permissive heterodimers with other nuclear receptors, such as PPAR and LXR-activation of transcription occurs with binding of ligand to either receptor. (3) RXR forms nonpermissive heterodimers with RAR, TR, or VDR. Activation of transcription occurs only with ligand binding on both receptors. DR elements, direct repeat elements; TR, Thyroid hormone receptor; VDR, vitamin D3 receptor. [a] Ligand.

promote the production of gap junctions, which are lost during malignant transformation, as well as their glycoproteins, which aid in cell communication, adhesion, and growth.[16]

Rexinoids, such as bexarotene, bind exclusively to the RXR, and its activation has been shown to induce apoptosis involving activation of the caspase pathway. Bexarotene has been shown to activate caspase-3, a key executor of the apoptotic pathway, with resultant apoptosis as evidenced by increased poly (ADP-Ribose) polymerase and downregulation of survivin (a suppressor of caspase-induced apoptosis).[8] Retinoids reduce expression of Bcl-2 protein and upregulate bax proteins, which also are involved in apoptotic pathways.[18] Activation of RXR receptor also has been associated with activation of p53, a tumor suppressor protein, by facilitating its binding to promoters leading to cell cycle arrest.[19] Other antitumor effects of rexinoids include reduction in matrix metalloproteinases, vascular endothelial growth factor, and epidermal growth factor, which are important factors in angiogenesis as well as tumor cell migration and invasion.[20]

Various investigators have reported the immunomodulatory effects of retinoids and rexinoids. RARs are constitutively expressed in human T and B lymphocytes. Activation of RAR γ has been shown to promote CD8+ T-cell responses.[15] Retinoids upregulate Langerhans cell antigen presentation and surface expression of HLA-DR and CD11c, which is important for T-cell activation.[21] Retinoids and rexinoids also have been shown to upregulate interleukin-2 receptor (IL-2R) expression with associated increase in interferon (IFN) γ levels.[22] Gorgun and Foss[4] reported elevation in IL-2R levels in human T-cell and B-cell leukemia cell lines after treatment with rexinoids. In the same study, they reported the upregulation of IL-2R in the malignant cells translated to increase sensitivity to denileukin diftitox (a fusion protein of diphtheria toxin bound to the ligand for the IL-2R previously used in the treatment of CTCL).[4,23]

RETINOIDS IN CUTANEOUS T-CELL LYMPHOMA

Currently all systemic retinoids in use for CTCL are oral agents (administered with food for optimal absorption). Isotretinoin was the first retinoid used for the off-label treatment of CTCL. In 1983, Kessler and colleagues[11] first reported activity in 4 patients with MF treated with isotretinoin at doses of 1 to 3 mg/kg per day with response seen in all patients, 1 patient with a complete response (CR). The investigator proceeded to study 21 additional patients with plaque, tumor, and erythrodermic MF, including 5 with SS using doses of 1 to 2 mg/kg per day.[24] Forty-four percent of patients were reported to have a clinical response, but most patients required dosage adjustment because of mucocutaneous side effects.[24] In 2005, Leverkus and colleagues[25] reported effective treatment of folliculotropic MF with isotretinoin at up to 1 mg/kg per day with specific regard to miniaturization of cysts and comedones associated with this subtype. This effect may be due to the strong affinity of isotretinoin for the pilosebaceous unit. Higher doses of isotretinoin (eg, >1 mg/kg per day) produced similar response rates with higher rates of toxicity compared with 1 mg/kg per day.[24] Overall, use of isotretinoin in MF/SS resulted in clinical responses of 43% to 100% with CR rates of typically less than 20% and short response duration ranging from 3 to 15 months.[3]

Etretinate was the second retinoid approved for clinical applications, originally approved for use in psoriasis. It is highly lipophilic and has a significantly longer half-life of more than 120 days compared with 21 hours with isotretinoin and requires 2 or more years to be completely eliminated from the body after completion of treatment. As such, it was replaced by its metabolite acitretin with a shorter half-life of 2 to 4 days and an elimination period of approximately 2 months (though alcohol ingestion can cause acitretin to convert to etretinate and should be avoided during acitretin use).[26] Before the withdrawal of etretinate from the market in 1998, several studies reported responses in patients with MF when used off-label. Claudy and colleagues[27] treated 12 patients with etretinate monotherapy using 0.8 to 1.0 mg/kg per day with response seen in all patients, but only 1 patient achieved a CR. Clinical response was seen in 55% of patients treated with etretinate in a larger study of 29 patients reported by Molin and colleagues[28] with CR seen in only 1 patient. The treatment response with etretinate appears to be similar to that reported with isotretinoin.

Cheeley and colleagues[29] reported a retrospective study on the use of acitretin in 32 patients with MF/SS. There was a 59% overall response rate with 1 patient achieving CR, but the interpretation of these results may be confounded by other concomitant treatments received by the patients. Acitretin was used as monotherapy in only 6 patients with MF in the study, with clinical response seen in approximately 25% of these patients. The investigators in the retrospective review attempted to compare response between acitretin and bexarotene in patients treated with both medications at different times in their treatment course, but timing of use in the disease course and other concomitant treatment may influence therapeutic

outcome, making comparison difficult. There is limited experience with acitretin in MF (doses used typically 10–50 mg daily), but anecdotal evidence suggests that it may be less effective in these patients than the other RAR agonists or bexarotene, but few comparative studies exist.[1] All-trans retinoic-acid has been shown in vitro to have beneficial effects in CTCL and has also been used off-label for CTCL.[30,31]

Bexarotene is a synthetic rexinoid with RXR selective binding. Unlike its predecessor retinoids, it was approved by the Food and Drug Administration (FDA) specifically for the treatment of CTCL in 1999. Bexarotene was investigated in 2 phase II-III trials in 58 patients with early-stage (I-IIA) MF and in 94 patients with advanced-stage (IIB-IVB) MF/SS.[32,33] In the early-stage trial, patients were treated at dosages ranging from 6.5, 300, and 650 mg/m^2 per day, but the 300 mg/m^2 per day dosage was found to be the ideal starting dose due to toxicity.[3] Clinical responses in this study were reportedly 20%, 54%, and 67% in the 6.5, 300, and 650 mg/m^2 per day treatment groups, respectively.[32] Of the advanced-stage patients, 56 were treated at a dosage of 300 mg/m^2 per day and 38 at a dosage of more than 300 mg/m^2 per day. Patients treated at 300 mg/m^2 per day had clinical responses in 45% (25 of 56) of patients compared with 55% (21 of 38) of patients in the higher-dose treatment group, suggesting that there is a dose-related treatment response. The CR rates for the 300 mg/m^2 per day group was 2% compared with 13% in the higher-dose group. The median time to response was 180 days and time to progression was projected to be 299 days for the lower-dose group and 385 days for the higher-dose group. Among patients with a history of previous retinoid therapy who had not previously responded to other retinoids or had previously responded but progressed, a large portion (54%) improved with bexarotene. More adverse reactions were reported in the higher-dose group with approximately 13% of patients in this group discontinuing treatment because of side effects compared with 7% in the lower-dose group.[33] Another large retrospective trial was reported by Abbott and colleagues[34] in 66 patients with MF and SS with most patients having advanced-stage MF/SS (IIB-IVB). Patients were included if they had received 150 to 300 mg/m^2 daily within the study period. Other treatment modalities, such as radiation or extracorporeal photopheresis (ECP), were used in some patients. Twenty-eight patients completed at least 1 month of treatment with bexarotene as monotherapy, and in these patients, 46% achieved a clinical response, with 14% (4 patients) achieving a CR and 32% (9 patients) achieving a partial response (PR). In patients treated with bexarotene in combination with other treatment modalities, the CR rate was 5% and PR rate was 37%. Bexarotene appears to have more potent activity in MF compared with its predecessors, but not all patients respond to monotherapy and some fail to maintain remission, prompting investigation into its use in combination with other agents. Bexarotene is available as a 75-mg capsule.

Alitretinoin is another synthetically derived retinoid (9-*cis* retinoic acid), which can bind to both RAR and RXR, hence its classification as a pan-retinoic receptor agonist.[1] It was approved in 1999 by the FDA for topical use in localized AIDS-related Kaposi sarcoma and has been available in Europe since 2008 as an oral formulation for the treatment of refractory severe chronic hand dermatitis.[35,36] Oral alitretinoin has been used for treatment of MF as reported in a case series of 2 patients, 1 with refractory disease, resulting in PRs and no significant side effects.[37] More recently, a retrospective study described efficacy of alitretinoin (10 or 30 mg daily) when combined with other therapies (including topical steroids, topical calcineurin inhibitors, phototherapy, IFN-alpha, and/or photopheresis) in 10 patients with MF (stages IA–IIB) and 1 patient with SS (4 CRs and 6 PRs). Side effects were uncommon and included headache, dyslipidemia, and low thyroid-stimulating hormone (TSH) without other thyroid abnormalities.[38] This drug holds significant promise for the treatment of MF/SS, but further studies are needed to investigate its efficacy and safety in this patient population.

Retinoids also have been studied in combination with other treatment modalities (both skin directed and other systemic agents) in MF/SS in an attempt to improve response rates, prolong remission, and decrease adverse effects by using lower doses with nonoverlapping toxicities. Of note, the limitation of these combination studies are that most of them were not controlled, were without comparator arm, had a limited number of patients, and were performed before International Society of Cutaneous Lymphomas (ISCL)/European Organization for the Research and Treatment of Cancer (EORTC) revisions in CTCL staging (2007) and ISCL/EORTC/US Cutaneous Lymphoma Consortium uniform response criteria definitions (2010), thus making it difficult to accurately compare response rates.[39,40] Furthermore, because of the paucity of data, it remains unclear if combination therapies are definitively superior to monotherapy.[41]

Systemic retinoids combined with skin-directed therapy, such as phototherapy (ultraviolet B [UVB]) or psoralen with ultraviolet A phototherapy (PUVA), referred to as Re-UVB or Re-PUVA are well-known combination therapies for many skin conditions (psoriasis, eczema). In MF/SS, isotretinoin was studied in combination with PUVA, with high response rates in 66 patients, with CR in 72% of patients. Although the clinical response was similar to PUVA alone, the study found that fewer UVA treatments were needed for response when the combination was used.[42] PUVA also was combined with acitretin in 42 patients with CTCL, producing a CR rate of 38%. This was significantly lower compared with the comparator arm of PUVA with IFN, which had a CR rate at 70%.[43]

Despite occasional association with photosensitivity in the early clinical studies, since its FDA approval in 1999, bexarotene has been combined successfully with phototherapy in patients with CTCL. In patients with MF stage IA-IIB, combination of low-dose bexarotene (75 mg per day) with PUVA led to clinical response in all patients with CR seen in 63% of patients.[44] In a prospective study of 14 patients with relapsed or treatment-refractory MF (stage IA-III), patients were treated with bexarotene at 150 to 300 mg per day concurrently with PUVA. Overall response rate was 67%, with 29% CRs.[45] In a large randomized controlled trial comparing PUVA versus bexarotene plus PUVA (EORTC 21011), 87 patients with stage IB/IIA MF were randomized to each treatment group but no significant difference in response rate (71% PUVA vs 77% combination arm) or response duration (9.7 PUVA vs 5.8 months combination) was found.[46]

Bexarotene also has been combined with narrow-band UVB (NBUVB) therapy in case reports. One patient with stage IB plaque-stage MF was treated successfully with low-dose bexarotene (75 mg daily) and NBUVB treatment 3 times weekly. The patient was previously treatment refractory and NBUVB was used in place of PUVA because of the history of multiple basal cell carcinomas.[47] Another case report in a patient with plaque-stage MF responded to a combination of bexarotene 300 mg daily with NBUVB. The disease flared when either bexarotene or NBUVB was discontinued, suggesting a possible synergistic or additive effect.[48]

Combination trials using retinoids with other systemics, such as IFNs, have been reported by various investigators. This combination is attractive because of synergistic effects of retinoid stimulation of Th1 activity through IL-12 production and inhibition of Th2 response by IFN-alpha and IFN-gamma.[49] Isotretinoin at 1 mg/kg per day was combined successfully with IFN-alfa-2b 2 million units (MU) 3 times weekly in 7 patients with clinical objective response (OR) seen in 57% of patients (29% achieving CR).[50] Isotretinoin also was studied in combination with IFN-alfa as induction therapy together with total-body electron beam radiation and chemotherapy in 28 patients. Overall response in this study was 82%, with 71% achieving CR.[51] Isotretinoin at 1 mg/kg per day has been investigated in combination with 3 MU daily of IFN-alfa in 18 patients with MF/SS.[52] Patients in this study had advanced-stage disease (IIB-IV) and were found to have OR rates of 33% with half the responders having SS. It appears that the combination was well tolerated.

Bexarotene has been investigated in a phase II trial in combination with IFN-alfa in 22 patients with MF/SS. Most of the patients in this study had advanced-stage disease (with 86% of patients having stage II-IV disease). Patients were treated initially with bexarotene 300 mg/m^2 per day alone for 8 weeks followed by the addition of IFN-alfa-2b at 3 to 5 MU 3 times weekly for 8 additional weeks if CR was not achieved with bexarotene alone. No patient achieved CR during the first 8 weeks of treatment with bexarotene alone. The overall response rate was 39%, with 1 patient achieving CR. Of note, 4 additional responses were observed with the addition IFN in the second stage of the study, with 1 patient initially having PR to bexarotene alone converting to CR.[53]

ECP is a treatment modality highly effective in patients with SS with treatment responses as a monotherapy reported at 60% and 19% CR.[54] Bexarotene at dosages ranging from 225 to 750 mg per day or up to 300 mg/m^2 daily in combination with ECP led to high response rates of 75% to 80% in small studies.[49,55] In another study in patients with SS, bexarotene at 150 mg per day was added, as part of a multimodality approach to treatment, to monthly ECP, PUVA with and without IFN-gamma or alfa 3 times weekly producing CRs in 3 of 5 patients and PR in the other 2 patients.[56]

Retinoids and rexinoids also have been used in combination with other biologic and chemotherapeutic agents active against MF/SS. The combination of bexarotene in combination with denileukin diftitox is believed to be synergistic, as retinoids have the ability to enhance the expression of high-affinity IL-2 receptor and thereby increase the susceptibility to denileukin diftitox.[4] This effect was observed at bexarotene dosages of 150 mg per day or higher. Fourteen patients with MF/SS treated with the combination of bexarotene 75 to 375 mg per day and denileukin diftitox 18 µg/kg per day 3 times every 21 days, had an overall response rate of 67%, including 29% with a CR.[57] Bexarotene was studied in combination with vorinostat, a histone deacetylase inhibitor, in

a combination phase I/II study in 23 patients with MF/SS in stages IB or higher. The maximum tolerated dosage in the phase I part of the study was 200 mg per day of vorinostat and 300 mg/m^2 per day of bexarotene. Patients in the phase II part of the study were treated with 400 mg per day of vorinostat and 150 mg/m^2 per day of bexarotene. Overall response was 26% (7% in phase I of the study and 33% in phase II). This OR rate was similar to patients treated with vorinostat monotherapy. However, improvement in pruritus was reported in several patients. More than 20% of patients required discontinuation from the trial because of adverse effects, but adverse effects reported (neutropenia, diarrhea, hypertriglyceridemia) did not appear to correlate with the higher dosages used in the second phase of the study.[58]

Bexarotene also has been studied in MF/SS in combination with chemotherapy agents, such as methotrexate (MTX) and pralatrexate. In a retrospective study of 12 patients with MF (stage IA-IIB) who were treated with bexarotene at dosages of 75 to 300 mg per day and MTX at 5 to 30 mg per week, overall response was 66% with 8% achieving CR.[59] Another study compared pralatrexate with the combination of bexarotene at 150 to 300 mg/m^2 daily and pralatrexate 15 mg/m^2 weekly. Overall response was seen in 33% of patients treated with pralatrexate alone compared with 50% in the combination group.[60] Clinical responses with the combination appear to be higher compared with the individual chemotherapy agents alone. However, not all combination trials demonstrate increased efficacy with the addition of retinoids. In a recently published study evaluating the combination of gemcitabine at 1000 mg/m^2 intravenously on days 1 and 8 every 21 days with oral bexarotene at 300 mg/m^2 per day in 35 predominantly advanced-stage (IB-IVA) CTCL, resulted in interruption of the trial when lower responses were revealed at interim analysis when compared with single-agent gemcitabine.[61] The prominent studies involving the retinoids and rexinoid for treatment of MF/SS are listed in **Table 2**.

Resistance to retinoids has been reported in the literature. In vitro evaluation of malignant T cells found that malignant cells from as high as 33% of patients with SS are intrinsically resistant to bexarotene.[62] The mechanism of bexarotene resistance was investigated in a patient who initially responded to treatment but later developed disease relapse. Malignant T cells obtained from this patient at baseline underwent apoptosis with exposure to bexarotene, but cells obtained at relapse did not. No genetic coding alterations in the RXR receptors were found to suggest that mutation of the receptor was responsible for loss

Table 2
Notable studies of retinoids and rexinoids in CTCL

Treatment	No. of Patients	Stage of CTCL	Dose	Response Rate	Author, Year
Isotretinoin	25	MF 20/SS 5	1–2 mg/kg/d	OR 44%; CR12%	Kessler et al,[24] 1987
Isotretinoin	7	NA	100 mg/m² daily	OR 43%; CR 14%	Warrell et al,[12] 1983
Isotretinoin	15	MF 10/SS 5	0.2–2 mg/kg/d	OR 59%; CR 21%	Molin et al,[28] 1987
Isotretinoin	20	MF 16/SS 4	1–2 mg/kg/d	OR 80%; CR 33%	Thomsen et al,[72] 1984
Isotretinoin	6	MF 6/SS 1	1–2 mg/kg/d	OR 100%; CR none	Neely et al,[73] 1987
Isotretinoin + interferon-alpha	7	MF 7	1 mg/kg/d (Isotretinoin) + 2 million units/d (interferon-alpha-2b)	OR 57%; CR 29%	Knobler et al,[50] 1991
Isotretinoin + interferon-alpha	18	MF 12/SS 6	1 mg/kg/d (Isotretinoin) + 3 million units/d (interferon-alpha-2b)	OR 33%; CR 6%	Tsimberidou et al,[52] 2004

(continued on next page)

Table 2
(continued)

Treatment	No. of Patients	Stage of CTCL	Dose	Response Rate	Author, Year
Isotretinoin + interferon-alpha + TSEB/CT	28	MF 23/SS 5	1 mg/kg/d (isotretinoin) + 5 million units/d (interferon-alpha-2b) followed by TSEB/CT	OR 82%; CR 71%	Duvic et al,[51] 1996
Isotretinoin + PUVA	69	MF 69	1 mg/kg/d isotretinoin + PUVA	CR 73%	Thomsen et al,[42] 1989
Etretinate	12	Parapsoriasis, MF, SS	0.8–1 mg/kg/d	OR 100%; CR 8%	Claudy et al,[27] 1983
Etretinate	29	MF/SS	NA	OR 55%; CR 21%	Molin et al,[28] 1987
Acitretin	32 (only 6 as monotherapy)	MF 29/SS 2/ Unspecified 1	10–50 mg daily	OR 25%; CR none (monotherapy)	Cheeley et al,[29] 2013
Bexarotene	94	MF 77/SS 17 Advanced stage	300 mg/m²/d and more than 300 mg/m²/d	OR 45%; CR 2% (300 mg/m²/d) vs OR 55%; CR 13% (>300 mg/m²/d)	Duvic et al,[33] 2001
Bexarotene	58	MF 58 (early stage)	6.5, 300, 650 mg/m²/d	OR 20%; CR none, OR 54%; CR 7%, and OR 67%; CR 27% in the 6.5, 300, and 650 mg/m²/d respectively	Duvic et al,[32] 2001
Bexarotene	66 (only 28 as monotherapy)	MF 25/SS 3	150–300 mg/m²/d	OR 46%; CR 14%	Abbott et al,[34] 2009
Bexarotene + interferon-alpha	22	CTCL (IB-IV)	300 mg/m²/d (Bexarotene) + interferon-alpha-2b 3 million units 3 times weekly	OR 39%; CR 6%	Straus et al,[53] 2007
Bexarotene + NBUVB	1	MF 1 (IB)	75 mg/d (Bexarotene) + NBUVB	Improvement	D'Acunto et al,[47] 2010
Bexarotene + NBUVB	1	MF 1 (1B)	150, increased to 300 mg/d + NBUVB	Improvement	Lokitz & Wong,[48] 2007
Bexarotene + PUVA	14	MF 12/SS 2	150–300 mg/d (Bexarotene) + PUVA	OR 67%; CR 29%	Papadavid et al,[45] 2008

Treatment	N	Stage/diagnosis	Dosage	Response	Reference
Bexarotene + PUVA	8	MF 8 (IA-IB)	75 mg/d (Bexarotene) + PUVA	OR 100%; CR 63%	Singh & Lebwohl et al,[44] 2004
Bexarotene + PUVA vs PUVA	87	MF 87 (IB-IIA)	Dosage not reported (Bexarotene) + PUVA	OR 71%; CR 22.2% (PUVA) vs OR 77%; CR 31.3% (Combination)	Whittaker et al,[46] 2012
Bexarotene + vorinostat	23	CTCL (stage IB or higher)	150–300 mg/m^2/d (Bexarotene) + 200–400 mg/d vorinostat	OR 26%;(CR not reported)	Dummer et al,[58] 2012
Bexarotene + ECP	5	MF 3/SS 2	300 mg/m^2/d (Bexarotene) + PUVA	OR 80%; CR 20%	Tsirigotis et al,[55] 2007
Bexarotene + ECP	8	MF/SS	100–300 mg/m^2/d (Bexarotene) + ECP	OR 75%; CR 13%	Talpur et al,[49] 2002
Bexarotene + denileukin diftitox	14	CTCL (IA-IVB)	75–375 mg/d (Bexarotene) + 18 μg/kg/d × 3 d q21 d	OR 67%; CR 29%	Foss et al,[57] 2005
Bexarotene + methotrexate	12	MF (Stage IA-IIB)	75–300 mg/d (Bexarotene) + methotrexate 5–30 mg/wk	OR 66%; CR 8%	Kannangara et al,[59] 2009
Bexarotene + gemcitabine	35	CTCL (IB-IVB)	300 mg/m^2/d (bexarotene) + 1000 mg/m^2 D1&8 q21 d (gemcitabine)	OR 31%; CR none Lower than single agent gemcitabine	Illidge et al,[61] 2013
Bexarotene + pralatrexate	14	MF	150–300 mg/m^2/d (bexarotene) + 15 mg/m^2/wk (pralatrexate)	OR 50%; CR none	Talpur et al,[60] 2014
Alitretinoin	2	MF 2	30 mg/d	OR/PR 100%	Coors & von den Driesch,[37] 2012
Alitretinoin	11	MF 10 (IA-IIB)/SS 1	10 or 30 mg daily	OR 91%; CR 40%	Kapser et al,[38] 2015

Abbreviations: CR, complete response; CT, chemotherapy; CTCL, cutaneous T-cell lymphoma; MF, mycosis fungoides; NA, not available; NBUVB, narrow band UVB; OR, objective response; PR, partial response; PUVA, psoralen plus UVA; SS, Sézary syndrome; TSEB, total-body skin electron beam radiation.

of activity. A decline in the levels of RXR receptor expression on cells, which is the receptor target for bexarotene, was found as a possible mechanism.[63]

ADVERSE EFFECTS

Retinoids have a unique side-effect profile compared with traditional cytotoxic agents. In clinical studies of bexarotene, the most common adverse effects are dyslipidemia, which has been reported to occur in 100% of patients, and secondary hypothyroidism, reported in 40% to 100% of patients taking bexarotene.[1] Other common side effects of bexarotene include liver function test abnormalities and dose-dependent leukopenia and neutropenia, and rarely, gastrointestinal disturbances. Dyslipidemia also is common in patients receiving isotretinoin. **Table 3** is a list of common side effects associated with bexarotene. In contrast to the adverse effects seen in RXR agonists, side effects associated with RAR agonists seen in clinical studies in patients with CTCL include xerosis (dose-limiting), cheilitis, headaches, and arthralgias/myalgias. See **Table 4** for side effects associated with isotretinoin. Because of teratogenic effects, all retinoids and rexinoids should be avoided in pregnant patients or in patients who wish to become pregnant.

Dyslipidemia is a dose-dependent and sometimes dose-limiting adverse reaction to both retinoids and rexinoids. This is typically manifested as hypertriglyceridemia and less commonly hypercholesterolemia. Activation of RAR leads to secretion and decreased catabolism of triglyceride particles leading to hypertriglyceridemia and resulting decrease in high-density lipopoprotein.[64] The binding of agonists to RXR has been shown to result in increased apoCIII synthesis, a hepatic protein that binds to lipids in the plasma and aids in hepatic uptake of triglyceride particles. It also

Side Effects	Prevalence/Moderate/ Severe, %
Xerosis	36/20
Chelitis	28/0
Conjunctivitis	36/0
Fatigue	12/8
Arthralgia/Myalgia	8/8
Mental status change	8/0
Headache	8/0

Table 4
Moderate to severe side effects of isotretinoin

Data from Kessler JF, Jones SE, Levine N, et al. Isotretinoin and cutaneous helper t-cell lymphoma (mycosis fungoides). Arch Dermatol 1987;123:201–4.

decreases lipoprotein lipase activity, which hydrolyzes triglycerides into fatty acids.[65] Peroxisome proliferator–activated receptors (PPARs) are nuclear hormone receptors that are part of the superfamily of receptors that also includes retinold receptors and others. These receptors are strongly expressed in the skin and sebaceous glands and are involved in oxidative pathways for fatty acids.[65] Retinoic X receptors form heterodimers with PPARs and transactivation by rexinoids are believed to influence lipid metabolism.[1] Triglyceride elevation also is regulated by transactivation of LXR (Liver X receptor)/RXR heterodimers by sterol regulatory element–binding proteins, which are transcription regulators involved in cholesterol biosynthesis.[1] The LXR acts by controlling cholesterol metabolism in the liver as well as reverse cholesterol transport from the peripheral tissues to the liver by increasing plasma lipids. Activation of LXR on RXR heterodimers may play only a small part in the complex pathway of the influence retinoids have on metabolism of not only lipids, but also of glucose and fatty acids.[1] In patients

Table 3
Side effects of bexarotene

Side Effect	Prevalence, %
Central hypothyroidism	29–100
Hypertriglyceridemia	82–100
Dyslipidemia (increased low-density lipoprotein; decreased high-density lipoprotein)	30
Liver toxicity	11–20
Headache	16–20
Skin rash, phototoxicity	8–13
Leucopenia	6–11

Adapted from Graeppi-Dulac J, Vlaeminck-Guillem V, Perier-Muzet M, et al. Endocrine side-effects of anti-cancer drugs: the impact of retinoids on the thyroid axis. Eur J Endocrinol 2014;170:R256.

receiving bexarotene as monotherapy at 300 mg/m^2 daily, hypertriglyceridemia was found in 83% of patients, with 2 of 70 patients developing pancreatitis due to the markedly elevated triglyceride levels.[49] Of interest, it was reported by Talpur and colleagues[49] in 2002 that higher response rates to bexarotene were associated with use of lipid-lowering agents, with the highest response rates seen in patients treated with atorvastatin and fenofibrate. The higher response rate in these patients may be merely a reflection of the higher doses of bexarotene used (as dyslipidemia is a dose-dependent phenomenon) or perhaps higher sensitivity to bexarotene, which parallels dose response. In contrast, patients who were treated with the lipid-lowering agent gemfibrozil had more severe hypertriglyceridemia and elevated bexarotene serum levels. Its use is contraindicated with bexarotene because it inhibits the oxidative metabolism of the drug, thereby increasing toxicity.[49] In one case series of 102 subjects on isotretinoin, patients with predisposing conditions, such as truncal obesity, hyperinsulinemia, or family history of hypertriglyceridemia, were more likely to develop retinoid-induced hypertriglyceridemia.[66] Patients receiving either isotretinoin or bexarotene should have baseline lipid evaluation before starting therapy and close monitoring should take place during treatment. In most patients treated with bexarotene, treatment with lipid-lowering agents and adherence to low-fat and low-cholesterol diet are recommended at the onset of treatment.

Central hypothyroidism also is commonly encountered in patients treated with bexarotene. This is caused by suppression of the pituitary production of the TSH. RXRγ is the subtype of receptor implicated in rexinoid-induced hypothyroidism and is strongly expressed in the pituitary. In contrast, isotretinoin and acitretin, RAR agonists, do not have effects on TSH levels and hypothyroidism.[2] Alitretinoin affects both RAR and RXR receptors, so it also may have effects on the thyroid hormone axis. Similar to retinoid-induced hyperlipidemia, bexarotene-induced hypothyroidism also appears to be dose dependent and reversible. In patients with normal thyroid function before starting treatment with bexarotene, serum TSH returns to normal in most patients as early as 8 days after stopping bexarotene.[67] Because bexarotene patients typically require doses higher than replacement thyroid doses used in hypothyroidism from other causes, it has been suggested that an increase in metabolism of thyroid hormone also may play a role, perhaps through induction of liver metabolic oxidative enzymes by retinoids.[2,68] Patients should be started on empiric thyroid supplementation at onset of treatment with bexarotene

(25–50 μg daily) and increased based on monthly serum-free thyroxine (free T4) levels. TSH remains suppressed while on bexarotene, even with adequate levothyroxine supplementation so the TSH should not be used as the basis by which one adjusts levothyroxine dose.

Dose-dependent leukopenia and neutropenia can be observed in 10% of patients, but in contrast to neutropenia observed after cytotoxic chemotherapy, bexarotene neutropenia is not typically associated with increased opportunistic infections because neutrophils are functionally normal. Given this, in our patients with MF/SS who have no previous history of cytotoxic chemotherapy, we do not dose reduce bexarotene unless absolute neutrophil count is less than 500/μL (Ellen Kim, personal communication, 2015).

Alitretinoin has been associated with a lower incidence of dyslipidemia and/or suppression of the thyroid axis as compared with isotretinoin or bexarotene, usually not requiring treatment for these side effects.[35] The mechanism explaining this difference in side-effect profile is not known.[37]

No definitive guidelines exist for monitoring or management of adverse effects associated with retinoids and rexinoids. Isotretinoin is contraindicated in patients who are pregnant and should be used with caution in patients who have history of uncontrolled psychiatric illness, inflammatory bowel disease, and osteoporosis. Patients who are being treated with isotretinoin in the United States should follow monitoring as per the iPLEDGE (a mandatory distribution program for isotretinoin in the United States) program. This includes pregnancy monitoring for female patients with childbearing potential at baseline and monthly. Patients receiving isotretinoin should avoid concomitant use of tetracycline class of antibiotics due to the increased risk of pseudotumor cerebri. We also recommend baseline laboratory testing such as complete blood count, liver function tests, and lipid profile while on therapy. Acitretin and bexarotene are also contraindicated in pregnancy and should be used with caution in patients with liver disease, history of alcohol abuse, or uncontrolled hyperlipidemia. Female patients should avoid becoming pregnant for at least 3 years after discontinuation of the acitretin. This should be considered before initiation of treatment in any female patient who is of childbearing age. Use of alcohol during treatment with acitretin results in conversion of acitretin to etretinate and can result in prolonged elimination of the retinoid.[69]

In patients on treatment with bexarotene, additional monitoring of free thyroxine (free-T4) levels and not TSH is required (TSH is typically suppressed in central hypothyroidism and is not

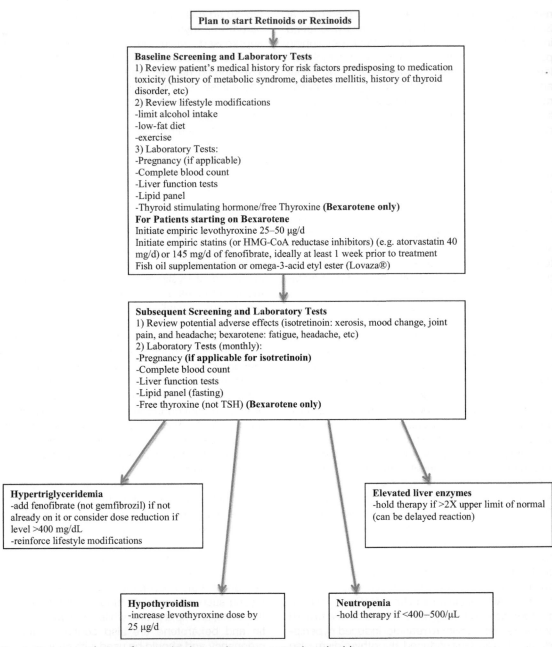

Fig. 2. Recommendations for monitoring patients on systemic retinoids.

reliable as a measure of thyroid function in patients on the medication). Bexarotene should not be given in combination with gemfibrozil because of increases in plasma concentration of bexarotene. It is metabolized in the liver via cytochrome p-450 3A4 and when used in combination with 3A4 inhibitors, such as azole class of antifungal agents (ketoconazole, itraconazole) or grapefruit juice or with 3A4 inducers, such as rifampin or phenytoin, alterations in plasma levels of the drug may occur.[70] In all patients receiving retinoids, lifestyle modifications, including exercise and dietary changes that include low-fat diet and limits on alcohol consumption should be advised. Recommended monitoring and management of adverse effects for patients on retinoids and rexinoids are shown in **Fig. 2**.[71]

SUMMARY

MF and SS subtypes of CTCL have a variable clinical course ranging from indolent disease that does not alter life expectancy to aggressive, rapidly progressive disease. Goals of treatment especially in patients with early-stage disease are to induce remission with agents that have a low toxicity profile. The systemic retinoids are an important component of the treatment options for all stages of this disease because of the ease of administration and relative low toxicity profile. Side effects appear to be dose related and should be monitored closely with hyperlipidemia observed with all retinoids, whereas other side effects are more drug or retinoid class specific. For example, central hypothyroidism appears to be limited to RXR agonists and mucocutaneous dryness to RAR agonists. Bexarotene is the only FDA-approved systemic retinoid approved specifically for CTCL but does require additional medications to treat the associated hyperlipidemia and hypothyroidism during the duration of bexarotene treatment. Combination treatment with retinoids and other agents with activity against MF/SS appear to be well tolerated and associated with high response rates in relapsed or treatment-refractory patients in small studies and series. Further high-quality clinical trials are needed in MF/SS patients to confirm whether combination therapies are superior to monotherapy.

REFERENCES

1. Sokołowska-Wojdyło M, Ługowska-Umer H, Maciejewska-Radomska A. Oral retinoids and rexinoids in cutaneous T-cell lymphomas. Postepy Dermatol Alergol 2013;30:19–29.

2. Graeppi-Dulac J, Vlaeminck-Guillem V, Perier-Muzet M, et al. Endocrine side-effects of anti-cancer drugs: the impact of retinoids on the thyroid axis. Eur J Endocrinol 2014;170:R253–62.

3. Zhang C, Duvic M. Treatment of cutaneous T-cell lymphoma with retinoids. Dermatol Ther 2006;19:264–71.

4. Gorgun G, Foss F. Immunomodulatory effects of RXR rexinoids: modulation of high-affinity IL-2R expression enhances susceptibility to denileukin diftitox. Blood 2002;100:1399–403.

5. Kempf W, Kettelhack N, Duvic M, et al. Topical and systemic retinoid therapy for cutaneous T-cell lymphoma. Hematol Oncol Clin North Am 2003;17:1405–19.

6. Tang X-H, Gudas LJ. Retinoids, retinoic acid receptors, and cancer. Annu Rev Pathol 2011;6:345–64.

7. Cheng AL, Su IJ, Chen CC, et al. Use of retinoic acids in the treatment of peripheral T-cell lymphoma: a pilot study. J Clin Oncol 1994;12:1185–92.

8. Zhang C, Hazarika P, Ni X, et al. Induction of apoptosis by bexarotene in cutaneous T-cell lymphoma cells: relevance to mechanism of therapeutic action. Clin Cancer Res 2002;8:1234–40.

9. Bradford PT, Devesa SS, Anderson WF, et al. Cutaneous lymphoma incidence patterns in the United States: a population-based study of 3884 cases. Blood 2009;113:5064–73.

10. National Comprehensive Cancer Network Guidelines. Non-Hodgkin's Lymphoma. Version 5.2014. Available at: http://www.nccn.org/professionals/physician_gls/PDF/nhl.pdf. Accessed February, 2015.

11. Kessler JF, Meyskens FL, Levine N, et al. Treatment of cutaneous T-cell lymphoma (mycosis fungoides) with 13-cis-retinoic acid. Lancet 1983;1:1345–7.

12. Warrell RP Jr, Coonley CJ, Kempin SJ, et al. Isotretinoin in cutaneous t-cell lymphoma. Lancet 1983;322:629.

13. Stadler R, Kremer A. Therapeutic advances in cutaneous T-Cell lymphoma (CTCL): from retinoids to rexinoids. Semin Oncol 2006;33(Supplement 3):7–10.

14. Layton A. The use of isotretinoin in acne. Dermatoendocrinol 2009;1:162–9.

15. Gordy C, Dzhagalov I, He Y-W. Regulation of CD8(+) T cell functions by RARgamma. Semin Immunol 2009;21:2–7.

16. Heller EH, Shiffman NJ. Synthetic retinoids in dermatology. Can Med Assoc J 1985;132:1129–36.

17. Boutwell RK. Retinoids and inhibition of ornithine decarboxylase activity. J Am Acad Dermatol 1982;6:796–800.

18. Burg G, Dummer R. Historical perspective on the use of retinoids in cutaneous T-cell lymphoma (CTCL). Clin Lymphoma 2000;1(Supplement 1):S41–4.

19. Nieto-Rementería N, Pérez-Yarza G, Boyano MD, et al. Bexarotene activates the p53/p73 pathway in human cutaneous T-cell lymphoma. Br J Dermatol 2009;160:519–26.

20. Yen W-C, Prudente RY, Corpuz MR, et al. A selective retinoid X receptor agonist bexarotene (LGD1069, targretin) inhibits angiogenesis and metastasis in solid tumours. Br J Cancer 2006;94:654–60.

21. Meunier L, Bohjanen K, Voorhees JJ, et al. Retinoic acid upregulates human Langerhans cell antigen presentation and surface expression of HLA-DR and CD11c, a beta 2 integrin critically involved in T-cell activation. J Invest Dermatol 1994;103:775–9.

22. Rook AH, Kubin M, Fox FE, et al. The potential therapeutic role of interleukin-12 in cutaneous T-cell lymphoma. Ann N Y Acad Sci 1996;795:310–8.

23. Sidell N, Chang B, Bhatti L. Upregulation by retinoic acid of interleukin-2-receptor mRNA in human T lymphocytes. Cell Immunol 1993;146:28–37.

24. Kessler JF, Jones SE, Levine N, et al. Isotretinoin and cutaneous helper T-cell lymphoma (mycosis fungoides). Arch Dermatol 1987;123:201–4.

25. Leverkus M, Rose C, Bröcker EB, et al. Follicular cutaneous T-cell lymphoma: beneficial effect of isotretinoin for persisting cysts and comedones. Br J Dermatol 2005;152:193–4.

26. Katz HI, Waalen J, Leach EE. Acitretin in psoriasis: an overview of adverse effects. J Am Acad Dermatol 1999;41:S7–12.

27. Claudy AL, Rouchouse B, Boucheron S, et al. Treatment of cutaneous lymphoma with etretinate. Br J Dermatol 1983;109:49–56.

28. Molin L, Thomsen K, Volden G, et al. Oral retinoids in mycosis fungoides and Sézary syndrome: a comparison of isotretinoin and etretinate. A study from the Scandinavian Mycosis Fungoides Group. Acta Derm Venereol 1987;67:232–6.

29. Cheeley J, Sahn RE, DeLong LK, et al. Acitretin for the treatment of cutaneous T-cell lymphoma. J Am Acad Dermatol 2013;68:247–54.

30. Fox FE, Kubin M, Cassin M, et al. Retinoids synergize with interleukin-2 to augment IFN-gamma and interleukin-12 production by human peripheral blood mononuclear cells. J Interferon Cytokine Res 1999;19:407–15.

31. Kim EJ, Hess S, Richardson SK, et al. Immunopathogenesis and therapy of cutaneous T cell lymphoma. J Clin Invest 2005;115:798–812.

32. Duvic M, Martin AG, Kim Y, et al. Phase 2 and 3 clinical trial of oral bexarotene (Targretin capsules) for the treatment of refractory or persistent early-stage cutaneous T-cell lymphoma. Arch Dermatol 2001; 137:581–93.

33. Duvic M, Hymes K, Heald P, et al. Bexarotene is effective and safe for treatment of refractory advanced-stage cutaneous T-cell lymphoma: multinational phase II-III trial results. J Clin Oncol 2001; 19:2456–71.

34. Abbott RA, Whittaker SJ, Morris SL, et al. Bexarotene therapy for mycosis fungoides and Sézary syndrome. Br J Dermatol 2009;160:1299–307.

35. Ruzicka T, Lynde CW, Jemec GB, et al. Efficacy and safety of oral alitretinoin (9-cis retinoic acid) in patients with severe chronic hand eczema refractory to topical corticosteroids: results of a randomized, double-blind, placebo-controlled, multicentre trial. Br J Dermatol 2008;158:808–17.

36. Cattelan AM, Trevenzoli M, Aversa SML. Recent advances in the treatment of AIDS-related Kaposi's sarcoma. Am J Clin Dermatol 2002;3:451–62.

37. Coors EA, von den Driesch P. Treatment of 2 patients with mycosis fungoides with alitretinoin. J Am Acad Dermatol 2012;67:e265–7.

38. Kapser C, Herzinger T, Ruzicka T, et al. Treatment of cutaneous T-cell lymphoma with oral alitretinoin. J Eur Acad Dermatol Venereol 2015;29(4):783–8.

39. Olsen E, Vonderheid E, Pimpinelli N, et al. Revisions to the staging and classification of mycosis fungoides and Sezary syndrome: a proposal of the International Society for Cutaneous Lymphomas (ISCL) and the cutaneous lymphoma task force of the European Organization of Research and Treatment of Cancer (EORTC). Blood 2007;110:1713–22.

40. Olsen EA, Whittaker S, Kim YH, et al. Clinical end points and response criteria in mycosis fungoides and Sézary syndrome: a consensus statement of the International Society for Cutaneous Lymphomas, the United States Cutaneous Lymphoma Consortium, and the Cutaneous Lymphoma Task Force of the European Organisation for Research and Treatment of Cancer. J Clin Oncol 2011;29: 2598–607.

41. Humme D, Nast A, Erdmann R, et al. Systematic review of combination therapies for mycosis fungoides. Cancer Treat Rev 2014;40:927–33.

42. Thomsen K, Hammar H, Molin L, et al. Retinoids plus PUVA (RePUVA) and PUVA in mycosis fungoides, plaque stage. A report from the Scandinavian Mycosis Fungoides Group. Acta Derm Venereol 1989;69:536–8.

43. Stadler R, Otte HG, Luger T, et al. Prospective randomized multicenter clinical trial on the use of interferon -2a plus acitretin versus interferon -2a plus PUVA in patients with cutaneous T-cell lymphoma stages I and II. Blood 1998;92:3578–81.

44. Singh F, Lebwohl MG. Cutaneous T-cell lymphoma treatment using bexarotene and PUVA: a case series. J Am Acad Dermatol 2004;51:570–3.

45. Papadavid E, Antoniou C, Nikolaou V, et al. Safety and efficacy of low-dose bexarotene and PUVA in the treatment of patients with mycosis fungoides. Am J Clin Dermatol 2008;9:169–73.

46. Whittaker S, Ortiz P, Dummer R, et al. Efficacy and safety of bexarotene combined with psoralen-ultraviolet A (PUVA) compared with PUVA treatment alone in stage IB-IIA mycosis fungoides: final results from the EORTC Cutaneous Lymphoma Task Force phase III randomized clinical trial (NCT00056056). Br J Dermatol 2012;167:678–87.

47. D'Acunto C, Gurioli C, Neri I. Plaque stage mycosis fungoides treated with bexarotene at low dosage and UVB-NB. J Dermatolog Treat 2010;21:45–8.

48. Lokitz ML, Wong HK. Bexarotene and narrowband ultraviolet B phototherapy combination treatment for mycosis fungoides. Photodermatol Photoimmunol Photomed 2007;23:255–7.

49. Talpur R, Ward S, Apisarnthanarax N, et al. Optimizing bexarotene therapy for cutaneous T-cell lymphoma. J Am Acad Dermatol 2002;47:672–84.

50. Knobler RM, Trautinger F, Radaszkiewicz T, et al. Treatment of cutaneous T cell lymphoma with a combination of low-dose interferon alfa-2b and retinoids. J Am Acad Dermatol 1991;24:247–52.

51. Duvic M, Lemak NA, Redman JR, et al. Combined modality therapy for cutaneous T-cell lymphoma. J Am Acad Dermatol 1996;34:1022–9.

52. Tsimberidou A-M, Giles F, Romaguera J, et al. Activity of interferon-alpha and isotretinoin in patients with advanced, refractory lymphoid malignancies. Cancer 2004;100:574–80.

53. Straus DJ, Duvic M, Kuzel T, et al. Results of a phase II trial of oral bexarotene (Targretin) combined with interferon alfa-2b (Intron-A) for patients with cutaneous T-cell lymphoma. Cancer 2007;109:1799–803.

54. Stadler R. Optimal combination with PUVA: rationale and clinical trial update. Oncology (Williston Park) 2007;21:29–32.

55. Tsirigotis P, Pappa V, Papageorgiou S, et al. Extracorporeal photopheresis in combination with bexarotene in the treatment of mycosis fungoides and Sézary syndrome. Br J Dermatol 2007;156: 1379–81.

56. McGinnis KS, Ubriani R, Newton S, et al. The addition of interferon gamma to oral bexarotene therapy with photopheresis for Sézary syndrome. Arch Dermatol 2005;141:1176–8.

57. Foss F, Demierre MF, DiVenuti G. A phase-1 trial of bexarotene and denileukin diftitox in patients with relapsed or refractory cutaneous T-cell lymphoma. Blood 2005;106:454–7.

58. Dummer R, Beyer M, Hymes K, et al. Vorinostat combined with bexarotene for treatment of cutaneous T-cell lymphoma: in vitro and phase I clinical evidence supporting augmentation of retinoic acid receptor/retinoid X receptor activation by histone deacetylase inhibition. Leuk Lymphoma 2012;53: 1501–8.

59. Kannangara AP, Levitan D, Fleischer AB. Evaluation of the efficacy of the combination of oral bexarotene and methotrexate for the treatment of early stage treatment-refractory cutaneous T-cell lymphoma. J Dermatolog Treat 2009;20:169–76.

60. Talpur R, Thompson A, Gangar P, et al. Pralatrexate alone or in combination with bexarotene: long-term tolerability in relapsed/refractory mycosis fungoides. Clin Lymphoma Myeloma Leuk 2014;14:297–304.

61. Illidge T, Chan C, Counsell N, et al. Phase II study of gemcitabine and bexarotene (GEMBEX) in the treatment of cutaneous T-cell lymphoma. Br J Cancer 2013;109:2566–73.

62. Budgin JB, Richardson SK, Newton SB, et al. Biological effects of bexarotene in cutaneous T-cell lymphoma. Arch Dermatol 2005;141:315–21.

63. Lin JH, Kim EJ, Bansal A, et al. Clinical and in vitro resistance to bexarotene in adult T-cell leukemia: loss of RXR-alpha receptor. Blood 2008;112:2484–8.

64. Staels B. Regulation of lipid and lipoprotein metabolism by retinoids. J Am Acad Dermatol 2001;45: S158–67.

65. Lilley JS, Linton MF, Fazio S. Oral retinoids and plasma lipids. Dermatol Ther 2013;26:404–10.

66. Rodondi N, Darioli R, Ramelet AA, et al. High risk for hyperlipidemia and the metabolic syndrome after an episode of hypertriglyceridemia during 13-cis retinoic acid therapy for acne: a pharmacogenetic study. Ann Intern Med 2002;136:582–9.

67. Sherman SI, Gopal J, Haugen BR, et al. Central hypothyroidism associated with retinoid X receptor-selective ligands. N Engl J Med 1999;340:1075–9.

68. Sherman SI. Etiology, diagnosis, and treatment recommendations for central hypothyroidism associated with bexarotene therapy for cutaneous T-cell lymphoma. Clin Lymphoma 2003;3:249–52.

69. Larsen F, Jakobsen P, Knudsen J, et al. Conversion of acitretin to etretinate in psoriatic patients is influenced by ethanol. J Invest Dermatol 1993;100:623–7.

70. Targretin [package insert]. Bridgewater, NJ: Valeant Pharmaceuticals NA LLC; 2013.

71. Scarisbrick JJ, Morris S, Azurdia R, et al. UK consensus statement on safe clinical prescribing of bexarotene for patients with cutaneous T-cell lymphoma. Br J Dermatol 2013;168:192–200.

72. Thomsen K, Molin L, Volden G, et al. 13-cis-retinoic acid effective in mycosis fungoides. A report from the Scandinavian Mycosis Fungoides Group. Acta Derm Venereol 1984;64:563–6.

73. Neely SM, Mehlmauer M, Feinstein DI. The effect of isotretinoin in six patients with cutaneous T-cell lymphoma. Arch Intern Med 1987;147:529–31.

The Use of Interferons in the Treatment of Cutaneous T-Cell Lymphoma

Natalie Spaccarelli, MD*, Alain H. Rook, MD

KEYWORDS

- Cutaneous T-cell lymphoma • Interferons • Interferon alfa • Interferon gamma • Mycosis fungoides
- Sézary syndrome

KEY POINTS

- Interferons (IFNs) have various immunomodulatory functions that are likely conducive to the treatment of cutaneous T-cell lymphoma (CTCL).
- IFN alfa and IFN gamma are the 2 types of IFNs that have primarily been used in the treatment of CTCL.
- IFNs can cause various laboratory abnormalities and side effects that do not typically necessitate cessation of therapy, but do require close monitoring on the part of the prescribing physician.
- Although there is a problematic lack of randomized controlled trials assessing the use of IFNs in CTCL, many studies have argued their efficacy in patients with various stages of CTCL.

INTRODUCTION

IFNs are polypeptides produced by stimulated eukaryotic cells and naturally occur in the human body as a part of the innate immune response.[1] Although IFNs were originally named in 1957 as a result of their ability to interfere with viral replication,[2] they have since been shown to also have cytostatic and immunomodulating functions.[3] Recognizing the potential for such functions to combat disease, researchers have used recombinant DNA technology to produce 3 major types of IFNs, which are commercially available products approved by the US Food and Drug Administration (FDA) in the United States. These products include IFN alfa, IFN beta, and IFN gamma. Although subsequent sections of this article focus almost entirely on the properties of the IFNs most commonly used in patients with CTCL, it first examines some of the basic attributes of the naturally occurring IFN counterparts.

Viruses, B-cell mitogens, foreign cells, and tumor cells stimulate leukocytes and lymphoblastoid cells to produce IFN alfa,[4] while T-cell mitogens, interleukin (IL)-2, and other antigens stimulate T cells and natural killer (NK) cells to make IFN gamma.[5] Viruses and foreign nucleic acids stimulate fibroblasts and epithelial cells to produce IFN beta.[4] As both are stable at the acidic pH of 2 and they bind to the same IFN surface receptors, IFN alfa and IFN beta are designated as type I IFNs.[5,6] In contrast, because IFN gamma is not stable at such an acidic pH and binds to a different IFN surface receptor, it is considered a type II IFN.[3]

As alluded to above, IFNs have demonstrated antiviral, cytostatic, and immunomodulatory functions. IFN seems to exert its antiviral impact via the stimulation of enzymes, which then induce the cleavage of viral RNA, the inhibition of protein synthesis, and the production of antiviral proteins.[7]

Author Conflicts of Interest: None.
Funding Sources: None.
Department of Dermatology, Hospital of the University of Pennsylvania, 3600 Spruce Street, Philadelphia, PA 19104, USA
* Corresponding author. Department of Dermatology, Perelman Center for Advanced Medicine, 3400 Civic Center Boulevard, 1st Floor, Suite 330S, Philadelphia, PA 19104.
E-mail address: Natalie.spaccarelli2@uphs.upenn.edu

Dermatol Clin 33 (2015) 731–745
http://dx.doi.org/10.1016/j.det.2015.05.008
0733-8635/15/$ – see front matter © 2015 Elsevier Inc. All rights reserved.

IFNs are cytostatic by their direct inhibition of cell cycle progression through the S phase[8] and possibly by stimulating enzymes that block protein synthesis.[9,10] The immunomodulatory functions of IFN alfa and IFN gamma therapies are discussed in detail in the Mechanism of Action sections. As literature has rarely addressed the use of therapeutic IFN beta in CTCL, the authors only discuss it briefly.

INTERFERON ALFA

Although alfa-type IFNs are primarily prescribed for the treatment of hepatitis C, the National Comprehensive Cancer Network guidelines have long included IFN alfa in its recommended treatments for the most common types of CTCL, mycosis fungoides (MF) and Sezary syndrome (SS).[11] Multiple studies have examined the use of commercially available IFN alfa in patients with all stages of MF/SS. Most studies assessing the efficacy of alfa-type IFNs in the management of MF/SS have considered 2 forms of recombinant IFN alfa, IFN alfa-2a (Roferon) and IFN alfa-2b (Intron-A), which are produced via genetically engineered *Escherichia coli*-containing DNA that codes for human protein.[10,12] Roferon is no longer manufactured in the United States. IFN alfa-2a and IFN alfa-2b share nearly identical structures because they only differ in their manners of purification and by a single amino acid[3]. These differences do not appear to impact their antigenicity as both of these IFNs seem to bind to an identical type I IFN receptor.

The pegylated forms of IFN alfa-2a and IFN alfa-2b are called Pegasys and PegIntron, respectively, and are larger in size than their nonpegylated counterparts.[14] Despite the lack of large studies or clinical trials assessing these pegylated IFNs in CTCL, the use of pegylated IFN alfa-2b for this indication has been reported, so the authors discuss it when possible. Other commercially available IFN alfa's (ie, IFN alfa-n3 and IFN alfacon-1), have not been used in the treatment of MF/SS[12,13] and are not discussed in this article.

Mechanism of Action

Although IFN alfa has cytostatic and antiviral properties like other IFNs, its immunomodulatory effects seem to be particularly conducive to combating the immune dysfunctions observed in CTCL. To provide a better foundation for understanding the properties that appear to make IFN alfa an effective therapy for MF/SS, it is helpful to first discuss the proposed mechanisms of immune dysregulation in these cancers.

The malignant T cells in MF/SS are typically mature skin-honing memory $CD4^+$ helper T cells, which exhibit a T-helper type 2 (T_H2) phenotype in

their release of elevated amounts of IL-4, IL-5, and IL-10 cytokines.[15–17] This increased T_H2 activity seems to create a cytokine imbalance that suppresses the host's T_H1-mediated immune activity[18]; this is consistent with research showing that factors produced by T_H2 cells counter T_H1 activity.[19,20] Studies have argued that decreased production of IFN gamma,[15] IL-12, and IFN alfa[15,21,22] provide evidence of decreased T_H1 activity in patients with MF/SS and that some of these immune abnormalities may underlie both the decreased activity and numbers of dendritic cells (DCs) observed in MF/SS.[22] In addition to diminished T_H1 immune activity and DC numbers and activity, other proposed mechanisms of deficient immune activity in MF/SS include decreased numbers and activities of both NK cells and $CD8^+$ T cells.[23,24] These immune defects could be means by which the cancer compromises the host immune system's abilities to not only combat infection but also mount an effective antitumor response.[25] Although not necessarily a marker of immune deficiency, peripheral eosinophilia and elevated serum immunoglobulin E levels are other immune abnormalities observed in MF/SS.[15,26] In addition to portending a worse prognosis in MF/SS,[27] peripheral eosinophilia in general has been associated with adverse events.[28]

IFN alfa seems to ameliorate several of the immune defects described above. Specifically, IFN alfa appears to activate $CD8^+$ T cells and NK cells[23] and to suppress the problematic increase in T_H2 activity by inhibiting Sézary cell and normal T-cell production of IL-4 and IL-5.[29–33] IFN alfa may further augment cytotoxicity by increasing the expression of class I molecules on lymphocytes.[34] In addition, culturing the peripheral blood of patients with SS with recombinant IFN alfa was observed to significantly inhibit the excess production of IL-5, a cytokine that stimulates the proliferation of eosinophils.[31] As noted above, peripheral eosinophilia has been associated with worse prognosis and adverse events. **Fig. 1** adapted from Kim and colleagues[25] summarizes these proposed targets of IFN alfa therapy in MF/SS.

It is worth mentioning in this section that some investigators have reported the development of resistance to IFN alfa.[35,36] Downregulation of IFN receptors,[37] production of neutralizing antibodies,[10,38] and loss of STAT1 expression in the malignant T cell[39] are purported mechanisms of resistance.[40]

Pharmacokinetics

IFN alfa is typically administered as a subcutaneous (SC) injection in patients with CTCL.

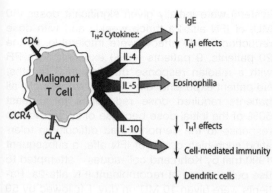

Fig. 1. Pathologic immune abnormalities in CTCL that likely serve as targets of IFN therapy. CCR4, chemokine (C-C Motif) receptor 4; CLA, cutaneous lymphocyte-associated antigen. (*Adapted from* Kim EJ, Hess S, Richardson SK, et al. Immunopathogenesis and therapy of cutaneous T cell lymphoma. J Clin Invest 2005;115(4):804; with permission.)

Nonpegylated IFN alfa administered through intramuscular (IM) or SC injections reaches peak serum concentration within 2 to 6 hours.[6] The elimination half-life of nonpegylated IFN alfa-2b is 2 to 3 hours and that of nonpegylated IFN alfa-2a is slightly longer. The pegylated forms of IFN alfa have much longer elimination half-lives than their nonpegylated counterparts. This prolonged half-life is because the addition of polyethylene glycol to their structures makes them more resistant to breakdown by proteolytic enzymes than the nonpegylated forms. The elimination half-life of pegylated IFN alfa-2a is approximately 80 hours, whereas that of pegylated IFN alfa-2b is approximately 40 hours.[3,40] In addition, pegylated IFN alpha-2b acts primarily as a prodrug with its slow IFN release.[14]

IFN alfa is metabolized by the liver, filtered through the glomeruli, and undergoes degradation during tubular resorption.[12] IFN alfa has also been administered intralesionally in MF. Although this method is safe, the systemic absorption of the IFN may be decreased.[41,42]

Typical Dosing

The following discussion focuses mostly on nonpegylated IFN alfa dosing and is gleaned from research on both IFN alfa-2a and IFN alfa-2b with the underlying assumption that because these types of IFN alfa are nearly biologically identical, they should behave almost equivalently. However, such an assumption is likely imperfect because some differences do exist between the 2 compounds.[3]

There is a wide range of doses reported in literature examining the use of IFN alfa in MF or SS. The maximally tolerated dose of nonpegylated IFN alfa has been reported to be 9 to 18 million units (MU) daily, but most clinicians seem to treat patients with 3 to 6 MU thrice weekly or daily.[35,43–45] It has been suggested that patients who are initially administered lower doses before being escalated to higher doses tolerate the higher doses better than individuals who are initially administered higher doses.[46] As discussed earlier, IFN alfa may also be administered intralesionally. If only aiming to treat the injected plaque or tumor, injecting 1 to 2 MU into the lesion 3 times a week until significant improvement is observed is reasonable.[41,42]

There is some suggestion that higher doses of IFN alfa, if tolerated, are more effective than lower doses.[35,47,48] Several patients in the study by Olsen and colleagues,[35] which randomized patients to 36 MU versus 3 MU per day, were able to achieve complete remission only after their dose was increased or the higher dose was continued for longer than the 10-week induction period.

Unlike nonpegylated IFN alfa, which is generally given as fixed doses unrelated to patient weight, pegylated IFN alfa-2b should be dosed according to the formula 1.5 μg/kg/wk. However, at the authors' center at the Hospital of the University of Pennsylvania, patients are typically initially administered approximately half of this dose and then the dose is eventually increased to 1.5 μg/kg/wk as tolerated. In contrast to the variable frequency of nonpegylated IFN alfa, pegylated IFN alfa-2b or IFN alfa-2a is given as a once-weekly injection because of its extended half-life.[49]

The lack of large-scale randomized controlled trials assessing IFN alfa in MF/SS has meant that its precise use, particularly in regard to duration of therapy, is highly institution dependent. For example, Elise Olsen of Duke University's Department of Dermatology has described her typical regimen as the following. Nonpegylated IFN alfa is usually started at 3 MU thrice weekly; half the dose is administered in elderly or debilitated patients for the first 2 weeks. Response is assessed at 3 months, and if at that time there is minimal to no response, then either the IFN is escalated to 3 MU daily or a retinoid is added. If the patient attains a complete response (CR), Olsen recommends continuing that dose for at least 3 months thereafter and then slowly reducing the dose or frequency over the following 6 to 12 months in the absence of relapse.[3] Although there is some evidence that the efficacy of IFN alfa could persist in patients who attain partial responses (PRs) on higher doses and are then administered lower doses for maintenance,[44,46] others contend that objective response (OR) could be compromised by a premature dose reduction before attaining a

CR.[35] If using pegylated IFN, because of the unavailability of multidose vials, Olsen either begins at 50 or 80 μg of pegylated alfa-2b (PegIntron) weekly taking into account the weight, age, and physical condition of the patient, escalating to 120 or 180 μg weekly, or instead uses 90 μg of pegylated IFN alfa-2a (Pegasys) weekly escalating to the higher dose vials of 135 or 180 μg weekly as tolerated—there is no preference for either pegylated forms, but one or the other may be preferred by a patient's insurance carrier.

In slight contrast to the approach described above, the authors' practice typically involves starting nonpegylated IFN alfa-2b, 1.5 MU thrice weekly, and then escalating the dose as tolerated to 3 MU thrice weekly. If the patient does not improve at such a dose after 3 months of therapy, the authors typically increase the frequency to 4 times weekly or increase the dose up to 5 MU. After 3 to 4 months without improvement on such a regimen, the authors add other therapies before altering the therapeutic approach. If using pegylated IFN alfa-2b, the authors administer 0.75 to 1.5 μg/kg/wk. However, if the patient does not show improvement after 3 to 4 months, the authors do not escalate the dose. Instead, they add an additional therapy and may either stop or continue the pegylated IFN alfa-2b.

Although a lack of clear recommendations regarding duration of therapy is frustrating, a benefit of IFN alfa therapy over many other systemic treatments for MF or SS is that it is not associated with chronic cumulative dose effects or secondary malignancies such that its long-term use seems safe in most patients.[3] However, there is a small risk of new or exacerbated autoimmune disease during long-term therapy (see sections Adverse Effects).

Response to Therapy

While there are many prospective studies and retrospective case series evaluating IFN alfa in MF/SS, there are few randomized controlled trials. Despite this, it is widely accepted that IFN alfa can be effective in all stages of MF or SS.[3] In this section, some of the largest published studies of IFN alfa in patients with MF/SS are detailed. Readers may refer to **Table 1** for a synopsis of published studies that assess IFN alfa in 20 or more subjects with MF or SS.

Interferon alfa alone

In 1984, Bunn and colleagues[13] first argued the efficacy of IFN alfa in CTCL. In this prospective trial, 20 patients with what was described as advanced-stage disease (5 with stage II, 2 with stage III, and 13 with stage IV MF using the TNM staging system) were initially given significant doses (50 MU) of IFN alfa-2a thrice weekly and with dose reduction if side effects were intolerable. Of the 20 patients, 9 patients (45%) experienced a PR with a median response duration of 5 months. No patient experienced a CR. Not surprisingly, all patients required dose reductions to at least 50% of the initial dose because of intolerance. In response to the demonstrated difficulty in tolerating such high doses of IFN alfa, a subsequent 1990 trial by Kohn and colleagues[50] attempted to use pulse doses of recombinant IFN alfa-2a. Patients were given 10 MU on day 1 followed by 50 MU on days 2 to 5 every 3 weeks. Of the 24 subjects enrolled in this trial, 1 patient had a CR and 6 subjects had PRs; this resulted in a 29% OR rate, and the median response duration was 8 months. Readers may refer to **Table 1** for study details. Since the study by Kohn and colleagues,[50] clinical trials have typically dosed IFN alfa 1 to 3 times weekly, not in a pulsed manner.

Papa and colleagues[45] prospectively analyzed 43 patients with stage I to IVB CTCL who received between 3 and 18 MU IFN alfa-2a (whatever dose each subject maximally tolerated) thrice weekly for 3 months, and responders were then continued on their maximally tolerated doses for 6 months. This study showed an impressive OR in 70% of patients with stage III or IV disease and in 80% of those at lesser stages. Among this study's subjects were 28 newly diagnosed and previously untreated patients. Not surprisingly, the study reported a greater overall response rate in the previously untreated subjects. However, the difference was not marked (79% or 22 of 28 previously untreated subjects vs 67% or 10 of 15 previously treated subjects). These findings complement those of the multicenter controlled trial by Olsen and colleagues,[35] which included patients with stage IA to IVA disease treated with IFN alfa-2a, 3 MU daily (n=8) or 36 MU daily (n=14). At the end of 10 weeks, all on the higher dose required a dose reduction, including decrease in dose in 6 of 14 patients to 3 to 3.6 MU/d; 10 patients (45.5%) had a PR (including 3 patients with stage IIB MF), 3 patients (13.6%) achieved a CR, 2 of which had stage IVA disease. An additional 3 patients achieved a CR with longer treatment times (27% overall) with a duration of CR in these 6 patients of 4 to 27.5 months. Overall response was greater in those receiving higher doses. Another prospective trial by Tura and colleagues[46] found that all 15 of its subjects (stage II–IV) experienced some reduction in skin lesions (3 CR, 9 PR, and 1 mild response) in response to IFN alfa-2a with a dosing protocol dispensing 3 to 18 MU daily for 3 months followed by 18 MU thrice

Table 1
Studies of at least 20 subjects assessing IFN alfa both alone and in combination with other treatments

Study, Year	Design	Treatment[a]	Number of Subjects, Stage Range of Subjects	Key Results
Bunn et al,[13] 1984	Prospective observational	IFN alfa-2a	20, stage II–IVB	9/20 (45%) achieved PR, 0/20 (0%) achieved CR, responses did not correlate with stage, extremely high (50 MU/wk) doses of IFN used, all subjects required dose reduction
Olsen et al,[35] 1989	Prospective observational	IFN alfa-2a	22, IA–IVA	3/22 (14%) achieved CR and 10/22 (45%) achieved PR after 10 wk, 2 patients with PR and 1 patient with stable response then went into CR with further treatment, remissions lasted 4–27.5 mo, response was greater at higher doses than at lower dose
Kohn et al,[50] 1990	Prospective observational	IFN alfa-2a	24, IA–IVB	1/24 (4%) achieved CR, 6/24 (25%) achieved PR, no improvement seen in 8 patients who received dose escalation
Papa et al,[45] 1991	Prospective observational	IFN alfa-2a	43, I–IVB	11/43 (26%) achieved CR, 21/43 (49%) achieved PR, greater response in previously untreated subjects
Stadler et al,[56] 1998	Randomized clinical trial	IFN alfa-2a with PUVA vs IFN alfa-2a with acitretin	98 randomized, 82 evaluable, stage IA–IIB	28/48 (70%) patients receiving IFN and PUVA achieved CR (26/31 stage I, 2/9 stage II), 16/42 (38%) receiving IFN and acitretin achieved CR (16/33 stage I, 0/9 stage II), median time to CR much shorter in IFN and PUVA group (18.6 wk) than IFN and acitretin group (21.8 wk)
Jumbou et al,[51] 1999	Retrospective observational	IFN alfa-2a	51, IA–IV	21/51 (41%) achieved CR (5/8 stage I, 1/1 stage IIA, 13/30 stage IIB, 2/11 stage III, 0/1 stage IV), 13/51 (25%) achieved PR (2/8 stage I, 0/1 stage IIA, 10/30 stage IIB, 1/11 stage III, 0/1 stage IV), mean time to CR was 4 mo and independent of stage
Kuzel et al,[36] 1995	Prospective observational	PUVA with IFN alfa-2a	39, IB–IVB	24/39 (62%) achieved CR, 11/39 (28%) achieved PR, median response duration was 28 mo
Chiarion-Sileni et al,[57] 2002	Prospective observational	PUVA with IFN alfa-2a	63, IA–IVA	51/63 (75%) achieved CR, 6/63 (10%) achieved PR, median response duration was 32 mo
Rupoli et al,[59] 2005	Prospective observational	PUVA with IFN alfa-2b	89, IA–IIA	75/89 (84%) of subjects achieved CR (82% of stage IA, 87% of stage IB, 73% of stage IIA), median time to CR was 6 mo
Nikolaou et al,[58] 2011	Retrospective observational	PUVA with IFN alfa-2b	22, IB–IVA	10/22 (45%) achieved CR, 5/22 (23%) achieved PR, more subjects in early stages (stage IA-IIA) achieved CR than those in later stage (IIB–IV) (96% vs 27%, P value .03)

(continued on next page)

Table 1
(continued)

Study, Year	Design	Treatment[a]	Number of Subjects, Stage Range of Subjects	Key Results
Wozniak et al,[60] 2009	Randomized clinical trial	PUVA vs PUVA with IFN alfa	29, IA–IIA	13/17 (76%) subjects on PUVA alone achieved CR, 9/12 (75%) on PUVA and IFN achieved CR, none of the 29 patients achieved PR
Hüsken et al,[62] 2012	Retrospective observational	PUVA with pegylated IFN alfa-2a vs PUVA with nonpegylated alfa-2b	17, IA–IV	4/9 (44%) achieved CR and 4/9 (44%) achieved PR in PUVA with pegylated IFN alfa-2b group, 3/8 (38%) achieved CR and 1/8 (13%) achieved PR in PUVA with IFN alfa-2a group, higher rate of myelosuppression and liver toxicity and lower rate of constitutional side effects in pegylated combination group
Wagner et al,[76] 2013	Retrospective observational	TSEBT alone vs TSEBT with IFN alfa-2b	41, IA–IVA	63% of subjects on combination achieved CR and 36% of subjects on TSEBT alone achieved CR but this difference was not statistically significant, no difference in overall survival and progression-free survival detected between the 2 groups

CR is the complete clearance of all skin lesions lasting at least 4 weeks and PR is at least 50% reduction of skin lesions lasting at least 4 weeks; wk ,weeks; mos, months.

Abbreviations: PUVA, psoralen plus ultraviolet A; TSEBT, total skin electron beam therapy.

[a] IFN administered is nonpegylated unless otherwise noted.

weekly for 6 months. However, this study also found that many patients could not tolerate 18 MU daily and suggested that future trials not give subjects older than 60 years doses greater than 9 MU/day.

A larger-scale retrospective study by Jumbou and colleagues[51] looked at 51 subjects with stage IA to IV CTCL who used IFN alfa-2a monotherapy at a mean dose of 2.7 MU daily for a mean duration of 15.8 months. The investigators reported 21 subjects with CRs, 13 with PRs, and 17 with stable or progressive disease. Although CRs were more common in lower stages, time to CR and the duration for which the CR was sustained were actually independent of stage. CRs were obtained within 6 months and lasted an average of 31 months. Readers may refer to **Table 1** for further study details.

There are numerous smaller-scale studies assessing the use of IFN alfa monotherapy in CTCL. Although Estrach and colleagues,[52] Dallot and colleagues,[53] and Vonderheid and colleagues[41] demonstrated good responses to IFN alfa-2b among patients with MF/SS, the positive results in Vonderheid and colleagues'[41] study were limited to the improvement of specific plaques with intralesional injections because the study patients did not seem to improve with subsequent IM injections of IFN alfa-2b. Other small-scale studies have reported responses in patients with MF/SS of all stages to IFN alfa-2a monotherapy.[43,44,54]

Interferon alfa in combination with psoralen plus ultraviolet light phototherapy

Several studies have examined the use of concomitant IFN alfa and psoralen plus ultraviolet A (PUVA) phototherapy. Kuzel and colleagues[36] and Stadler and Otte[55] argued in their 1995 trials of 39 and 16 subjects, respectively, that the CR rates they demonstrated with the combination of IFN alfa-2a and PUVA were superior to those demonstrated in previous studies with IFN or PUVA alone. While neither study compared the combination treatment groups directly to monotherapy groups, a later prospective randomized study of 98 subjects with stage IA to IIB disease by Stadler and colleagues[56] compared the efficacy of IFN alfa-2a (9 MU thrice weekly) and PUVA (5 times weekly during first 4 weeks, 3 times weekly during weeks 5 through 23, 2 times weekly during weeks 24 through 48) with that of IFN alfa-2a (9 MU thrice weekly) and acitretin (25 mg daily during week 1, 50 mg during weeks 2 through 48). The combination of PUVA and IFN resulted in CR in 70% of subjects, whereas only 38.1% of subjects in the IFN and acitretin group experienced CR. **Table 1** provides further study details. A later study by Chiarion-Sileni and

colleagues[57] found an impressive CR rate of 75% (mean response duration of 37 months) in 63 patients with stage IA to IVA disease treated with PUVA and IFN alfa-2a, but did not directly compare these results with those of subjects undergoing monotherapy. However, CRs were obtained in all stages of disease. Like Chiarion-Sileni and colleagues,[57] a case series by Nikolaou and colleagues[58] showed an impressive overall response rate of 68%. In a phase 2 prospective trial of 89 patients with stage IA to IIA CTCL by Rupoli and colleagues[59] reported an impressive overall response rate of 98% for IFN (6–18 MU weekly) and PUVA but it did not compare these results to those of patients treated with monotherapy. **Table 1** provides details of the studies by Chiarion-Sileni and colleagues,[57] Nikolaou and colleagues[58] and Rupoli and colleagues.[59]

In contrast to the results of Rupoli and colleagues'[59] study, Wozniak and colleagues[60] did not demonstrate significant differences in response to PUVA alone versus PUVA and IFN alfa in their randomized controlled trial of 29 patients with similar low-stage disease (IA–IIA). Humme and colleagues[61] conducted an overall assessment of the many trials looking at the combination of IFN alfa and PUVA including that by Wozniak and colleagues.[60] This review pooled the results of 11 selected trials that investigated the combination of PUVA and IFN alfa, including 3 randomized controlled trials, 3 prospective cohort studies, 2 retrospective case series, 2 undefined trials, and a study that included data from a retrospective analysis as well as a prospective randomized trial. Although this review calculated a mean overall response rate of 79% ± 15% across all trials, it concluded that the addition of IFN alfa did not increase the efficacy of PUVA in patch- or plaque-stage MF. The study did not address whether the time to response was decreased or unchanged with the addition of IFN to PUVA.

Although there is little mention of the use of pegylated IFN alfa in CTCL, a retrospective cohort study by Hüsken and colleagues[62] compared 9 patients with stages IA to IV CTCL (2 stage IA, 3 stage IB, 2 stage IIA/B, 1 stage III, 1 stage IV) treated with PUVA and pegylated IFN alfa-2b (1.5 µg/kg weekly) to 8 patients (2 stage IA, 4 stage IB, 1 stage IIA/B, and 1 stage III) treated with PUVA and nonpegylated IFN alfa-2a (9 MU thrice weekly). While this study concluded that myelosuppression and liver toxicity occurred more frequently in the pegylated group, it also found that overall response was much higher in the pegylated group than in the nonpegylated group (89% vs 50%). However, like many of the studies described above, its conclusions are limited by its small size.

Interferon alfa in combination with oral retinoids

Several small studies have suggested that oral retinoids and IFN alfa are more effective together than as monotherapy in the treatment of MF/SS. Straus and colleagues[63] conducted a prospective trial in which 22 patients with stage IB to IV disease were first treated with oral bexarotene (300 mg/m^2/d for 8 weeks), and then those who had not improved on bexarotene alone were given IFN alfa-2b (3–5 MU thrice weekly) in addition to bexarotene. Of the 8 of 22 subjects who had not responded to bexarotene alone and were given IFN alfa-2b, there was a 38% overall response rate (3/8) after the IFN alfa-2b was added. Other literature has suggested that combinations of IFN alfa-2b with bexarotene,[64] isotretinoin,[65] or etretinate[44,66] are effective, but such studies are limited by their small size and their failure to directly compare their results to those of monotherapy.

Interferon alfa in combination with extracorporeal photopheresis

Multiple small-scale studies have attempted to determine the efficacy of IFN alfa and extracorporeal photopheresis (ECP). One of the larger analyses was by Dippel and colleagues[67] who retrospectively compared the responses of 9 patients who received both ECP and IFN alfa-2a (3–18 MU thrice weekly) with those of 10 patients who received ECP alone and found a better response rate in the subjects on combination therapy. A prospective controlled study by Wollina and colleagues[68] assessed the use of twice-monthly ECP and IFN alfa-2a (6–18 MU thrice weekly) in 14 patients with stage IIA and IIB CTCL. After 6 months, 60% patients with stage IIA and 25% patients with stage IIB CTCL had some response (either CR or PR) to therapy. Although other case reports also promote the efficacy of IFN alfa in combination with ECP,[69–71] a pilot study by Vonderheid and colleagues[72] of 6 patients with SS did not find a significant response to treatment with ECP and IFN alfa-2b. Similarly, the only prospective study in patients with various stages of MF/SS comparing IFN alfa alone to the combination of IFN alfa and ECP failed to show an improved response of the combination regimen over IFN alone.[10] This finding is echoed by Humme and colleagues[61] who compared the findings of Wollina and colleagues[68] with those of trials assessing IFN alfa monotherapy and concluded that the combination of IFN alfa and ECP are not superior to IFN alone. This observation has raised the question as articulated by Zackheim and colleagues[73] of whether there is genuinely an additive or synergistic effect with the combination of ECP and IFN alfa

and underscores the necessity of a prospective randomized clinical trial to address this.[40] Nevertheless, at the authors' center, patients with SS are routinely treated with IFN alfa and ECP, and this approach is found to be effective.[74]

Interferon alfa in combination with total skin electron beam therapy

Although there are many published examples of total skin electron beam therapy (TSEBT) being used in conjunction with IFN therapy,[74] the evidence supporting the notion that the combination of the 2 therapies is more effective than either treatment alone is lacking. A study by Roberge and colleagues[75] compared the outcomes of 31 patients with various stages of MF treated with TSEBT alone with those of 19 patients with various stages of MF treated with both TSEBT and IFN alfa. In those 19 subjects, IFN was given both concurrently with TSEBT and after the completion of the entire course of TSEBT. This study concluded that there was not a significant difference in CR, disease-free survival, or overall survival between the 2 groups (median follow-up for living patients was 70 months). Similarly, a later retrospective study by Wagner and colleagues[76] assessed 41 patients who received TSEBT either alone or in combination with IFN alfa-2b and found CRs in 63% of patients receiving the combination regimen versus in 35% of patients receiving TSEBT alone. However, this difference was not statistically significant and the study did not show a statistically significant difference in overall survival or progression-free survival between the combination and monotherapy groups. Despite such a lack of published evidence, the authors' center feels justified in concomitantly treating patients with both TSEBT and IFN given the ability of electron beam radiation to induce apoptosis in malignant T cells[77] and the probable ability of IFNs to enhance the immune system's processing of apoptosed cells.

Interferon alfa in combination with chemotherapeutics

The use of IFN alfa in conjunction with chemotherapeutics is not common. Studies by Foss and colleagues[78,79] showed an objective response in only 41% of patients with stage I to IVB MF/SS treated with pentostatin (4 mg/m^2 on days 1 through 3 every 42 days) and IFN alfa-2a (10 MU/m^2 on day 22 and 50 MU/m^2 on days 23 through 26) and in 51% of patients with stage I to IVB MF/SS treated with fludarabine (25/m^2 on days 1 through 5 every 28 days) and IFN alfa-2a (5–7.5 MU/m^2 SC thrice weekly). In marked contrast, the study by Avilés and colleagues[80] reported an impressive CR in 74% of 158 patients with stage IIB to IVA CTCL treated with methotrexate (MTX, 10 mg/m^2 biweekly) and IFN alfa-2b (9 MU thrice weekly). The investigators did not provide a mean duration of response, but the 10-year estimated survival was 69%. It seems that a possible mechanism for this efficacy could be that MTX and IFN together enhance the expression of Fas (CD95), which augments Fas/Fas ligand-induced apoptosis of the malignant T-cell population.[81] However, the shortage of reported adverse effects in Aviles and colleagues study was unusual considering the toxicities usually associated with both MTX and IFN alfa monotherapy.[40]

Interferon alfa as part of multimodality treatment

It is perhaps most difficult to assess the efficacy of IFN alfa as part of multimodality treatment, which the authors define as 3 or more systemic CTCL agents given concurrently. In addition to IFN alfa, agents most often included in multimodality treatment include PUVA, oral retinoids, and ECP. Although there are reports of successful responses to the combinations of vorinostat/IFN alfa-2a/ECP,[82] IFN alfa-2a/ECP/PUVA,[83] and IFN alfa/ECP/IL-2[84] and retrospective cohort analyses that promote the multimodality approach,[75,85] none of the available literature includes trials that directly compare multimodality regimens to either each other or to regimens consisting of 1 to 2 treatments. Nevertheless, the authors' center routinely treats more advanced stages of CTCL with multimodality regimens that most often include IFN, an oral retinoid, skin-directed therapy, and/or ECP.

Adverse Effects

The most common acute side effects of IFN alfa are described as flulike and include fever, fatigue, chills, myalgias, arthralgias, and headache. Patients most frequently experience these symptoms during the hours immediately after the IFN injection and usually only during the first 2 weeks of treatment. Taking acetaminophen before the IFN injection can mitigate these discomforts. The most common chronic side effects of IFN alfa include fatigue, appetite loss, and weight loss (usually 2.3–4.5 kg).[3] These common side effects generally are dose related, decline in severity over time, and do not usually require dose reduction or cessation of therapy. Dose-related cytopenias (most commonly anemia, thrombocytopenia, and leukopenia) are relatively frequent side effects that may require dose reduction or stoppage of therapy if severe.[40] However, in the absence of prior chemotherapy or known primary immunosuppressive disorder, the authors' center usually does not alter dose when neutrophil counts are above 500 per mm.

While other possible side effects of IFN alfa are less common than those mentioned above, they are nonetheless worth discussing because they can become dangerous if they go unrecognized and may require dose reduction or cessation of therapy. Depressed mood and increased irritability have been reported with IFN alfa, and physicians should proceed with caution particularly in patients with a history of mood disorders. Impaired cognitive function is also possible and is usually more marked in the elderly. Thyroid dysfunction (most often hypothyroidism, but thyroiditis has been noted as well) can occur in up to 20% of patients using IFN alfa. Prescribing physicians should have a low threshold to draw thyroid function blood tests in patients with worsening fatigue despite being on a stable IFN dose. Altered taste, diarrhea, and elevated values of liver function tests may also occur but are usually mild and do not typically require dose modification. Peripheral neuropathy has been reported and, if severe, may require dose reduction or stoppage of therapy. Visual and auditory impairments, including the development of retinal cotton wool spots, are rare side effects, but such patients should immediately be referred to the appropriate specializing physicians to best assess the cause of the visual or auditory dysfunction. If IFN is deemed the likely culprit of visual or auditory impairment, the drug is usually stopped.[40]

There have also been reported cases of IFN alfa both inducing and worsening autoimmune disorders.[86] As a result, prescribers may be hesitant to use IFN alfa in patients with known autoimmune disease. In addition, IFN alfa is thought to possibly have antiangiogenic properties[87] such that the authors' center routinely stops IFN for 1 week before scheduled surgery and does not restart IFN until 1 week after surgery. Since IFN alfa was first introduced, various forms of cardiac toxicity have been reported and have included cardiac arrhythmias, cardiomyopathy, myocarditis, and myocardial infarction. However, some research has argued against the association of IFN alfa with these cardiac toxicities.[88] In addition, it seems that these events occurred at higher doses of IFN alfa than those generally used in the treatment of MF or SS. Nonetheless, patients with a history of coronary artery disease should be carefully monitored while on IFN.[40]

Although the list of possible side effects of IFN alfa is long, the vast majority of these adverse events seem reversible once IFN alfa is stopped. That there seem to be no long-range cumulative dose effects in most patients likely makes the drug safe for long-term use if tolerated.[40]

INTERFERON GAMMA

In contrast to the use of recombinant IFN alfa, there is much less literature regarding the use of IFN gamma in systemic diseases. IFN gamma-1b (Actimmune) is the only commercially available recombinant form of IFN gamma and is approved by the FDA for the treatment of chronic granulomatous disease and osteoporosis.[3] Although there is a lack of large-scale cohort studies and trials evaluating the use of IFN gamma in patients with CTCL, there are some reports of its utility for this indication. Because there is little literature addressing IFN gamma in MF or SS, the authors' examination of the use of IFN gamma in these conditions is limited. Nevertheless, the authors' program has administered IFN gamma to more than 200 patients with MF or SS during the past 20 years and has found it to be a promising modality.

Mechanism of Action

IFN gamma has many important functions in both the innate and adaptive immune responses including, but not limited to, the stimulation of DCs and macrophages to upregulate major histocompatibility complexes leading to enhanced antigen presentation, activation of NK cells, and increasing expression of costimulatory molecules. In addition, IFN gamma is considered essential for the T_H1 immune response.[89] Researchers have postulated that many of these functions could underlie the utility of IFN gamma in MF/SS. Specifically, enhancement of cytotoxicity mediated by $CD8^+$ T cells and NK cells, priming of DCs, inhibition of tumor cell proliferation, reduced T_H2 immune activity, increased T_H1 immune activity, and inhibition of T regulatory cells are proposed mechanisms of IFN gamma's efficacy in MF/SS.[40]

Pharmacokinetics and Dosing

Like recombinant IFN alfa, recombinant IFN gamma-1b is most often administered as an SC injection in patients with MF/SS; it has also been given intralesionally but less commonly than IFN alfa in patients with MF/SS. The recommended dosage is 50 $\mu g/m^2$ (1 MU/m^2) for patients whose body surface area is greater than 0.5 m^2 and 1.5 $\mu g/kg/dose$ for patients whose body surface area is equal to or less than 0.5 m^2. The mean elimination half-lives of IM and SC doses equivalent to 100 $\mu g/m^2$ are 2.9 and 5.9 hours, respectively. Peak plasma concentrations occur 4 hours after IM dosing and 7 hours after SC dosing.[90] IFN gamma injections seem to be most frequently prescribed as daily to thrice-weekly injection in patients with MF/SS. At the authors' center, typically patients are first administered 1 MU thrice weekly and then the dose is increased as tolerated to 2 MU thrice weekly.

Response to Therapy

Interferon gamma alone

The first report of using recombinant IFN gamma-1b in patients with MF/SS was published in 1990. In this prospective phase 2 study by Kaplan and colleagues,[91] 16 patients with MF/SS of various stages (IB–IVB) received recombinant IFN gamma for at least 8 weeks. The investigators reported an objective PR in 31% of patients and noted that 1 of 5 subjects with an objective PR had previously progressed after an initial PR to IFN alfa-2a. Although this study offered that IFN gamma may be effective in patients with MF or SS, its very small size and lack of control arm limited its ability to compare such efficacy to the efficacy of other treatments such as IFN alfa. The authors' group has found some success in using recombinant IFN gamma-1b in patients who have failed to respond to IFN alfa. Although on a smaller scale and via a different mechanism of IFN delivery than used by Kaplan and colleagues,[91] another trial in 2004 by Dummer and colleagues[92] also assessed the use of IFN gamma alone in subjects with CTCL. A total of 5 subjects with CTCL in this phase 1 prospective study received intralesional injections of IFN gamma complementary DNA contained in an adenoviral vector. The local intralesional injections resulted in impressive improvement of individual lesions in these patients. In addition, elevated serum levels of IFN gamma were observed, which seemed to be associated with regression of uninjected lesions.[25]

The most recent study investigating the use of recombinant IFN gamma-1b in patients with MF/SS was published in 2013 by Sugaya and colleagues.[93] This prospective phase 2 study administered IFN gamma-1b (2 MU daily for 5 days each week for 4 weeks followed by intermittent injections) to 15 patients with stage IA to IIIA CTCL. The investigators reported that 11 of 15 subjects had PRs including 9 of 10 subjects with stage IA to IIA CTCL, 1 of 4 subjects with stage IIB CTCL, and 1 of 1 subject with stage IIIA CTCL. There was no CR.

Interferon gamma as part of combination treatment

Although there are no trials comparing IFN gamma-1b directly to other CTCL treatments, several case reports and series have recorded patients with MF/SS responding to IFN gamma-1b administered in conjunction with other therapies such as bexarotene, ECP, TSEBT, and vorinostat.[74,94,95] A prospective study by Shimauchi and colleagues[96] treated 12 patients with MF (4 with erythroderma and the rest with plaque disease) with recombinant IFN gamma or natural IFN gamma for 5 days weekly for 4 weeks in conjunction with narrowband ultraviolet B (NBUVB) therapy three times weekly. Of the 12 patients, 6 had a PR and 4 had a CR. This study also measured particular T_H1 and T_H2 cytokine levels in all 12 subjects who received the combination of IFN gamma and NBUVB and an additional 3 patients who received NBUVB alone. It was found that T_H1 chemokine levels were elevated and T_H2 chemokine levels were depressed in the combination group when compared with those receiving NBUVB alone.

The authors' center has used IFN gamma extensively as a component of multimodality treatment. The authors surmise that an advantage of IFN gamma over IFN alfa could be the former's ability to prime and enhance antigen-presenting cell functions. The authors think this could be particularly advantageous when used in conjunction with treatments such as ECP, PUVA, or TSEBT, which induce apoptosis of malignant T cells. Use of the IFN gamma can presumably enhance the afferent immune response to the apoptotic tumor cells leading to a more effective efferent immune response mediated by cytotoxic T cells.

Although not published in large case series or studies, the authors' practice has occasionally used IFN gamma and IFN alfa (usually not administering both on the same day) simultaneously in patients who have failed to achieve adequate control on a single IFN and have found that this regimen can be helpful if tolerated.

Adverse Effects

The adverse effects of IFN gamma-1b are nearly identical to those of IFN alfa. Side effects are most often flulike and include low-grade fever, myalgias, fatigue, and arthralgias. Like IFN alfa, IFN gamma can also induce nausea, headache, weight loss, dose-dependent cytopenias, liver function enzyme abnormalities, nonscarring alopecia, and the triggering of autoimmune phenomena.[91] One of the advantages cited in using IFN gamma over IFN alfa is that it does not seem to impair the cognitive or mood functions of elderly patients as often as IFN alfa.[40] The authors' group has found IFN gamma to be less frequently associated with autoimmune side effects and peripheral neuropathy than IFN alfa.

INTERFERON BETA

Although there are 2 commercially available beta-type IFNs, IFN beta-1b (Betaseron) and IFN beta-1a (Avonex), they are almost exclusively used in the treatment of multiple sclerosis so the authors summarize their attributes in an abbreviated manner. These IFNs are administered via IM or SC injections, and their side effect profile is very similar to that of IFN alfa.[12] Although there are no sizable studies or trials assessing the use of IFN beta in CTCL, a notable study is that by Zinzani and colleagues.[97] This group analyzed the use of daily IFN beta injections for 4 months in 5 patients with treatment-refractory stage III MF and 3 patients with previously untreated stage I and II MF and reported only a single OR (12.5%).[3]

TREATMENT PEARLS FOR PRESCRIBING PHYSICIANS

- It is reasonable to start nonpegylated IFN alfa, 1.5 to 3 MU, thrice weekly and increase the dose to 5 MU thrice weekly as tolerated. If the patient does not respond, increasing the frequency of the tolerated dose is an option, but the authors typically do not exceed 4 times weekly.
- Many patients experience constitutional side effects with IFNs, but these usually diminish over time. Starting at a lower dose and escalating the dose as tolerated and taking acetaminophen immediately before injection likely increase the tolerability of the drug.
- Laboratory abnormalities including cytopenias and elevated values of liver function tests can occur with IFNs, so prescribing physicians should monitor complete metabolic panels and complete blood cell counts. Mild abnormalities are typically tolerated without dose modification. If moderate or severe abnormalities occur, one should consider dose reduction or stopping the drug and referral to the appropriate specializing physician (hematologist or gastroenterologist) to address whether IFNs are contraindicated in the patient.
- Although the long-term use of IFNs seems safe, they should be used with caution in patients with history of autoimmune, mood, cognitive, and/or cardiovascular disorders.

SUMMARY

Although the available literature demonstrating the utility of recombinant IFN alfa in the treatment of CTCL is convincing, more randomized controlled trials directly comparing it both as a monotherapy and as part of combination therapy, particularly its pegylated form, to other systemic modalities used in CTCL are necessary. In addition, larger-scale studies evaluating IFN gamma both alone and in comparison to other systemic CTCL treatments including IFN alfa would greatly enhance the understanding of its efficacy in CTCL.

REFERENCES

1. Strander H. Interferon treatment of human neoplasia. Adv Cancer Res 1986;46:1–265.
2. Isaacs A, Lindenmann J. Virus interference. I. the interferon. Proc R Soc Lond B Biol Sci 1957;147:258–67.
3. Olsen EA. Interferon in the treatment of cutaneous T-cell lymphoma. Dermatol Ther 2003;16(4):311–21.
4. Roth MS, Foon KA. Alpha interferon in the treatment of hematologic malignancies. Am J Med 1986;81(5):871–82.
5. Ross C, Tingsgaard P, Jorgensen H, et al. Interferon treatment of cutaneous T-cell lymphoma. Eur J Haematol 1993;51(2):63–72.
6. Koeller JM. Biologic response modifiers: the interferon alfa experience. Am J Hosp Pharm 1989;46(11 SUPPL. 2):S11–5.
7. Rotstein H, Butler JM, Czarnecki DB, et al. The treatment of mycosis fungoides with PUVA. Australas J Dermatol 1980;21(2):100–4.
8. Tamm I, Jasny BR, Pfeffer LM. Antiproliferative action of interferons. Mechanisms of Interferon Actions 1987;2:25–58.
9. Ganeshaguru K, De Mel WC, Sissolak G, et al. Increase in 2',5'-oligoadenylate synthetase caused by deoxycoformycin in hairy cell leukaemia. Br J Haematol 1992;80(2):194–8.
10. Olsen EA, Bunn PA. Interferon in the treatment of cutaneous T-cell lymphoma. Hematol Oncol Clin North Am 1995;9(5):1089–107.
11. Horwitz SM, Olsen EA, Duvic M, et al. Review of the treatment of mycosis fungoides and Sézary syndrome: a stage-based approach. J Natl Compr Canc Netw 2008;6(4):436–42.
12. Medical Economics, editor. Physicians' desk reference. 57th edition. Montvale (NJ): Medical Economics, Inc; 2003.
13. Bunn PA Jr, Foon KA, Ihde DC, et al. Recombinant leukocyte A interferon: an active agent in advanced cutaneous T-cell lymphomas. Ann Intern Med 1984;101(4):484–7.
14. Lai L, Hui CK, Leung N, et al. Pegylated interferon alpha-2a (40 kDa) in the treatment of chronic hepatitis B. Int J Nanomedicine 2006;1(3):255–62.
15. Vowels BR, Cassin M, Vonderheid EC, et al. Aberrant cytokine production by Sezary syndrome patients: cytokine secretion pattern resembles murine TH2 cells. J Invest Dermatol 1992;99(1):90–4.
16. Vowels BR, Lessin SR, Cassin M, et al. Th2 cytokine mRNA expression in skin in cutaneous T-cell lymphoma. J Invest Dermatol 1994;103(5):669–73.
17. Asadullah K, Döcke WD, Haeuler A, et al. Progression of mycosis fungoides is associated with increasing cutaneous expression of interleukin-10 mRNA. J Invest Dermatol 1996;107(6):833–7.
18. Guenova E, Watanabe R, Teague JE, et al. TH2 cytokines from malignant cells suppress TH1 responses and enforce a global TH2 bias in leukemic cutaneous T-cell lymphoma. Clin Cancer Res 2013;19(14):3755–63.
19. Fiorentino DF, Bond MW, Mosmann TR. Two types of mouse T helper cell. IV. Th2 clones secrete a factor that inhibits cytokine production by Th1 clones. J Exp Med 1989;170(6):2081–95.
20. Hsieh CS, Heimberger AB, Gold JS, et al. Differential regulation of T helper phenotype development by interleukins 4 and 10 in an aß T-cell-receptor transgenic system. Proc Natl Acad Sci U S A 1992;89(13):6065–9.
21. French LE, Huard B, Wysocka M, et al. Impaired CD40L signaling is a cause of defective IL-12 and TNF-α production in Sézary syndrome: circumvention by hexameric soluble CD40L. Blood 2005;105(1):219–25.
22. Wysocka M, Zaki MH, French LE, et al. Sézary syndrome patients demonstrate a defect in dendritic cell populations: effects of CD40 ligand and treatment with GM-CSF on dendritic cell numbers and the production of cytokines. Blood 2002;100(9):3287–94.
23. Yoo EK, Cassin M, Lessin SR, et al. Complete molecular remission during biologic response modifier therapy for Sézary syndrome is associated with enhanced helper T type 1 cytokine production and natural killer cell activity. J Am Acad Dermatol 2001;45(2):208–16.
24. Wysocka M, Benoit BM, Newton S, et al. Enhancement of the host immune responses in cutaneous T-cell lymphoma by CpG oligodeoxynucleotides and IL-15. Blood 2004;104(13):4142–9.
25. Kim EJ, Hess S, Richardson SK, et al. Immunopathogenesis and therapy of cutaneous T cell lymphoma. J Clin Invest 2005;115(4):798–812.
26. Molin L, Thomsen K, Volden G. Serum IgE in mycosis fungoides. Br Med J 1978;1(6117):920–1.
27. Tancrède-Bohin E, Ionescu MA, De La Salmonière P, et al. Prognostic value of blood eosinophilia in primary cutaneous T-cell lymphomas. Arch Dermatol 2004;140(9):1057–61.
28. Ogbogu PU, Bochner BS, Butterfield JH, et al. Hypereosinophilic syndrome: a multicenter, retrospective analysis of clinical characteristics and response to therapy. J Allergy Clin Immunol 2009;124(6):1319–25.e3.
29. Axelrod PI, Lorber B, Vonderheid EC. Infections complicating mycosis fungoides and Sézary syndrome. J Am Med Assoc 1992;267(10):1354–8.
30. Goldgeier MH, Cohen SR, Braverman IM, et al. An unusual and fatal case of disseminated cutaneous herpes simplex. Infection in a patient with cutaneous

T cell lymphoma (mycosis fungoides). J Am Acad Dermatol 1981;4(2):176–80.

31. Suchin KR, Cassin M, Gottleib SL, et al. Increased interleukin 5 production in eosinophilic Sézary syndrome: regulation by interferon alfa and interleukin 12. J Am Acad Dermatol 2001;44(1):28–32.

32. Sieling PA, Modlin RL. T cell and cytokine patterns in leprosy skin lesions. Springer Semin Immunopathol 1992;13(3–4):413–26.

33. Rook AH, Heald P. The immunopathogenesis of cutaneous T-cell lymphoma. Hematol Oncol Clin North Am 1995;9(5):997–1010.

34. Dinarello CA, Mier JW. Current concepts: lymphokines. N Engl J Med 1987;317(15):940–5.

35. Olsen EA, Rosen ST, Vollmer RT, et al. Interferon alfa-2a in the treatment of cutaneous T cell lymphoma. J Am Acad Dermatol 1989;20(3):395–407.

36. Kuzel TM, Roenigk HH Jr, Samuelson E, et al. Effectiveness of interferon alfa-2a combined with phototherapy for mycosis fungoides and the Sézary syndrome. J Clin Oncol 1995;13(1):257–63.

37. Kirkwood JM, Ernstoff MS. Interferons in the treatment of human cancer. J Clin Oncol 1984;2(4):336–52.

38. Rajan GP, Seifer B, Prümmer O, et al. Incidence and in-vivo relevance of anti-interferon antibodies during treatment of low-grade cutaneous T-cell lymphomas with interferon alpha-2a combined with acitretin or PUVA. Arch Dermatol Res 1996;288(9):543–8.

39. Sun WH, Pabon C, Alsayed Y, et al. Interferon-α resistance in a cutaneous T-cell lymphoma cell line is associated with lack of STAT1 expression. Blood 1998;91(2):570–6.

40. Olsen EA, Rook AH, Zic J, et al. Sézary syndrome: immunopathogenesis, literature review of therapeutic options, and recommendations for therapy by the united states cutaneous lymphoma consortium (USCLC). J Am Acad Dermatol 2011;64(2):352–404.

41. Vonderheid EC, Thompson R, Smiles KA, et al. Recombinant interferon alfa-2b in plaque-phase mycosis fungoides. Arch Dermatol 1977;113:454–62.

42. Wolff JM, Zitelli JA, Rabin BS, et al. Intralesional interferon in the treatment of early mycosis fungoides. J Am Acad Dermatol 1985;13(4):604–12.

43. Dreno B, Godefroy WY, Fleischmann M, et al. Low-dose recombinant interferon-α in the treatment of cutaneous T-cell lymphomas. Br J Dermatol 1989; 121(4):543–4.

44. Thestrup-Pedersen K, Hammer R, Kaltoft K, et al. Treatment of mycosis fungoides with recombinant interferon-α2a2 alone and in combination with etretinate. Br J Dermatol 1988;118(6):811–8.

45. Papa G, Tura S, Mandelli F, et al. Is interferon alpha in cutaneous T-cell lymphoma a treatment of choice? Br J Haematol 1991;79(Suppl 1):48–51.

46. Tura S, Mazza P, Zinzani PL, et al. Alpha recombinant interferon in the treatment of mycosis fungoides (MF). Haematologica 1987;72(4):337–40.

47. Bunn PA Jr, Ihde DC, Foon KA. The role of recombinant interferon alfa-2a in the therapy of cutaneous T-cell lymphomas. Cancer 1986;57(8 SUPPL): 1689–95.

48. Mughal TI. Role of interferon alfa-2b in the management of patients with advanced cutaneous T-cell lymphoma. Eur J Cancer Clin Oncol 1991;27(SUPPL 4): S39–40.

49. PegIntron [package insert]. Kenilworth, NJ: Schering-Plough; 2013.

50. Kohn EC, Steis RG, Sausville EA, et al. Phase II trial of intermittent high-dose recombinant interferon alfa-2a in mycosis fungoides and the Sézary syndrome. J Clin Oncol 1990;8(1):155–60.

51. Jumbou O, Guyen JM, Tessier MH, et al. Long-term follow-up in 51 patients with mycosis fungoides and Sezary syndrome treated by interferon-alfa. Br J Dermatol 1999;140(3):427–31.

52. Estrach T, Marti R, Lecha M. Treatment of cutaneous T-cell lymphoma with recombinant alfa 2B interferon. J Invest Dermatol 1989;93:549.

53. Dallot A, Feyeux C, Gorin I. Interferon treatment in cutaneous lymphomas. Proceedings of the International Society of Haematology Conference. 1988. p. 267.

54. Nicolas JF, Balblanc JC, Frappaz A, et al. Treatment of cutaneous T cell lymphoma with intermediate doses of interferon alpha 2a. Dermatologica 1989; 179(1):34–7.

55. Stadler R, Otte HG. Combination therapy of cutaneous T cell lymphoma with interferon alpha-2a and photochemotherapy. Recent Results Cancer Res 1995;139:391–401.

56. Stadler R, Otte HG, Luger T, et al. Prospective randomized multicenter clinical trial on the use of interferon α-2a plus acitretin versus interferon α-2a plus PUVA in patients with cutaneous T-cell lymphoma stages I and II. Blood 1998;92(10):3578–81.

57. Chiarion-Sileni V, Bononi A, Fornasa CV, et al. Phase II trial of interferon-α-2a plus psoralen with ultraviolet light A in patients with cutaneous T-cell lymphoma. Cancer 2002;95(3):569–75.

58. Nikolaou V, Siakantaris MP, Vassilakopoulos TP, et al. PUVA plus interferon a2b in the treatment of advanced or refractory to PUVA early stage mycosis fungoides: a case series. J Eur Acad Dermatol Venereol 2011;25(3):354–7.

59. Rupoli S, Goteri G, Pulini S, et al. Long-term experience with low-dose interferon-a and PUVA in the management of early mycosis fungoides. Eur J Haematol 2005;75(2):136–45.

60. Wozniak MB, Tracey L, Ortiz-Romero PL, et al. Psoralen plus ultraviolet A ± interferon-α treatment resistance in mycosis fungoides: the role of tumour microenvironment, nuclear transcription factor-κB and T-cell receptor pathways. Br J Dermatol 2009; 160(1):92–102.

61. Humme D, Nast A, Erdmann R, et al. Systematic review of combination therapies for mycosis fungoides. Cancer Treat Rev 2014;40(8):927–33.

62. Hüsken AC, Tsianakas A, Hensen P, et al. Comparison of pegylated interferon a-2b plus psoralen PUVA versus standard interferon a-2a plus PUVA in patients with cutaneous T-cell lymphoma. J Eur Acad Dermatol Venereol 2012;26(1):71–8.

63. Straus DJ, Duvic M, Kuzel T, et al. Results of a phase II trial of oral bexarotene (Targretin) combined with interferon alfa-2b (Intron-A) for patients with cutaneous T-cell lymphoma. Cancer 2007; 109(9):1799–803.

64. McGinnis KS, Junkins-Hopkins JM, Crawford G, et al. Low-dose oral bexarotene in combination with low-dose interferon alfa in the treatment of cutaneous T-cell lymphoma: clinical synergism and possible immunologic mechanisms. J Am Acad Dermatol 2004;50(3):375–9.

65. Knobler RM, Trautiger F, Radaszkiewicz T, et al. Treatment of cutaneous T cell lymphoma with a combination of low-dose interferon alfa-2b and retinoids. J Am Acad Dermatol 1991;24(2I):247–52.

66. Stavrianeas N, Katsambas A, Vareltzides A, et al. Treatment of mycosis fungoides with recombinant alpha 2B interferon in combination with etretinate. J Invest Dermatol 1989;93(3):580.

67. Dippel E, Schrag H, Goerdt S, et al. Extracorporeal photopheresis and interferon-α in advanced cutaneous T-cell lymphoma. Lancet 1997;350(9070): 32–3.

68. Wollina U, Looks A, Meyer J, et al. Treatment of stage II cutaneous T-cell lymphoma with interferon alfa-2a and extracorporeal photochemotherapy: a prospective controlled trial. J Am Acad Dermatol 2001;44(2):253–60.

69. Ferenczi K, Yawalkar N, Jones D, et al. Monitoring the decrease of circulating malignant T cells in cutaneous T-cell lymphoma during photopheresis and interferon therapy. Arch Dermatol 2003;139(7):909–13.

70. Rook AH, Prystowsky MB, Cassin M, et al. Combined therapy for Sezary syndrome with extracorporeal photochemotherapy and low-dose interferon alfa therapy. Clinical, molecular, and immunologic observations. Arch Dermatol 1991;127(10):1535–40.

71. Haley HR, Davis DA, Sams WM. Durable loss of a malignant T-cell clone in a stage IV cutaneous T-cell lymphoma patient treated with high-dose interferon and photopheresis. J Am Acad Dermatol 1999;41(5 II):880–3.

72. Vonderheid EC, Bigler RD, Greenberg AS, et al. Extracorporeal photopheresis and recombinant interferon alfa 2b in Sezary syndrome: use of dual marker labeling to monitor therapeutic response. Am J Clin Oncol 1994;17(3):255–63.

73. Zackheim HS, Fimiani M, Rubegni P, et al. Evidence is lacking for a synergistic or additive effect of combination extracorporeal photopheresis with interferon alfa for cutaneous T-cell lymphoma [2] (multiple letters). J Am Acad Dermatol 2000;42(6): 1087–8.

74. Raphael BA, Shin DB, Suchin KR, et al. High clinical response rate of Sézary syndrome to immunomodulatory therapies: prognostic markers of response. Arch Dermatol 2011;147(12):1410–5.

75. Roberge D, Muanza T, Blake G, et al. Does adjuvant alpha-interferon improve outcome when combined with total skin irradiation for mycosis fungoides? Br J Dermatol 2007;156(1):57–61.

76. Wagner AE, Wada D, Bowen G, et al. Mycosis fungoides: the addition of concurrent and adjuvant interferon to total skin electron beam therapy. Br J Dermatol 2013;169(3):715–8.

77. Kacinski BM, Flick M, editors. Apoptosis and cutaneous T cell lymphoma. New York (NY): Annals of the New York Academy of Sciences; 2001. No. 941.

78. Foss FM, Ihde DC, Breneman DL, et al. Phase II study of pentostatin and intermittent high-dose recombinant interferon alfa-2a in advanced mycosis fungoides/Sézary syndrome. J Clin Oncol 1992; 10(12):1907–13.

79. Foss FM, Ihde DC, Linnoila IR, et al. Phase II trial of fludarabine phosphate and interferon alfa-2a in advanced mycosis fungoides/Sézary syndrome. J Clin Oncol 1994;12(10):2051–9.

80. Avilés A, Nambo MJ, Neri N, et al. Interferon and low dose methotrexate improve outcome in refractory mycosis fungoides/Sézary syndrome. Cancer Biother Radiopharm 2007;22(6):836–40.

81. Nihal M, Wu J, Wood GS. Methotrexate inhibits the viability of human melanoma cell lines and enhances Fas/Fas-ligand expression, apoptosis and response to interferon-alpha: rationale for its use in combination therapy. Arch Biochem Biophys 2014;563:101–7.

82. Sanli H, Akay BN, Anadolu R, et al. The efficacy of vorinostat in combination with interferon alpha and extracorporeal photopheresis in late stage mycosis fungoides and Sézary syndrome. J Drugs Dermatol 2011;10(4):403–8.

83. Booken N, Weiß C, Utikal J, et al. Combination therapy with extracorporeal photopheresis, interferon-a, PUVA and topical corticosteroids in the management of Sézary syndrome. J Dtsch Dermatol Ges 2010;8(6):428–38.

84. Fritz TM, Kleinhans M, Nestle FO, et al. Combination treatment with extracorporeal photopheresis, interferon alfa and interleukin-2 in a patient with the Sezary syndrome. Br J Dermatol 1999;140(6): 1144–7.

85. Richardson SK, Lin JH, Vittorio CC, et al. High clinical response rate with multimodality immunomodulatory therapy for Sézary syndrome. Clin Lymphoma Myeloma 2006;7(3):226–32.

86. Amos SM, Duong CP, Westwood JA, et al. Autoimmunity associated with immunotherapy of cancer. Blood 2011;118(3):499–509.

87. Indraccolo S. Interferon-a as angiogenesis inhibitor: learning from tumor models. Autoimmunity 2010; 43(3):244–7.

88. Kadayifci A, Aytemir K, Arslan M, et al. Interferon-alpha does not cause significant cardiac dysfunction in patients with chronic active hepatitis. Liver 1997; 17(2):99–102.

89. Miller CH, Maher SG, Young HA. Clinical use of interferon-γ. Ann N Y Acad Sci 2009;1182:69–79.

90. Actimmue [package insert]. Roswell, GA: Vidara Therapeutics; 2013.

91. Kaplan EH, Rosen ST, Norris DB, et al. Phase II study of recombinant human interferon gamma for treatment of cutaneous T-cell lymphoma. J Natl Cancer Inst 1990;82(3):208–12.

92. Dummer R, Hassel JC, Fellenberg F, et al. Adenovirus-mediated intralesional interferon-γ gene transfer induces tumor regressions in cutaneous lymphomas. Blood 2004;104(6):1631–8.

93. Sugaya M, Tokura Y, Hamada T, et al. Phase II study of i.v. interferon-gamma in Japanese patients with mycosis fungoides. J Dermatol 2014;41(1):50–6.

94. McGinnis KS, Ubriani R, Newton S, et al. The addition of interferon gamma to oral bexarotene therapy with photopheresis for Sézary syndrome. Arch Dermatol 2005;141(9):1176–8.

95. Gardner JM, Introcaso CE, Nasta SD, et al. A novel regimen of vorinostat with interferon gamma for refractory Sézary syndrome. J Am Acad Dermatol 2009;61(1):112–6.

96. Shimauchi T, Sugita K, Nishio D, et al. Alterations of serum Th1 and Th2 chemokines by combination therapy of interferon-γ and narrowband UVB in patients with mycosis fungoides. J Dermatol Sci 2008;50(3):217–25.

97. Zinzani PL, Mazza P, Gherlinzoni F. Beta interferon in the treatment of mycosis fungoides. Haematologica 1988;73(6):547–8.

Methotrexate and Pralatrexate

Gary S. Wood, MD*, Jianqiang Wu, MD, PhD

KEYWORDS

- Methotrexate • Pralatrexate • Dihydrofolate reductase • Folate • Folic acid • Purine synthesis
- S phase • Apoptosis

KEY POINTS

- Methotrexate (MTX) and pralatrexate (PDX) are competitive inhibitors of folate metabolism that block dihydrofolate reductase, thereby preventing thymidylate and purine synthesis and resulting in cell cycle arrest in the S phase.
- MTX and other folate inhibitors also reduce cellular levels of S-adenosylmethionine, the principal methyl donor for methyltransferases, thereby inhibiting DNA methylation.
- In CTCL, this derepresses tumor suppressor genes such as the death receptor, Fas (CD95), thereby enhancing apoptosis.
- These properties make folate antagonists useful for the treatment of lymphomas, either as single agents or in combination with other therapies that enhance or complement their effects.

INTRODUCTION

Methotrexate (MTX) is a well-known antimetabolite that blocks the action of dihydrofolate reductase, thereby inhibiting the metabolism of folic acid. It has been used widely since the 1950s to treat a variety of neoplastic and inflammatory diseases. Recently, a more potent analog, pralatrexate (PDX), has been developed and approved by the Food and Drug Administration (FDA) for the treatment of peripheral T-cell lymphomas (PTCLs). This article discusses some emerging concepts relevant to the optimal use of folate antagonists and reviews these drugs in regard to the therapy for cutaneous T-cell lymphomas (CTCLs), including clinical indications, mechanism of action, pharmacokinetics, dosing regimens, response rates, and adverse effects. According to convention, MTX will be used as the abbreviation for methotrexate. In keeping with prior publications, pralatrexate will be abbreviated as PDX, a designation derived from its alternative name: 10-propargyl-10-deazaaminopterin.[1]

EMERGING CONCEPTS RELEVANT TO THE OPTIMAL USE OF FOLATE ANTAGONISTS
The Role of Folate Antagonists in the Epigenetic Regulation of Gene Expression

The products of at least 5 tumor suppressor genes generally known to be silenced by promoter methylation have been reported to be deficient in mycosis fungoides (MF) and Sézary syndrome (SS), FAS/CD95, FAS-ligand, p16, p21, and protein phosphatase 4 regulatory subunit-1 (PP4R1).[2–11] These and other genes are also known to be silenced by promoter methylation in many other cancers (eg, TRAIL-R1, TRAIL-R2, p16, p21, hMLH1, MGMT, and RASSF1A).[12,13] These findings suggest that demethylating agents

The project described was supported by the Biomedical Laboratory Research & Development Service of the VA Office of Research and Development, award number I01BX002204.
The authors have no conflicts of interest to disclose.
Department of Dermatology, University of Wisconsin and VA Medical Center, 7th Floor, One South Park, Madison, WI 53715, USA

* Corresponding author. Department of Dermatology, University of Wisconsin and VA Medical Center, 7th Floor, One South Park, Madison, WI 53715.
E-mail address: gwood@dermatology.wisc.edu

Dermatol Clin 33 (2015) 747–755
http://dx.doi.org/10.1016/j.det.2015.05.009

derm.theclinics.com

could benefit MF/SS patients by derepressing silenced tumor suppressor genes. Although FDA-approved for use in other diseases, traditional demethylating agents such as 5-azacytidine and decitabine have a toxicity profile that discourages their use for the treatment of chronic cutaneous lymphomas such as MF/SS. One of the most exciting aspects of folate antagonists is the recent realization that, in addition to their well-established role as S phase cell cycle inhibitors, they can also act as DNA methylation inhibitors.[2,14] Most of the relevant experiments have been performed using MTX; however, all related folate antagonists should share the same basic properties (see later discussion).

The Importance of Combination Therapy for Cancer

Inhibition of DNA methylation constitutes a novel mechanism of action and rationale for the use of MTX and related compounds in the management of cutaneous lymphomas. It also provides a new justification for their use in combination with other treatments that produce effects complementary to those of folate antagonists. The advantages of combination therapy relative to monotherapy for cancer treatment have been calculated recently by Bozic and colleagues.[15] In brief, they used mathematical modeling to show that by the time a tumor reaches a few millimeters in diameter it is likely to harbor hundreds to thousands of mutant cells that are resistant to any particular monotherapy. This typically results in short-term clinical benefit followed by treatment failure because resistant mutant tumor clones proliferate in response to the selection pressures of monotherapy. In contrast, dual therapy results in long-term disease control in most cases, if there are no mutations in a single cell that cause cross-resistance to both agents. The chances of cross-resistance are diminished if the 2 agents target different pathways. For patients with large disease burden in which the number of resistant mutants is greater, triple therapy is needed. The mathematical models also showed that simultaneous therapy with 2 agents is much more effective than when they are used as sequential therapies.

The implications of these mathematical models are relevant to folate antagonists because these drugs can be used in combination with other treatments that have different mechanisms of action and affect multiple cellular pathways. **Table 1** summarizes examples of MTX in combination with other modalities. Using this combination therapy approach, the likelihood of a favorable therapeutic outcome can be enhanced.

TREATMENT
Indications

MTX and PDX have been used to treat a wide variety of cancers. Among the cutaneous lymphomas, MTX has been used primarily to treat MF/SS and primary cutaneous CD30+ lymphoproliferative disorders (LPDs) such as lymphomatoid papulosis (LyP) and anaplastic large cell lymphoma (cALCL). PDX is FDA-approved for refractory or relapsed PTCLs. Among the cutaneous lymphomas, it has proven efficacy for advanced stages of MF/SS, including MF with large cell transformation (LCT).[16,17] It has also been used to treat other rarer forms of primary CTCLs.[18–20] Folate antagonists have not been used widely to treat cutaneous B-cell lymphomas. In fact, MTX has been associated with the development of cutaneous B-cell LPDs (sometimes related to Epstein-Barr virus), many of which regress when MTX is reduced or discontinued.[21,22]

Mechanism of Action

MTX and PDX are folic acid analogues that block cell division in the S phase.[23,24] They are competitive inhibitors of dihydrofolate reductase with an affinity for this enzyme that is several logs greater than that of its natural substrate, folate. Dihydrofolate reductase converts dihydrofolate to tetrahydrofolate, which is required for synthesis of thymidylate and purine nucleotides involved in DNA and RNA synthesis. It also inhibits the folate-dependent enzymes of purine and thymidylate synthesis such as glycinamide ribonucleotide transformylase, aminoimido-caboxyamido-ribonucleotide transformylase, and thymidylate synthase. MTX also inhibits methionine synthase, thereby reducing S-adenosyl methionine (SAM) levels. Because SAM is the principal methyl donor for DNA methyltransferases (DNMTs),[25,26] the authors propose that MTX can act as a demethylating agent by depleting DNMTs of their SAM methyl donor supply. The mechanism underlying this effect is illustrated in **Fig. 1**. Recently, the authors reported in vitro and ex vivo evidence that MTX acts as a demethylating agent for the promoter of the FAS/CD95 death receptor by blocking the synthesis of SAM.[14] When CTCL cell lines and freshly isolated leukemic CTCL cells were treated with MTX, it resulted in decreased SAM levels, decreased FAS promoter methylation, and increased FAS protein expression. This enhanced FAS expression was accompanied by a major increase in sensitivity to FAS pathway apoptosis, especially for leukemic cells. In strong support of the authors' hypothesis regarding MTX's mechanism of action, experiments using CTCL lines with high baseline FAS

Table 1
Novel combination therapies for cutaneous T-cell lymphomas involving methotrexate

Other Agent	Rationale
Interferon	In addition to effects promoting a TH1 immune response, IFN-α also upregulates Fas (CD95) by a STAT-1–dependent mechanism that is distinct from the effects of MTX on Fas. This combination is effective for advanced MF/SS; 74% complete response rate at 1 year among subjects with advanced CTCL (stage IIB–IVB).[34]
HDAC	There is well recognized interaction between DNMTs and HDACs, which collaborate to silence tumor suppressor genes. HDAC inhibitors and demethylating agents have shown synergistic reactivation of genes silenced by methylation.[49] Recent findings showed that the class III HDAC, SIRT1, is overexpressed in CTCL and that its knock-down or inhibition induced growth arrest and apoptosis.[50] Combination therapy with vorinostat is effective for controlling SS.
Photodynamic therapy	Photodynamic therapy upregulates Fas-ligand. Combined with MTX, both Fas and Fas-ligand are increased, resulting in greater apoptosis than with either agent alone (ePDT).[51]
UV phototherapy	Narrow-band UVB upregulates Fas-ligand. Combination therapy is effective in treating generalized patch and plaque MF.
Ionizing radiation	In addition to its direct cytotoxic effects associated with DNA and other cell damage, local radiation therapy increases Fas-ligand. Combined with MTX, it is postulated that both Fas and Fas-ligand are increased, resulting in greater apoptosis. Combination therapy induces a durable complete local response in follicular MF extensively involving both ears and external ear canals (associated with an enhanced but transient inflammatory reaction to radiation therapy).
c-CBL inhibitor	Agents that block c-CBL (an E3 ubiquitin ligase) upregulate Fas-ligand. When combined with MTX, both Fas and Fas-ligand are increased resulting in extensive apoptosis (still under investigation).[52]

Abbreviations: DNMT, DNA methyltransferase; ePDT, epigenetically enhanced photodynamic therapy; HDAC, histone deacetylase inhibitor; IFN-α, alpha-interferon; SIRT1, silent information regulator type-1; STAT, signal transducer and activator of transcription; TH1, type 1 helper T cell.

promoter methylation showed that the addition of SAM reversed both the decreased FAS promoter methylation and the increased FAS protein expression induced by MTX. Representative results are shown in **Figs. 2** and **3**, respectively. In aggregate, these in vitro and ex vivo data consistently support not only our hypothesis but also its clinical relevance. Other folate antagonists that we have tested (eg, pemetrexed) showed similar results. Therefore, we expect the same will be true of PDX.

In addition to its effects on DNA methylation, MTX (and related compounds) likely inhibit protein methylation because SAM is also the principal methyl donor for protein methyltransferases. For example, MTX was able to inhibit carboxyl methylation of Ras (possibly by inhibiting isoprenylcysteine carboxylmethyltransferase), thereby down-regulating Ras signaling, which is a major inducer of DNA methylation in many cancers.[13,27,28] Like acetylation, methylation of histones plays a key role in gene regulation. MTX is likely to reduce the activity of histone methyltransferases such as SETDB1 and SUV39. Histone methylation at H3K9 and H3K27 is associated with gene silencing,

whereas methylation at H3K4 is associated with gene activation.[12] There is a recent report that MTX can inhibit the expression of methionine S-adenosyltransferase-1 and -2 genes.[29] This would also reduce SAM levels by blocking the conversion of methionine to SAM.

Pharmacokinetics

Therapeutic levels of MTX (1 μM) are reached at 1 to 5 hours after an oral dose of 20 mg/m². Levels remain greater than 0.1 μM for about 6 hours. Inhibition of DNA synthesis ends at levels below 0.01 μM. Inhibition of protein synthesis ends at levels below 0.1 μM.[30] In the plasma, about 50% to 70% of MTX is protein-bound (mainly to albumin). In the dose range generally used for cutaneous lymphomas, little MTX enters the central nervous system. There is a triphasic disappearance of MTX that depends on drug distribution, renal clearance, and the enterohepatic circulation. The mean terminal half-life is about 10 hours.

Relative to MTX, PDX has preferential uptake in cells due to its increased affinity for the reduced

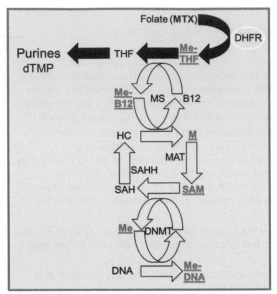

Fig. 1. MTX inhibits DNA methylation by depleting SAM. Chain of methyl group (Me) transfer is shown underlined from N-Me-tetrahydrofolate (Me-THF) to Me-vitamin B12 to methionine (M) to SAM to Me-DNA. MTX competitively inhibits dihydrofolate reductase (DHFR) which is involved in the multistep conversion of folate to Me-THF and inhibits methionine synthase (MS) and subsequent downstream methyl transfers that normally generate SAM. Other factors shown: homocysteine (HC), methionine adenosyltransferase (MAT), S-adenosylhomocysteine (SAH), SAH hydrolase (SAHH). The upper portion of the diagram is simplified and does not show that the immediate product of DHFR is THF, which is then converted into methylene THF before generation of Me-THF, which is then converted back to THF. Methylene THF is the more proximate precursor of deoxythymidine monophosphate (dTMP) and purines. DNMT, DNA methyltransferase.

folate carrier type 1 (RFC-1). This may give PDX greater selectivity for cancer cells because many tumors overexpress RFC-1. At an intravenous (IV) PDX dose of 150 mg/m^2 biweekly, the mean area under the curve (AUC) was 20.6 μM times hours, and the mean terminal half-life was 8 hours.[1] Exposure to IV PDX (AUC) is controlled with dosing based on body size. Pretreatment with folic acid and vitamin B12 can diminish the incidence and severity of mucositis while retaining drug efficacy.[31]

MTX and PDX are metabolized intracellularly into polyglutamates by folylpolyglutamyl synthetase.[16,32] These polyglutamates are preferentially retained in cells, thereby making them less susceptible to efflux-based drug resistance. The extent of polyglutamylation depends on both drug concentration and the duration of drug exposure. This process may be enhanced for PDX. Polyglutamylation is often upregulated in cancer cells,

providing another potential form of relative selectivity for PDX.

Most of an MTX dose is excreted unchanged in the urine within 24 hours. A minority is metabolized during enterohepatic circulation. There are many genes that can affect the processing of folate antagonists, including RFC-1 (influx), ABCC1 and ABCG2 (efflux), adenosine receptors 1 and 2, and folate polyglutamates. For example, a single nucleotide polymorphism in exon 28 of the ABCC1 gene alters cellular efflux of MTX and affects its efficacy.[33] In addition to these variables, younger age correlates with enhanced distribution and elimination of these agents.

Typical Dosing

For CTCLs, MTX is usually administered orally once weekly at a dose of 10 to 25 mg, although higher doses have been used. The total dose is often divided into 2 or 3 portions taken 12 hours apart to enhance drug absorption and decrease gastrointestinal (GI) side effects.[30] Higher doses of MTX are sometimes used (for example, 10 mg/m^2 biweekly in combination with alpha-interferon [IFN-α]).[34] LyP is often quite sensitive to MTX and sometimes responds well to weekly doses as low as 5 mg. Oral folic acid supplementation (1–5 mg daily) ameliorates GI symptoms[35]; however, the dose or dosing of folic acid might affect efficacy.[36] When high-dose MTX (60–240 mg/m^2 IV) has been used to treat advanced MF/SS, it has been accompanied by leucovorin (folinic acid) rescue to minimize damage to normal tissues and to counteract acute toxicity.[37] Currently, such high-dose IV regimens are rarely used for cutaneous lymphomas.

Although higher and lower doses have been used successfully for various CTCLs, PDX is usually administered IV at 15 mg/m^2/wk for 3 weeks out of every 4 week cycle.[16] The total number of cycles depends on clinical response and toxicity. In addition to daily folic acid supplementation (1 mg orally), patients receive vitamin B12 supplementation (1 mg intramuscular [IM] every 8–10 weeks).

Response to Therapy

Methotrexate

Despite its longstanding and fairly common use in the management of MF/SS patients, relatively few clinical studies of MTX have been published. The response of MF/SS subjects to low-dose MTX (defined commonly as <100 mg/wk but often limited to doses ≤30 mg/wk that do not require folic acid to prevent toxicity) ranges from "definite improvement" in 9 out of 16 (using 2.5–10 mg/d)[38]

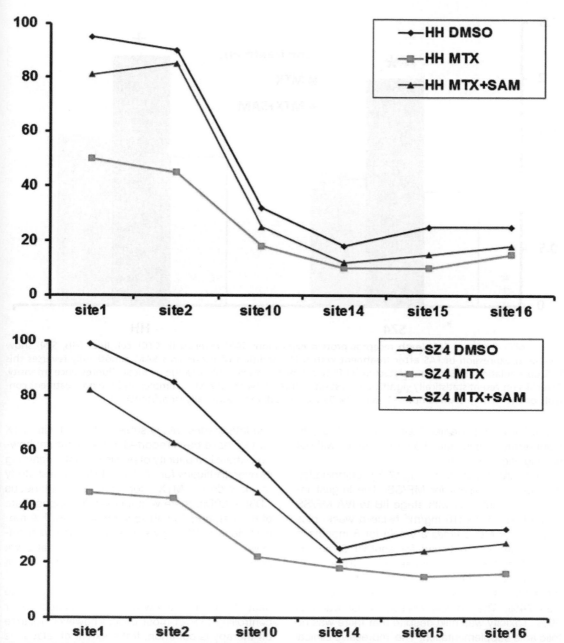

Fig. 2. MTX reduces FAS promoter methylation. SAM reverses it. Demethylation of 6 CpG sites in the FAS promoter was detected by pyrosequencing after treatment with MTX in Fas promoter methylation-high CTCL cell lines (SZ4, HH). The y-axis shows the percentage of the methylation. The upper lines are the dimethyl sulfoxide (DMSO) controls. The lower lines show the demethylating effect of MTX. The middle lines show that exogenous SAM can reverse the demethylating effect of MTX.

to an overall response (complete response [CR] plus partial response [PR]) in 17 out of 29 with erythrodermic MF (E-MF) and 20 out of 60 with plaque MF (using a median dose of 25 mg/wk).[39,40] Although rarely used currently, MF/SS subjects treated with high-dose MTX (up to 240 mg/m^2 IV) showed 9 out of 11 with greater than 80% clearing including 7 of these with CR.[37] An overall response

rate to MTX monotherapy in SS is difficult to estimate because of the small number of cases reported. There is one published phase I-II study of subjects with stage IA or IB MF treated topically with 1% MTX compounded in a hydrophilic gel containing laurocapram to enhance percutaneous absorption. After every-other-day application for 24 weeks, 7 out of 9 subjects showed "slight

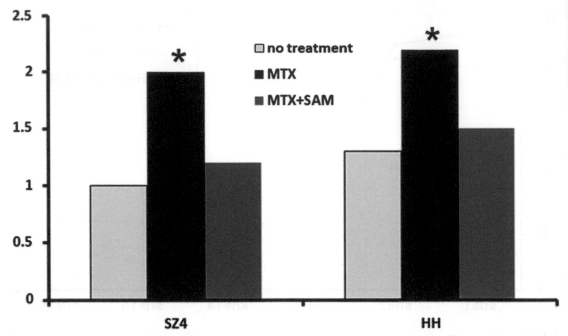

Fig. 3. MTX increases FAS death receptor protein expression; SAM reverses it. CTCL cell lines (HH, SZ4) show increased expression of FAS after treatment with MTX. Addition of exogenous SAM almost fully reverses this FAS upregulation. FAS protein detected by flow cytometry. Y-axis: fold change in mean fluorescence intensity. Asterisks represent statistically significant *t* test differences between the MTX samples and the no-treatment controls or the MTX + SAM samples (2-tailed *P*<.05 was considered statistically significant).

to moderate improvement" with statistically significant reductions in induration and pruritus without any significant toxicity.[41]

There are also studies using MTX in combination with other therapies for MF/SS. The largest involves 158 subjects with stage IIB to IVA MF/SS treated with MTX (10 mg/m^2 twice a week) plus IFN-α-2a (9 MU 3 times a week) for 6 months.[34] Those with PR continued for another 6 months on IFN and MTX and those with CR at 6 or 12 months continued only on IFN. At 6 months, there was 49% CR and at 12 months, the CR was 74%. The 10-year estimated survival was 69%. Toxicity was mild despite that there was no folic acid supplementation. The impressive clinical efficacy observed in this study is supported by the authors' own in vitro and ex vivo data that demonstrated greater MF/SS tumor cell killing with the combination of MTX and IFN-α than with either agent alone.[34] A small study of IV MTX 60 mg/m^2 IV followed by 5-fluorouracil 20 mg/kg with leucovorin rescue showed at least 80% clearing in 2 out of 2 SS subjects and 1 out of 2 E-MF subjects.[42] A single SS subject had a durable (>4 year) PR following combination therapy with MTX (10 mg/wk) and etoposide (25 mg/d).[43]

Low-dose MTX (5–25 mg/wk) is recommended by expert consensus for the treatment of primary cutaneous CD30+ LPDs, including LyP, cALCL,

and intergrades. Many subjects treated with MTX for LyP have been reported in the literature; however, there is a paucity of published data regarding its overall efficacy for cALCL.[44] In the largest study of low-dose MTX for primary cutaneous CD30+ LPDs, there was an overall response rate of 87% among 45 subjects (mostly LyP).[45] A median dose of 20 mg/wk was given for 1 year followed by maintenance therapy typically at 2 wk intervals. After treatment was discontinued, about one-quarter of the responders remained disease-free for at least 2 years. From the aggregate data, it is clear that low-dose MTX is effective for controlling LyP in most cases; however, relapse off therapy is common. If the extent of relapse is clinically significant, maintenance therapy may be needed for an extended period. There is a case report of LyP responding to local application of topical MTX.[46]

Pralatrexate Regarding treatment of advanced MF/SS with PDX, there is a dose deescalating study in which the starting dose was 30 mg/m^2/wk IV for 3 weeks of every 4-week cycle.[16] The dose was progressively reduced to find the optimal balance between efficacy and toxicity. Overall, 54 subjects were treated, 29 with the optimized schedule of 15 mg/m^2/wk IV for 3 of 4 weeks (median of 4 cycles). The overall response among these 29 cases was 45%, mostly PRs with 2 CRs. Another study of subjects with relapsed or refractory PTCLs included 12 subjects with MF and LCT.[20] The overall response rate was 58% by investigator assessment and 25% by central review.

PDX therapy for cALCL or other rare types of CTCL is not well reported. However, a few cases are contained in larger studies of PTCLs and showed some objective responses, including CRs.[16,18–20] In addition, 17 subjects with the systemic CD30+ cALCL showed an overall response of rate of 35%.[20]

Trimetrexate Finally, there is a study of trimetrexate (another MTX-related folate antagonist) administered IV at a dose of 200 mg/m^2 biweekly. There was a 47% overall response rate among 15 MF/SS cases (most with LCT).[47]

Adverse Effects

MTX side effects include GI (nausea, vomiting, stomatitis, ulcers, diarrhea), bone marrow (leukopenia, anemia, thrombocytopenia), liver (increased transaminases, hepatitis, fibrosis, cirrhosis; the latter 2 related to cumulative dose), lung (pneumonitis, fibrosis), pregnancy (abortifacient, teratogen), and miscellaneous (alopecia, anaphylaxis, oligospermia, photosensitivity, radiation recall, reactivation sunburn). Several MTX-induced LPDs have been reported, including in a patient with SS.[48]

PDX has a toxicity profile similar to MTX; however, in the dose ranges commonly used, PDX side effects tend to be more common and severe, thereby limiting its use to more advanced stages of MF/SS and other aggressive types of CTCLs. The most common PDX side effects (≥10%) include mucositis (17% grade 3), fatigue, nausea, vomiting, anorexia, skin toxicity, epistaxis, and anemia.[16]

Toxicity of MTX and PDX can be enhanced by interactions with other folate antagonists (dapsone, sulfonamides, trimethoprim), hepatotoxins (ethanol, retinoids), preexisting liver disease and other conditions or drugs (eg, nonsteroidal antiinflammatory drugs, probenecid) that result in increased blood levels (reduced renal excretion, displacement from binding proteins).

PEARLS TO HELP MANAGEMENT USING METHOTREXATE AND PRALATREXATE

It is important to remember that LyP does not need to be treated if mild. In fact, it is useful to titrate the dose of MTX close to the point at which a few small lesions will still occur. In this way, excessively large doses can be avoided. If oral MTX induces problematic GI side effects, it can be administered intramuscularly instead. This also results in a

higher, more prolonged level of MTX in the serum relative to the same dose given orally. The IM route may also be useful in those patients who are suspected of poor uptake of MTX from the GI tract and may be used to enhance compliance when delivered at a physician's office. When administering IV PDX, the dosing schedule can be modified by delaying or reducing doses as needed to help manage severe adverse events such as mucositis. Side effects of both MTX and PDX can be ameliorated by avoiding concomitant use of the many other drugs that can potentiate their toxicity.

SUMMARY

This article reviews the use of MTX and its more recently developed analog, PDX, for the treatment of cutaneous T-cell LPDs. Although traditionally regarded principally as proliferation inhibitors that block the S phase of the cell cycle, folate antagonists are now known to inhibit DNA methylation by depleting cellular stores of S-adenosylmethionine, the main methyl donor for DNMTs. This has led to their novel use as agents that can derepress silenced tumor suppressor genes. Furthermore, recent mathematical modeling of cancer cell mutational dynamics provides a rationale for the use of all anticancer agents as part of combination therapy regimens rather than as monotherapies. A strategic advantage of combination regimens is the ability to attack multiple cell signaling pathways simultaneously, thereby preventing the emergence of drug-resistant tumor clones. Together, these recent advances hold new promise for the use of folate antagonists in combination with other modalities such as IFNs, histone deacetylase inhibitors, photodynamic therapy, narrow band UVB phototherapy, and ionizing radiation (see **Table 1**). Clinical validation for this approach comes from the impressive 74% CR at 1 year observed among subjects with advanced stage CTCL who were treated with a combination of low-dose MTX and IFN-α-2b.[34] In aggregate, these advances are ushering in a new era for the use of folate antagonists in the management of cutaneous lymphomas.

REFERENCES

1. Krug LM, Ng KK, Kris MG, et al. Phase I and pharmacokinetic study of 10-propargyl-10-deazaaminopterin, a new antifolate. Clin Cancer Res 2000; 6(9):3493–8.
2. Wu J, Nihal M, Siddiqui J, et al. Low FAS/CD95 expression by CTCL correlates with reduced sensitivity to

apoptosis that can be restored by FAS upregulation. J Invest Dermatol 2009;129(5):1165–73.

3. Scarisbrick JJ, Woolford AJ, Calonje E, et al. Frequent abnormalities of the p15 and p16 genes in mycosis fungoides and sezary syndrome. J Invest Dermatol 2002;118(3):493–9.

4. Lamprecht B, Kreher S, Mobs M, et al. The tumour suppressor p53 is frequently nonfunctional in Sézary syndrome. Br J Dermatol 2012;167(2):240–6.

5. Manfe V, Biskup E, Johansen P, et al. MDM2 inhibitor nutlin-3a induces apoptosis and senescence in cutaneous T-cell lymphoma: role of p53. J Invest Dermatol 2012;132(5):1487–96.

6. Stutz N, Johnson RD, Wood GS. The Fas apoptotic pathway in cutaneous T-cell lymphomas: frequent expression of phenotypes associated with resistance to apoptosis. J Am Acad Dermatol 2012; 67(6):1327.e1–10.

7. Kanavaros P, Ioannidou D, Tzardi M, et al. Mycosis fungoides: expression of C-myc p62 p53, bcl-2 and PCNA proteins and absence of association with Epstein-Barr virus. Pathol Res Pract 1994; 190(8):767–74.

8. Zhang C, Toulev A, Kamarashev J, et al. Consequences of p16 tumor suppressor gene inactivation in mycosis fungoides and Sézary syndrome and role of the bmi-1 and ras oncogenes in disease progression. Hum Pathol 2007;38(7):995–1002.

9. Gallardo F, Esteller M, Pujol RM, et al. Methylation status of the p15, p16 and MGMT promoter genes in primary cutaneous T-cell lymphomas. Haematologica 2004;89(11):1401–3.

10. Navas IC, Algara P, Mateo M, et al. p16(INK4a) is selectively silenced in the tumoral progression of mycosis fungoides. Lab Invest 2002;82(2):123–32.

11. Brechmann M. Identification and characterization of protein phosphatase 4 regulatory subunit 1 (PP4R1) as a suppressor of NF-kappaB in T lymphocytes and T cell lymphomas [PhD Thesis]. Heidelberg (Germany): Faculty of Biosciences, Ruperto-Carola University; 2010.

12. Hopkins-Donaldson S, Ziegler A, Kurtz S, et al. Silencing of death receptor and caspase-8 expression in small cell lung carcinoma cell lines and tumors by DNA methylation. Cell Death Differ 2003; 10(3):356–64.

13. Patra SK, Szyf M. DNA methylation-mediated nucleosome dynamics and oncogenic Ras signaling: insights from FAS, FAS ligand and RASSF1A. FEBS J 2008;275(21):5217–35.

14. Wu J, Wood GS. Reduction of Fas/CD95 promoter methylation, upregulation of Fas protein, and enhancement of sensitivity to apoptosis in cutaneous T-cell lymphoma. Arch Dermatol 2011;147(4):443–9.

15. Bozic I, Reiter JG, Allen B, et al. Evolutionary dynamics of cancer in response to targeted combination therapy. Elife 2013;2:e00747.

16. Horwitz SM, Kim YH, Foss F. Identification of an active, well-tolerated dose of pralatrexate in patients with relapsed or refractory cutaneous T-cell lymphoma. Blood 2012;119(18):4115–22.

17. Foss F, Horwitz SM, Coiffier B, et al. Pralatrexate is an effective treatment for relapsed or refractory transformed mycosis fungoides: a subgroup efficacy analysis from the PROPEL study. Clin Lymphoma Myeloma Leuk 2012;12(4):238–43.

18. O'Connor OA, Hamlin PA, Portlock C, et al. Pralatrexate, a novel class of antifol with high affinity for the reduced folate carrier-type 1, produces marked complete and durable remissions in a diversity of chemotherapy refractory cases of T-cell lymphoma. Br J Haematol 2007;139:425–8.

19. O'Connor OA, Horwitz S, Hamlin P, et al. Phase II-I-II study of two different doses and schedules of pralatrexate, a high-affinity substrate for the reduced folate carrier, in patients with relapsed or refractory lymphoma reveals marked activity in T-cell malignancies. J Clin Oncol 2009;27:4357–64.

20. O'Connor OA, Pro B, Pinter-Browen L, et al. Pralatrexate in patients with relapsed or refractory peripheral T-Cell lymphoma: results from the pivotal PROPEL study. J Clin Oncol 2011;29:1182–9.

21. Clarke LE, Junkins-Hopkins J, Seykora JT, et al. Methotrexate-associated lymphoproliferative disorder in a patient with rheumatoid arthritis presenting in the skin. J Am Acad Dermatol 2007;56:686–90.

22. Maurani A, Wierzbicka E, Machet M-C, et al. Reversal of multifocal cutaneous lymphoproliferative disease associated with Epstein-Barr virus after withdrawal of methotrexate therapy for rheumatoid arthritis. J Am Acad Dermatol 2007;57:S69–71.

23. Spurgeon S, Yu M, Phillips JD, et al. Cladribine: not just another purine analogue? Expert Opin Investig Drugs 2009;18(8):1169–81.

24. Beardsley GP, Moroson BA, Taylor EC, et al. A new folate antimetabolite, 5,10-dideaza-5,6,7,8-tetrahydrofolate is a potent inhibitor of de novo purine synthesis. J Biol Chem 1989;264(1):328–33.

25. Jurkowska RZ, Jurkowska TP, Jeltsch A. Structure and function of mammalian DNA methyltransferases. Chembiochem 2010;12(2):206–22.

26. Hermann A, Gowher H, Jeltsch A. Biochemistry and biology of mammalian DNA methyltransferases. Cell Mol Life Sci 2004;61(19–20):2571–87.

27. Philips MR. Methotrexate and Ras methylation: a new trick for an old drug? Sci STKE 2004;2004(225):pe13.

28. Morgan MA, Ganser A, Reuter CW. Targeting the RAS signaling pathway in malignant hematologic diseases. Curr Drug Targets 2007;8(2):217–35.

29. Wang YC, Chiang EP. Low-dose methotrexate inhibits methionine S-adenosyltransferase in vitro and in vivo. Mol Med 2012;18(1):423–32.

30. Olsen EA. The pharmacology of methotrexate. J Am Acad Dermatol 1991;25:306–18.

31. Mould DR, Sweeney K, Duffull SB, et al. A population pharmacokinetic and pharmacodynamics evaluation of pralatrexate in patients with relapsed or refractory non-Hodgkin's or Hodgkin's lymphoma. Clin Pharmacol Ther 2009;86(2):190–6.

32. Calabresi P, Parks RE Jr. Antiproliferative agents and drugs used for immunosuppression. In: Gilman AG, Goodman LS, Rail TW, et al, editors. The pharmacological basis of therapeutics. 7th edition. New York: Macmillan; 1985. p. 1263–7.

33. Warren RB, Smith RL, Campalani E, et al. Genetic variation in efflux transporters influences outcome to methotrexate therapy in patients with psoriasis. J Invest Dermatol 2008;128(8):1925–9.

34. Aviles A, Nambo MJ, Neri N, et al. Interferon and low dose methotrexate improve outcome in refractory mycosis fungoides/Sézary syndrome. Cancer Biother Radiopharm 2007;22(6):836–40.

35. Duhra P. Treatment of gastrointestinal symptoms associated with methotrexate therapy for psoriasis. J Am Acad Dermatol 1993;28:466–9.

36. Salim A, Tan E, Ilchyshyn A, et al. Folic acid supplementation during treatment of psoriasis with methotrexate: a randomized, double-blind, placebo-controlled trial. Br J Dermatol 2006;154:1169–74.

37. McDonald CJ, Bertino JR. Treatment of mycosis fungoides lymphoma: effectiveness of infusions of methotrexate followed by oral citrovorum factor. Cancer Treat Rep 1978;62:1009–14.

38. Wright JC, Lyons MM, Walker DG, et al. Observations on the use of cancer chemotherapeutic agents in patients with mycosis fungoides. Cancer 1964;17: 1045–62.

39. Zackheim HS, Kashani-Sabet M, Hwang ST. Low-dose methotrexate to treat erythrodermic cutaneous T-cell lymphoma: results in twenty-nine patients. J Am Acad Dermatol 1996;34:626–31.

40. Zackheim HS, Kashani-Sabet M, McMillan A. Low-dose methotrexate to treat mycosis fungoides: a retrospective study in 69 patients. J Am Acad Dermatol 2003;49:873–8.

41. Demierre M-F, Vachon L, Ho V, et al. Phase 1/2 pilot study of methotrexate-laurocapram topical gel for the treatment of patients with early-stage mycosis fungoides. Arch Dermatol 2003;139:624–8.

42. Schappell DL, Alper JC, McDonald CJ. Treatment of advanced mycosis fungoides and Sézary syndrome with continuous infusions of methotrexate followed by fluorouracil and leucovorin rescue. Arch Dermatol 1995;131:307–13.

43. Hirayama Y, Nagai T, Ohta H, et al. Sézary syndrome showing a stable clinical course for more than four years after oral administration of etoposide and methotrexate. Rinsho Ketsueki 2000;41:750–4 [in Japanese].

44. Kempf W, Pfaltz K, Vermeer MH, et al. EORTC, ISCL, and USCLC consensus recommendations for the treatment of primary cutaneous CD30-positive lymphoproliferative disorders: lymphomatoid papulosis and primary cutaneous anaplastic large-cell lymphoma. Blood 2011;118(15):4024–35.

45. Vonderheid EC, Sajjadian A, Kadin ME. Methotrexate is effective therapy for lymphomatoid papulosis and other primary cutaneous CD30-positive lymphoproliferative disorders. J Am Acad Dermatol 1996;34:470–81.

46. Bergstrom JS, Jaworsky C. Topical methotrexate for lymphomatoid papulosis. J Am Acad Dermatol 2003;49:937–9.

47. Sarris AH, Phan A, Duvic M, et al. Trimetrexate in relapsed T-cell lymphoma with skin involvement. J Clin Oncol 2002;20:2876–80.

48. Rodrigues M, Westerman D, Lade S, et al. Methotrexate-induced lymphoproliferative disorder in a patient with Sézary syndrome. Leuk Lymphoma 2006;47:2257–9.

49. Strathdee G, Brown R. Aberrant DNA methylation in cancer: potential clinical interventions. Expert Rev Mol Med 2002;4(4):1–17.

50. Nihal M, Ahmad N, Wood GS. SIRT1 is upregulated in cutaneous T-cell lymphoma and its inhibition induces growth arrest and apoptosis. Cell Cycle 2014;l13:632–40.

51. Salva KA, Nihal M, Wu J, et al. Epigenetically enhanced photodynamic therapy (ePDT) is superior to conventional PDT for inducing apoptosis in cutaneous T-cell lymphoma (CTCL) [abstract]. J Invest Dermatol 2014;134:S117.

52. Wu J, Salva K, Wood GS. c-CBL E3 ubiquitin ligase is over-expressed in cutaneous T-cell lymphoma: its inhibition promotes activation-induced cell death. J Invest Dermatol 2015;135(3):861–8.

Histone Deacetylase Inhibitors for Cutaneous T-Cell Lymphoma

Madeleine Duvic, MD

KEYWORDS

- T-cell lymphoma • Histone deacetylase • Histone deacetylase inhibitors
- Cutaneous T-cell lymphomas

KEY POINTS

- Romidepsin and vorinostat are the only histone deacetylase (HDAC) inhibitors currently approved for cutaneous T-cell lymphomas (CTCL), and belinostat is also approved for peripheral T-cell lymphoma.
- There is little information regarding combinations of HDAC inhibitors with other CTCL therapies. There are no data to exclude combining HDAC inhibitors with skin-directed therapies.
- Although there are now several approved treatments available, the field is still in need of newer drugs and approaches for this disease with poor prognosis.

INTRODUCTION

Cutaneous T-cell lymphomas (CTCLs) are non-Hodgkin's T-cell lymphomas that present as skin lesions. The most common is mycosis fungoides (MF) and its leukemic variant, Sézary syndrome (SS). CTCLs are currently rarely cured and may have an indolent clinical course. MF with large cell transformation, defined as greater than 25% atypical lymphocytes with nuclei 4 times the normal size, has poor survival, similar to that of peripheral T-cell lymphoma (PTCL) with a 5-year overall survival of only 32% with involved skin and 7% with extracutaneous involvement.[1] The failure of MF with large cell transformation and PTCL to respond to multiagent chemotherapy with cytoxan, adriamycin, oncovin, and prednisone (CHOP) or CHOP-based chemotherapy has resulted in a search for novel targeted agents including antibodies and gene modulators. Histone deacetylase (HDAC) inhibitors are small molecules that seem to be particularly active for T-cell lymphoma.[2]

MECHANISM OF ACTION OF HISTONE DEACETYLASE INHIBITORS

Histone acetyltransferases and HDACs are enzymes capable of modifying histone and nonhistone acetylation sites in proteins. Histone acetyltransferases and HDACs regulate a broad range of pathways and processes that are dysregulated in cancer, including the cell cycle, apoptosis, and protein folding. The balance between histone acetylation effected by acetylases and deacetylation is mediated by HDAC inhibitors and is abnormal in cancer cells.[3,4] Acetylation of histones promotes opened chromatin, transcription factor binding to promoters, and initiation of mRNA synthesis encoding genes.[5] The action of deacetylase inhibitors is not limited to histones and can prevent deacetylation of other proteins, such as the tumor promoter p53.

HDAC inhibitors are small molecules that interact with HDAC's catalytic sites preventing the removal of acetyl groups, counteracting the effects of HDACs. Valproic acid was the first HDAC

Division of Internal Medicine, Department of Dermatology, University of Texas MD Anderson Cancer Center, Houston, TX 77030, USA
E-mail address: mduvic@mdanderson.org

Dermatol Clin 33 (2015) 757–764
http://dx.doi.org/10.1016/j.det.2015.05.010
0733-8635/15/$ – see front matter

inhibitor investigated for malignancy followed by development of pan-HDAC and more selective inhibitors to improve efficacy and safety. Whether HDAC inhibitors with selected specificity are more effective with fewer side effects and thus are superior to pan-inhibitors is still under debate.[6] Wells and colleagues[6] showed that selective HDAC3 inhibition by the first HDAC3 inhibitor, RGFP966, resulted in decreased cell growth in CTCL lines owing to increased apoptosis associated with DNA damage and impaired S phase progression. HDAC3 was present around the DNA replication forks and significantly decreased the speed of replication.

The 18 known HDACs are classified into 4 main groups based on their homology to yeast HDACs and dependence on the essential cofactor, zinc, present at the active sites. Zinc-dependent HDACs include those of class I that target histones and includes HDACs 1, 2, 3, and 8; class IIa HDACs that target both histones and nonhistone proteins and includes HDACs 4, 5, 7, 9; Class IIb HDAC 6, which targets the mitogen-activated protein kinase pathway,[7] and 10; and class IV HDAC targeting only HDAC 11. The class 3 HDACs, called sirtulins (1–7), are zinc independent and nicotinamide adenine dinucleotide dependent.[5,8]

HDAC inhibitors have been classified by 4 major chemical structures and their ability to interact with specific HDACs. By clinical structure, HDAC inhibitors are short-chain fatty acids (valproic acid), hydroxamic acids (vorinostat [suberoylanilide hydroxamic acid (SAHA)], panobinostat [LBH589], and quisinostat [JNJ-26481585]), depsipeptide (romidepsin [FK228]), and benzamides (entinostat [MS-275] and mocetinostat [MGCD-0103]). The chemical structures of the hydroxamic acids and romidepsin are shown in **Fig. 1**. Vorinostat was the first HDAC inhibitor approved by US Food and Drug Administration (FDA) for use in cancer based on 2 phase II studies in refractory CTCL patients.[9,10] In a study of 45 PTCL patients, HDAC 1, 2, and 6 were overexpressed compared with normal lymphoid tissue making T-cell lymphoma a logical target for HDAC inhibition.[11]

HDAC inhibitors inhibit cell cycle progression by upregulating p21, p27, and p16, which bind to and deactivate CDK2 and CDK4 leading to G1 arrest.[12] HDAC inhibitors may also inhibit S-phase progression through inhibition of cytidine triphosphate synthase and thymidylate synthetase, involved in DNA synthesis.[13] They also induce generation of reactive oxygen species while inhibiting DNA repair.[6]

The balance between proapoptotic and antiapoptotic factors is influenced by HDAC inhibitors. HDAC inhibitors increase expression of genes encoding death receptors and their respective ligands (Fas and Apo 2 L/TRAIL receptors, DR4 and DR5). They also downregulate c-FLIP (a negative regulator of caspase-8), and modulate the mitogen-activated protein kinase pathway, a possible mechanism of resistance.[12–14] HDAC inhibitors also upregulate expression of proapoptic BH3 domain proteins while downregulating the antiapoptotic proteins BCL-2, BCL-XL, and MCL-1.[12] In leukemia cells, apoptosis-involved pathways independent of p53, regulated by Bcl-2/Bxl-XL, c-Jun, and p21CIP1.[15]

The STAT family of transcription factors (STAT-3, -4, -5, and -6) are thought to have a key role in driving T-cell proliferation in CTCL.[16] STAT-4, associated with a T helper cell (Th) 1 phenotype, is downregulated in CTCL cell lines, whereas STAT-6, which is associated with Th2 phenotype, is upregulated. Change in STAT expression could contribute to the TH1 to TH2 phenotype switch seen in disease progression. Increasing STAT-5 signaling may upregulate Th2 cytokines and synergize to promote the malignancy. Downregulation of STAT-4 may be owing to upregulation of STAT 5 signaling during the early stages of CTCL. HDAC inhibitors may act through STATs to increase the Th1>TH2 response.

Growing evidence shows that STAT5 is important for the expression of anti-apoptotic proteins (including bcl-2 and bcl-x), cell cycle genes (Cyclin D and c-myc), and the oncogenic miR-155 microRNA (which has a putative binding site on the STAT4 3'UTR). Evidence suggests that with STAT5 upregulation early in CTCL, the resulting miR-155 increase promotes proliferation of malignant T-cells and may be responsible for STAT-4 decline and conversion to TH2 phenotype.[16,17] The imbalance between STAT-4 and STAT-6 is thought to be owing to aberrant histone acetylation. MyLa cells treated with romidepsin or vorinostat, show downregulation of STAT-6 and upregulation of STAT-4, which is beneficial for CTCL. HDAC inhibitors may restore this balance because treatment with HDAC inhibitors have been shown to upregulate STAT-4 and decrease STAT-6 in vitro.[16]

VORINOSTAT (ZOLINZA; SUBEROYLANILIDE HYDROXAMIC ACID)

The mechanisms of action of vorinostat have been studied extensively with complexity related to the ability of HDAC inhibitors to modulate multiple genes and cell types.[3] Vorinostat induces differentiation and growth arrest in a wide range of cancer cells studied.[18,19]

We reported that CTLC lines treated in vitro with vorinostat underwent apoptosis selectively compared with normal T cells.[9] The level of acetylated histone protein does not predict response,

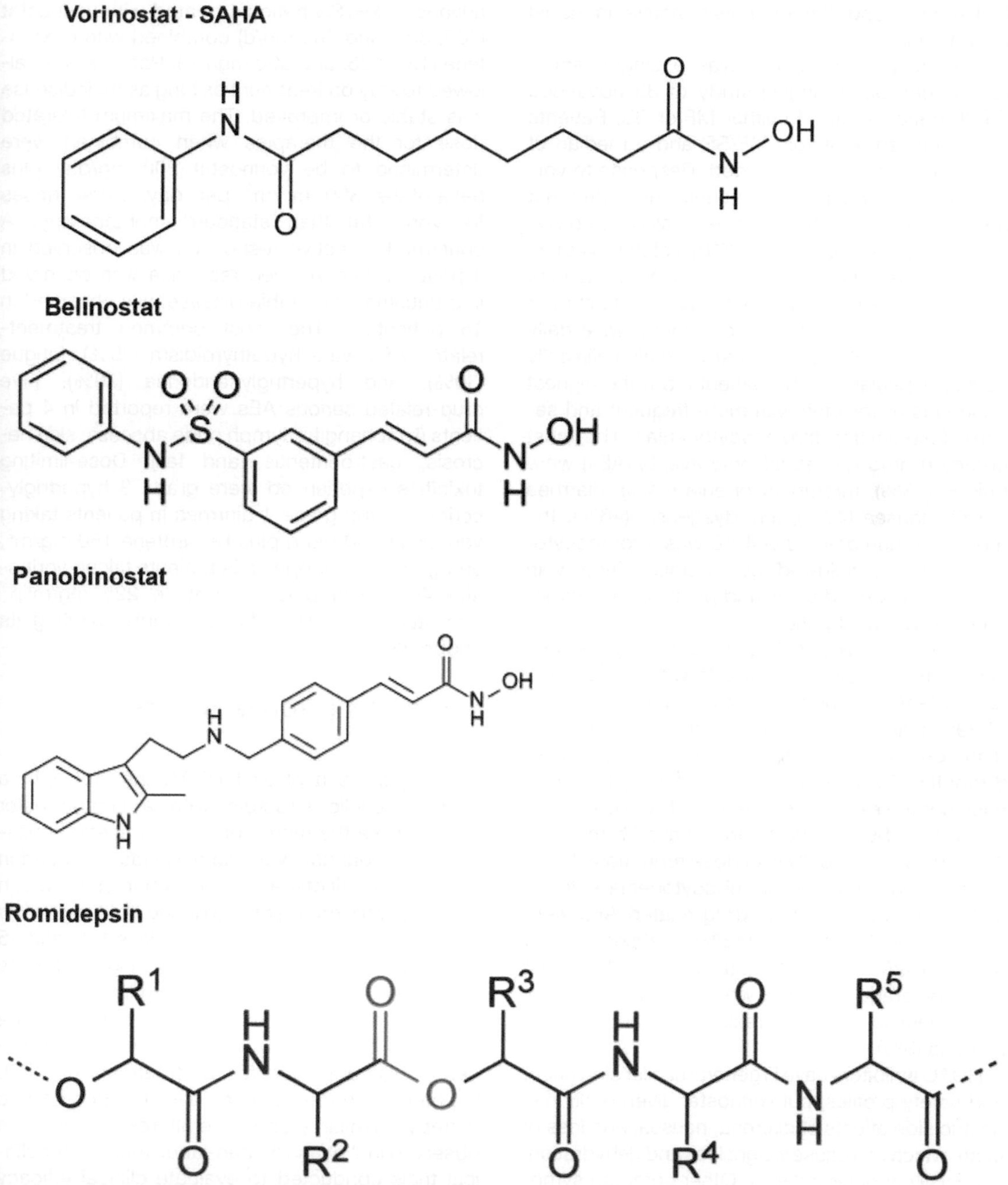

Vorinostat - SAHA

Belinostat

Panobinostat

Romidepsin

Fig. 1. Chemical structures of histone deacetylase inhibitors.

but did increase in duration with higher doses of vorinostat. In MF skin lesions, phospho-stat 3 localized in the cytoplasm at baseline became nuclear in distribution in patients who had clinical responses to vorinostat.[9] Vorinostat and romidepsin were reported to downregulate expression of interleukin-10 (a Th2 cytokine) in CTCL cells.[20]

Vorinostat (suberoyl + anilide + hydroxamic acid or SAHA),[21] is a class I/II HDAC inhibitor with a hydroxamic structure. After activity was

shown in cancer cell lines,[18] vorinostat was evaluated in phase I trials as both an oral and intravenous formulation with initial responses seen in hematopoietic malignancies, including T-cell lymphoma.[19] Vorinostat was the first HDAC inhibitor to receive FDA approval in 2006 for the treatment of relapsed/refractory CTCL.[22] Approval was based on the overall response seen in 2 phase II single-arm clinical trials.[23,24] A phase I study was also completed in patients with advanced leukemia,[25] and the drug was active in nodal lymphoma.[19]

The initial phase II trial was a single-center, open-label, dose-ranging study of 33 advanced CTCL patients, all with either MF or SS. Patients with relapsed/refractory MF/SS and a median of 5 prior therapies were included. Response to vorinostat in the first group of patients suggested that an optimal dose of 400 mg given orally once daily[9] and an overall response rate (ORR) of 24% with no complete remissions (CR). The median duration of response was only about 4 months.[9] Intermittent dose schedules of 300 mg by mouth twice daily for 2 weeks with a 2 week rest were also clinically active, especially for SS patients, but the highest dose was associated with more frequent and severe dose-limiting thrombocytopenia.[9] The most common drug-related adverse events (AEs) were fatigue (73%), thrombocytopenia (54%), diarrhea (49%), nausea (49%), and dysgeusia (46%); the most common grade 3 or 4 AE was thrombocytopenia (19%), followed by anemia, deep vein thrombosis, dehydration, and pyrexia (each experienced by 8% of patients).

The second phase II multicenter, open-label, clinical trial enrolled 74 patients with MF/SS who had at least 2 prior systemic therapies. The ORR of 29% was similar to the first study and the median duration of response was longer than 6 months. Of note, 6 patients had long-term disease control exceeding 2 years.[10] The recommended dose of vorinostat for the phase IIb trial was 400 mg by mouth daily with dose reductions taken for gastrointestinal or thrombocytopenia side effects. The most common drug-related AEs were diarrhea (49%), fatigue (46%), nausea (43%), anorexia (26%), and dysgeusia (24%); the most common grade 3 or 4 AEs were thrombocytopenia (5%), nausea (4%), anorexia (3%), and muscle spasms (3%).

HDAC inhibitors have in general similar side effect and safety profiles, but vorinostat given orally has gastric side effects of diarrhea, nausea, and loss of taste, which can cause weight loss and dehydration, especially in older patients. Other common symptoms of HDAC inhibitors are fatigue and thrombocytopenia owing to platelet maturation arrest. The initial warning of alterations in cardiac rhythm with HDAC inhibitors was removed based on lack of evidence. Elimination is primarily hepatic, with total mean plasma clearance and elimination half-life of 1240 mL/min and 1.1 hours, respectively.[26]

Vorinostat has been combined with other agents, especially with protease inhibitors and lenolidamide, in the setting of multiple myeloma. With respect to CTCL, a single phase I safety and efficacy multicenter clinical trial evaluated 23 advanced MF/SS patients treated with vorinostat (200, 300, and 400 mg/d) combined with bexarotene (150, 225, and 300 mg/m^2). Patients were allowed to stay on treatment as long as their disease was stable or improved. The maximum tolerated dose for the therapies when combined were determined to be vorinostat 200 mg/day plus bexarotene 300 mg/m^2 per day, lower doses for vorinostat than standard monotherapy. A confirmed objective responses was observed in 4 patients, unconfirmed response was observed in 2 patients, and stable disease was observed in 15 patients.[27] The most common treatment-related AEs were hypothyroidism (35%), fatigue (30%), and hypertriglyceridemia (30%). Five drug-related serious AEs were reported in 4 patients (lymphangitis, lymph node abscess, skin necrosis, gastroenteritis, and fall). Dose-limiting toxicities experienced were grade 3 hypertriglyceridemia and grade 1 diarrhea in patients taking vorinostat 300 mg/d plus bexarotene 150 mg/m^2, and grade 3 neutropenia in patients taking vorinostat 400 mg/d plus bexarotene 225 mg/m^2.[27] The study was discontinued before meeting its endpoints.

ROMIDEPSIN (ISTODAR, DEPSIPEPTIDE, FK228)

Romidepsin is a class I HDAC inhibitor with a unique bicyclic structure with a central ester bond. Unlike the more common synthetic benzamide compounds, cyclic compounds are found in nature.[28] For all of the T-cell lymphomas for which it is approved, romidepsin is dosed at 14 mg/m^2 as a 4-hour intravenous infusion on days 1, 8, and 15 every 28 days.[29] Potassium and magnesium are recommended to be normal before infusion.

Romidepsin is the second HDAC inhibitor to be approved by the FDA. In September 2009, romidepsin was approved for the treatment of CTCL in patients who received at least 1 prior systemic therapy. Similar global overall responses were observed in 2 phase II open-label, multicenter clinical trials conducted to evaluate clinical efficacy and safety of romidepsin in patients with CTCLs (specifically MF or SS)[30,31] and accelerated approval for PTCL.[30–34] The global response rate in the multicenter CTCL trial was 34%.[30] This trial used a global evaluation of the skin composed of assessments of skin lesions by the modified skin weighted assessment tool, lymph nodes, and visceral compartments (by CT) and blood (by flow cytometry), setting a new higher standard for evaluation of CTCL patients' response in clinical trials.[30,35] Approval was based not on overall response, but on improvement in the duration of response and pruritus over conventional therapies. An ORR of 34% and CR rate of 6% was also notable. Nausea, vomiting, fatigue, or myelosuppression were the most commonly encountered AEs. QT interval changes on electrocardiography that were insignificant clinically did not correlate with decreased left ventricular ejection fraction, or elevated laboratory markers of myocardial damage.[36]

Romidepsin was given accelerated approval for patients with PTCLs who had received 1 or more prior therapies. Approval was based on 2 single-arm phase II studies. The first study included 45 patients with relapsed/refractory PTCL and a median of 3 prior therapies.[31] The ORR of 38% (CR 18%) was achieved with a median duration of response of 9 months.[31] A second multinational phase II study enrolled 130 patients with relapsed/refractory PTCL and a median of 2 (range, 1–8) prior therapies. The primary endpoint was the number of CRs or unconfirmed responses assessed by independent review.[29] The trial achieved an ORR of 25% (CR or complete response unspecified [CRU]) of 15%, with a median duration of response of 17 months.[29] Of 19 patients with CR/CRUs, 17 (89%) had not experienced disease progression at a median follow-up of 13.4 months.[29]

The safety profile of romidepsin in patients with PTCL is similar to patients with CTCL. The most common AEs in PTCL patients were nausea, fatigue, and transient thrombocytopenia and granulocytopenia. In the pivotal PTCL trial, severe grade 3 or higher AEs experienced by patients included thrombocytopenia, neutropenia, and infections. The ORR was 25% (33/130) with 15% of patients (19/130) achieving a CR or unconfirmed CR.[31] Based on these trials, romidepsin was approved by the FDA in 2011 for the treatment of PTCL in patients who have received at least 1 prior therapy.[29,31,36]

BELINOSTAT (BELEODAQ; PXD101 MECHANISM OF ACTION)

Belinostat [(2E)-N-hydroxy-3-[3-(phenylsulfamoyl) phenyl]prop-2-enamide] is a pan- HDAC inhibitor with a sulfonamide-hydroxamide structure and high affinity for the class I, II and IV HDACs. In vitro, belinostat causes accumulation of acetylated histones, restores expression of epigenetically silenced tumor suppressor genes (transforming growth factor β receptor II), represses survivin (an antiapoptotic protein), and causes cell-cycle arrest and apoptosis of malignant cells.[37] Belinostat is active at nanomolar concentrations (<250 nmol/L) and shows preferential cytotoxicity toward malignant cells.

Belinostat was granted orphan drug and accelerated designation in September 2014 by the FDA for use in patients with relapsed or refractory PTCL.[38,39] Belinostat is included in the National Comprehensive Cancer Network guidelines as second-line therapy (category 2B) for patients with relapsed PTCL.

A small, multicenter, phase II study was conducted in 24 adults with relapsed/refractory PTCL and 29 adults with MF/SS.[39] Patients had received a median of 3 and 4 prior systemic therapies, respectively. PTCL patients' prior treatments included an autologous stem cell transplant in 21%; 40% and 55% of patients had stage IV disease, respectively. Belinostat was administered at 1000 mg/m² intravenously on days 1 through 5 every 3 weeks, with dose escalation to 1200 mg/m² and 1400 mg/m² permitted in cycles 2 and 3. The primary endpoint, overall response, was 25% (8% CR) in PTCL patients. ORR in MF/SS patients was 14% with 10% CRs and did not meet the predetermined ORR needed to continue the study. The median duration of response in the 2 groups was 109 and 83 days, respectively. AEs were reported in 77% of patients included nausea (62%), vomiting (26%), fever (21%), and dizziness (21%).

A phase I study of patients with advanced hematologic malignancies enrolled 16 patients, none of whom had MF or SS.[19] Belinostat doses were 600, 900, and 1000 mg/m² per day given by intravenous infusion. Phase I studies were conducted to determine the optimal dose and route of administration.[26,40,41] The most common treatment related AEs were nausea (50%), vomiting (31%), fatigue (31%), and flushing (31%). Two patients with multiple myeloma experienced acute renal injury from tumor lysis. Based on this study, the dose of 1000 mg/m² intravenously, days 1 through 5 of a 21- to 128-day cycle was selected for subsequent phase II clinical trials. Studies have investigated continuous dosing and oral formulation; an optimal dose and schedule has not yet been established.[26,40]

The phase II BELIEF study led to accelerated approval of belinostat.[40] This phase II multicenter study was conducted at 62 sites enrolling 129 adults with relapsed/refractory PTCL and median age of 64 years who had had a median of 2 prior lines of therapies. All patients had received at least one prior systemic treatment (96% CHOP or CHOP-like regimens, including an autologous stem cell transplant in 23%). Belinostat was administered 1000 mg/m² intravenously on days 1 through 5 every 3 weeks and was continued as long as belinostat was effective and tolerated. The primary endpoint, overall response, was

26% with 11% CRs in 120 evaluable patients. The median time to response was 5.6 weeks, but late responses, beyond 6 months, were also seen. Responses were generally durable, with a median duration of response of 8.4 months and 7.5% of patients went on to receive a stem cell transplant. Treatment was well-tolerated, with AE-related discontinuation reported only in 7% of patients. The most frequent grades III or IV AEs were thrombocytopenia (13%), neutropenia (13%), and anemia (10%). In the BELIEF trial, QTc interval prolongation was observed in 4% of patients and grades 3 and 4 cytopenias in 10% to 15% of patients.

After this accelerated approval, the FDA has required the sponsor to conduct a dose-finding trial of belinostat combined with CHOP (Bel-CHOP), followed by a phase III trial of Bel-CHOP versus CHOP as frontline treatment of PTCL. The first study is currently active and recruiting patients (NCT01839097), with the primary endpoint of finding the maximum tolerated dose for belinostat to be combined with CHOP. In this study, belinostat will be administered to 5 cohorts of patients at 1000 mg/m^2 on day 1, days 1 to 2, days 1 to 3, days 1 to 4, and days 1 to 5 of each 21-day cycle.

Pharmacogenomic studies found reduced UGT1A1 activity in individuals with the UGT1A1*28 polymorphism, which is most prevalent among black individuals with 20% homozygosity. Thus, dose reduction to 750 mg/m^2 is recommended in patients homozygous for UGT1A1*28 to minimize toxicity.

PANOBINOSTAT (LBH-589, FARYDAK)

Panobinostat is a potent and broad spectrum hydroxamic acid HDAC inhibitor that was recently approved by the FDA in February 2015 for the treatment of multiple myeloma. Panobinostat is dosed orally 3 times weekly. CTCL patients with SS had remarkable responses that were durable in a phase I study conducted by Sharma and colleagues.[42] The clinical trials for hematologic malignancies including those involving patients with CTCL were reviewed recently.[43]

A phase II, multicenter, open-label, clinical trial was conducted in 79 MF/SS patients who had formerly been treated with bexarotene and 60 bexarotene-naïve patients.[44] The dose was 20 mg orally 3 days per week. The overall response by the modified skin weighted assessment tool assessment of skin involvement was only 17% in all patients, 15.2% for bexarotene exposed, and 20% in the bexarotene-naïve patients. The median progression-free survival was 4.2 and 3.7 months in the bexarotene or no bexarotene groups, respectively. The duration of response in the bexarotene exposed group was 5.6 months. Reductions of the modified skin weighted assessment tool score were observed in 103 patients (74.1%). The study design did not take into consideration tumor flares so patients were taken off prematurely for "progressive disease."[44] The most common AEs were thrombocytopenia, diarrhea, fatigue, and nausea. Thrombocytopenia and neutropenia were the only grade 3 or 4 AEs in greater than 5% of patients and were manageable.

SUMMARY

Although romidepsin and vorinostat are the only HDAC inhibitors currently approved for CTCL (MF/SS), belinostat is also approved for PTCL. Their efficacy and side effects were similar in the pivotal trials. The overall response (OR) rate for Vorinostat was 30% with no CRs and the OR rate for romidepsin was 34% with a 6% CRS. Vorinostat has the advantage of oral administration, but has more associated gastrointestinal side effects such as intolerable diarrhea and loss of taste in some patients. Romidepsin can only be administered intravenously over 4 hours and has more fatigue and nausea, which are the most frequent reasons for stopping therapy. Thrombocytopenia can occur with either and is dose related. QTc prolongation is a rare but potentially serious adverse effect of the class, occurring in fewer than 5% of patients treated. Romidepsin and vorinostat responders have continued therapy for over a year with dose reductions taken in some cases for toxicity or convenience.

There is little information regarding combinations of HDAC inhibitors with other CTCL therapies. Vorinostat added to electron beam therapy did not increase the response rate or add to the toxicity (Kim, unpublished, ASH abstract, 2014). There are no data to exclude combining HDAC inhibitors with skin-directed therapies. Belinostat is a new intravenous and Pabinostat a new oral HDAC inhibitor approved for other indications but in which phase II exploratory trials in CTCL patients have shown ORs of less than 20%.

Finally, although there are now several approved treatments available for patients with advanced MF/SS, the field is still in need of newer drugs and approaches for this disease with poor prognosis.

ACKNOWLEDGMENTS

The authors thank Ashley Turkeltaub, MS Baylor College of Medicine for her help with references and the Blanche Bender Professorship in Cancer Research (MD).

REFERENCES

1. Vergier B, de Muret A, Beylot-Barry M, et al. Transformation of mycosis fungoides: clinicopathological and prognostic features of 45 cases. French Study Group of Cutaneous Lymphomas. Blood 2000;95:2212–8.
2. Rangwalla S, Zhang C, Duvic M. HDAC Inhibitors for the treatment of cutaneous T-cell lymphomas. Future Med Chem 2012;4:471–86.
3. Lakshmaiah KC, Jacob LA, Aparna S, et al. Epigenetic therapy of cancer with histone deacetylase inhibitors. J Cancer Res Ther 2014;10:469–78.
4. Bose P, Dai Y, Grant S. Histone deacetylase inhibitor (HDACI) mechanisms of action: emerging insights. Pharmacol Ther 2014;143:323–36.
5. Meier K, Brehm A. Chromatin regulation: how complex does it get? Epigenetics 2014;9:1485–95.
6. Wells CE, Bhaskara S, Stengel KR, et al. Inhibition of histone deacetylase 3 causes replication stress in cutaneous T cell lymphoma. PLoS One 2013;8(7):e68915.
7. Haakenson J, Wu JY, Xiang S, et al. HDAC6-dependent functions in tumor cells: crossroad with the MAPK pathways. Crit Rev Oncog 2015;20:65–81.
8. Parbin S, Kar S, Shilpi A, et al. Histone deacetylases: a saga of perturbed acetylation homeostasis in cancer. J Histochem Cytochem 2014;62:11–33.
9. Duvic M, Talpur R, Ni X, et al. Phase II trial of oral vorinostat (suberoylanilide hydroxamic acid, SAHA) for refractory cutaneous T-cell lymphoma (CTCL). Blood 2007;109:31–9.
10. Olsen E, Kim YH, Kuzel T, et al. A phase IIb multicenter trial of vorinostat (suberoylanilide hydroxamic acid, SAHA) in patients with persistent, progressive, or treatment refractory mycosis fungoides or sezary syndrome subtypes of cutaneous T-cell lymphoma. J Clin Onc 2007;25:3109–15.
11. Marquard L, Poulsen CB, Gjerdrum LM, et al. Histone deacetylase 1, 2, 6 and acetylated histone H4 in B- and T-cell lymphomas. Histopathology 2009;54:688–98.
12. Jain S, Zain J, O'Connor O. Novel therapeutic agents for cutaneous T-Cell lymphoma. J Hematol Oncol 2012;5:5–24.
13. Luchenko VL, Litman T, Chakraborty AR, et al. Histone deacetylase inhibitor-mediated cell death is distinct from its global effect on chromatin. Mol Oncol 2014;8:1379–92.
14. Irmler M, Thome M, Hahne M, et al. Inhibition of death receptor signals by cellular FLIP. Nature 1979;388(6638):190–5.
15. Vrana JA, Decker RH, Johnson CR, et al. Induction of apoptosis in U937 human leukemia cells by suberoylanilide hydroxamic acid (SAHA) proceeds through pathways that are regulated by Bcl-2/Bcl-XL, c-Jun, and p21CIP1, but independent of p53. Oncogene 1999;18:7016–25.
16. Litvinov IV, Cordeiro B, Fredholm S, et al. Analysis of STAT4 expression in cutaneous T-cell lymphoma (CTCL) patients and patient-derived cell lines. Cell Cycle 2014;13:2975–82.
17. Netchiporouk E, Litvinov IV, Moreau L, et al. Deregulation in STAT signaling is important for cutaneous T-cell lymphoma (CTCL) pathogenesis and cancer progression. Cell Cycle 2014;13:3331–5.
18. Richon VM. Cancer biology: mechanism of antitumour action of vorinostat (suberoylanilide hydroxamic acid), a novel histone deacetylase inhibitor. Br J Cancer 2006;95:S2–6.
19. O'Connor OA. Clinical experience with the novel histone deacetylase inhibitor vorinostat (suberoylanilide hydroxamic acid) in patients with relapsed lymphoma. Br J Cancer 2006;95:S7–12.
20. Tiffon C, Adams J, van der Fits L, et al. The histone deacetylase inhibitors vorinostat and romidepsin downmodulate IL-10 expression in cutaneous T-cell lymphoma cells. Br J Pharmacol 2011;162:1590–602.
21. Marks PA, Jiang X. Histone deacetylase inhibitors in programmed cell death and cancer therapy. Cell Cycle 2005;4:549–51.
22. Mann BS, Johnson JR, Cohen MH, et al. FDA approval summary: vorinostat for treatment of advanced primary cutaneous T-cell lymphoma. Oncologist 2007;12:1247–52.
23. Duvic M, Vu J. Vorinostat in cutaneous T-cell lymphoma. Drugs Today (Barc) 2007;43:585–99.
24. Duvic M, Vu J. Update on the treatment of cutaneous T-cell lymphoma (CTCL): focus on vorinostat. Biol Targets Ther 2007;1:377–92.
25. Garcia-Manero G, Yang H, Bueso-Ramos C, et al. Phase 1 study of the histone deacetylase inhibitor vorinostat (suberoylanilide hydroxamic acid [SAHA]) in patients with advanced leukemias and myelodysplastic syndromes. Blood 2008;111:1060–6.
26. Steele NL, Plumb JA, Vidal L, et al. A phase 1 pharmacokinetic and pharmacodynamic study of the histone deacetylase inhibitor belinostat in patients with advanced solid tumors. Clin Cancer Res 2008;14:804–10.
27. Dummer R, Beyer M, Hymes K, et al. Vorinostat combined with bexarotene for treatment of cutaneous T-cell lymphoma: in vitro and phase I clinical evidence supporting augmentation of retinoic acid receptor/retinoid X receptor activation by histone deacetylase inhibition. Leuk Lymphoma 2012;53:1501–8.
28. Kitagaki J, Shi G, Miyauchi S, et al. Cyclic depsipeptides as potential cancer therapeutics. Anticancer Drugs 2015;26:259–71.
29. Coiffier B, Pro B, Prince HM, et al. Results from a pivotal, open-label, phase II study of romidepsin in

relapsed or refractory peripheral T-cell lymphoma after prior systemic therapy. J Clin Oncol 2012;30: 631–6.

30. Whittaker SJ, Demierre MF, Kim EJ, et al. Final results from a multicenter, international, pivotal study of romidepsin in refractory cutaneous T-cell lymphoma. J Clin Oncol 2010;28:4485–91.

31. Piekarz RL, Frye R, Prince HM, et al. Phase 2 trial of romidepsin in patients with peripheral T-cell lymphoma. Blood 2011;117:5827–34.

32. Kim YH, Reddy S, Kim EJ, et al. Romidepsin (depsipeptide) induces clinically significant responses in treatment-refractory CTCL: an international study. Blood 2007;110.

33. Piekarz RL, Frye R, Turner M, et al. Phase II multi-institutional trial of the histone deacetylase inhibitor romidepsin as monotherapy for patients with cutaneous T-cell lymphoma. J Clin Oncol 2009;27: 5410–7.

34. Piekarz RL, Robey RW, Zhan Z, et al. T-cell lymphoma as a model for the use of histone deacetylase inhibitors in cancer therapy: impact of depsipeptide on molecular markers, therapeutic targets, and mechanisms of resistance. Blood 2004; 103:4636–43.

35. Olsen E, Vonderheid E, Pimpinelli N, et al, ISCL/ EORTC. Revisions to the staging and classification of mycosis fungoides and Sezary syndrome: a proposal of the International Society for Cutaneous Lymphomas (ISCL) and the cutaneous lymphoma task force of the European Organization of Research and Treatment of Cancer (EORTC). Blood 2007;110: 1713–22.

36. Kim M, Thompson LA, Wenger SD, et al. Romidepsin: a histone deacetylase inhibitor for refractory cutaneous T-cell lymphoma. Ann Pharmacother 2012;46:1340–8.

37. Chowdhury S, Howell GM, Teggart CA, et al. Histone deacetylase inhibitor belinostat represses surviving expression through reactivation of transforming growth factor beta (TGFbeta) receptor II leading to cancer cell death J Biol Chem 2011;286:30937–48.

38. Poole RM. 1543-1554 Belinostat: first global approval. Drugs 2014;74:1543–54.

39. Foss F, Advani R, Duvic M, et al. Phase II trial of belinostat (PXD101) in patients with relapsed or refractory peripheral or cutaneous T-cell lymphoma. Br J Haematol 2015;168(6):811–9.

40. Zain JM, Foss F, Kelly WK, et al. Final results of a phase I study of oral belinostat (PXD101) in patients with lymphoma. J Clin Oncol 2009;27.

41. Kelly WK, Yap T, Lee J, et al. A phase I study of oral belinostat (PXD101) in patients with advanced solid tumors. J Clin Oncol 2007;25:299.

42. Sharma S, Beck J, Mita M, et al. A phase I dose-escalation study of intravenous panobinostat in patients with lymphoma and solid tumors. Invest New Drugs 2013;31:974–85.

43. Khot A, Dickinson M, Prince HM. Panobinostat in lymphoid and myeloid malignancies. Expert Opin Investig Drugs 2013;22(9):1211–23.

44. Duvic M, Dummer R, Becker JC, et al. Panobinostat activity in both bexarotene-exposed and -naïve patients with refractory cutaneous T-cell lymphoma: results of a phase II trial. Eur J Cancer 2013;42: 386–94.

Extracorporeal Photopheresis in the Treatment of Mycosis Fungoides and Sézary Syndrome

John A. Zic, MD

KEYWORDS

- Extracorporeal photopheresis • Cutaneous T-cell lymphoma • Sézary syndrome
- Mycosis fungoides • Photochemotherapy

KEY POINTS

- Extracorporeal photopheresis induces an immune response to mycosis fungoides (MF)/Sézary syndrome (SS).
- Extracorporeal photopheresis alone or in combination with other immunostimulatory agents leads to a response rate ranging from 40% to 60% in patients with various stages of MF/SS.
- Extracorporeal photopheresis is a safe procedure with few side effects and no induction of immunosuppression.

INTRODUCTION

Cutaneous T-cell lymphoma (CTCL) is a broad term describing cancers of the T cell whereby the skin is the primary organ of involvement. Although the disease was first recognized in 1806 by Alibert,[1] it was not until the 1970s when investigators discovered the T-cell origin of this malignancy.[2] Extracorporeal photopheresis (ECP) or photopheresis is one of many treatment modalities to treat the cutaneous T-cell lymphomas. It is unique among those treatment modalities, however, in that it is the only treatment, aside from allogeneic stem cell transplantation, that specifically induces an immune reaction directed against the malignant T cell.

ECP is an apheresis procedure whereby a leukocyte-enriched fraction of blood spiked with 8-methoxypsoralen (8-MOP) is exposed to a UV-A light source and then returned to patients. ECP is similar to the psoralen followed by UV-A exposure (PUVA) form of phototherapy in that both take advantage of the photoactivated drug 8-MOP and are classified as photochemotherapies. In 1988, the US Food and Drug Administration (FDA) approved the use of a new medical device for the treatment of CTCL. The UVAR instrument (Therakos Inc, Exton, PA) combined, for the first time, leukapheresis with a modified phototherapy chamber.

HISTORICAL ASPECTS

In 1921, J.F. Heymans[3] first published the concept of treating blood by exposing it to physical agents, such as cold, heat, or radiation, as it flows through an extracorporeal shunt. A better understanding of lymphocyte function and life span emerged in the late 1950s leading to the development of procedures to deplete the body of lymphocytes to study

Disclosure: No conflicts of interest.

Division of Dermatology, Vanderbilt University School of Medicine, 701 Thompson Ln, Ste 26300, Nashville, TN 37204, USA

E-mail address: john.zic@vanderbilt.edu

Dermatol Clin 33 (2015) 765–776
http://dx.doi.org/10.1016/j.det.2015.05.011
0733-8635/15/$ – see front matter Published by Elsevier Inc.

lymphocyte kinetics and ultimately treat disease.[4] In the early 1960s, Eugene Cronkite, MD, while at the Brookhaven National Laboratory in Upton, New York, developed an extracorporeal system using a venovenous shunt to expose whole blood to gamma rays generated by a [60]cobalt irradiator.[5] This modality, called extracorporeal irradiation of the blood (ECIB), was based on the difference between the radiosensitivity of lymphocytes and the radioresistance of erythrocytes.[6] By 1970, at least 150 patients with acute and chronic leukemias were treated with ECIB; but remissions were short lived.[7] Although most authorities thought only gamma radiation could kill activated lymphocytes and leukemic cells, a French team in the late 1960s led by J.L. Binet investigated the effects of using UV radiation (UVR) produced by mercury arc lamps.[8] Their UVR ECIB system was tested on lymphocyte function and ultimately in several patients with chronic lymphocytic leukemia leading to transient clinical remission.[9]

In the mid-1970s, Barbara Gilchrest and colleagues[10,11] at Massachusetts General Hospital discovered that PUVA phototherapy was effective in treating the early skin lesions of mycosis fungoides (MF), the most common subtype of CTCL. At about the same time, Richard L. Edelson,[12] MD, while at the National Cancer Institute, worked with colleagues to treat several patients with Sézary syndrome (SS) using leukapheresis to debulk the circulating tumor load of malignant T cells.[12] The question arose whether the malignant circulating lymphocytes in SS would respond to PUVA phototherapy if the energy could be directed at blood cells. Initial experiments performed in Edelson's laboratory found evidence that an anti-idiotypic response to disease-specific T-cell receptors could be found after exposing autoreactive T cells from rats to 8-MOP and UV-A in an ex vivo system inspired by Cohen and colleagues[13–15] at the Weizmann Institute. With the help of engineers at Therakos, Inc, a subsidiary of Johnson and Johnson, Edelson[16] designed a device that could expose a fraction of leukocyte-enriched blood, removed from patients after they had taken psoralen, to UV-A light in an extracorporeal system before returning the treated blood products back to the patients. After a promising phase I clinical trial, a multicenter clinical trial was performed from 1982 to 1986 testing the efficacy of ECP after ingestion of 8-MOP in the management of refractory erythrodermic patients with MF/SS. In 1987, the landmark report was published that found a significant response in 27 of 37 patients treated with ECP.[17]

In 2000, the FDA approved a sterile liquid formulation of 8-MOP to replace the oral formulation.

The liquid formulation (UVADEX) is added directly to the collection bag in the extracorporeal circuit, thus avoiding the gastrointestinal intolerance and unreliable blood levels of the oral formulation.[15] The latest fourth-generation photopheresis instrument, the CELLEX System (Therakos, Inc, Raritan, NJ), was approved in 2009 by the FDA and combines state-of-the-art cell collection, photoactivation, and reinfusion technologies in a single, integrated, closed system.[18]

MECHANISM OF ACTION

Despite the safe and effective use of ECP for more than 25 years, the precise mechanism of action continues to be explored. There is good evidence that ECP induces an immune-mediated response to the malignant T-cell clone.[17] This is supported, in part, by the clinical observation that, although less than 10% of the total population of white blood cells is treated during one ECP treatment, there is often a larger reduction of malignant T cells in the peripheral circulation.[19] The proposed mechanism of action involves the following processes: (1) the induction of apoptosis of malignant T cells, (2) the conversion of circulating monocytes to immature dendritic cells (DCs), (3) the presentation of tumor-loaded DCs to cytotoxic T cells, and (4) expansion of a population of cytotoxic T cells against the malignant T-cell clone.

Because they lack nuclei, the radioresistance of erythrocytes and platelets may be expected. However, the differences in the radiosensitivity of peripheral blood mononuclear cells (PBMCs) are more difficult to explain. Why are lymphocytes more radiosensitive than other peripheral blood mononuclear cells?[20,21] Also intriguing are the results of Spary and colleagues[22] demonstrating enhancement of the Th1 T-cell responses as a result of synergy between lower doses of ionizing radiation (0.6–2.4 Gy) and T-cell stimulation. Further studies are needed that focus on the impact of ECP (UV energy) on enhancement of Th1 T-cell responses of normal T cells. ECP and PUVA induce apoptosis in CD4+ and CD8+ lymphocytes but not monocytes, and the apoptosis is likely attributed to dysregulation in the expression of the apoptotic genes Bcl-2 and Bax.[23–26] But what about the surviving malignant T cells exposed to UV-A energy and psoralen? Studies using ionizing radiation demonstrate alteration in the biology of surviving tumor cells from patients with solid organ carcinomas, rendering them more susceptible to T cell–mediated killing possibly via increased cell-surface expression of calreticulin.[27]

It has been established that monocytes differentiate to immature DCs in the presence of interleukin (IL)-4 and granulocyte-macrophage colony stimulating factor (GM-CSF).[28] In 2001, Berger and colleagues[29] published their observation of the conversion of monocytes to immature DCs during overnight incubation in gas-permeable bags of ECP-treated leukocytes from 5 patients with refractory CTCL. Further observations confirmed that both the initial leukapheresis step and subsequent passage through the narrow plastic photoactivation plate initiated and contributed to the monocyte to immature dendritic cell differentiation. Edelson proposed that the frequent encounters of monocytes with the plastic surface of the photoactivation plate activated the cells to begin differentiation to immature DCs.[30] The adsorption of fibronectin on the photoactivation plate may be a convincing candidate for influencing monocyte biology during ECP and participating in the early events of monocyte-to-DC conversion.[31] Recently, Berger and colleagues[32] demonstrated that ECP-derived DCs are maturationally synchronized and show a reproducible distinctive molecular signature, common to ECP-processed monocytes from normal subjects and those from patients.

There are 2 major subsets of DCs in human peripheral blood: myeloid (mDC) and plasmacytoid (pDC).[33] It is known that mDCs primarily polarize naïve T cells toward a Th1 phenotype, whereas pDCs primarily result in a Th2/Treg phenotype.[34] Recently, Shiue and colleagues[35] found increased mDC populations, increased mDC/pDC ratios, and upregulation of HLA-DR expression on DCs following ECP in two-thirds of patients with MF and B1/B2 blood stage or SS. Their results suggest that ECP treatment is associated with favorable mDC modulation.

Inducing a Th1 phenotype produces a cell-mediated T-cell response capable of launching a cytotoxic T-cell response against a malignant clone. Clinical improvements after ECP in patients with MF/SS are associated with a shift from Th2 to IL-12/Th1 phenotype.[36]

Using an animal model of ECP, investigators identified the induction of a CD8+ T-cell response against expanded clones of pathogenic T cells.[14] Moor and Schmitt[37] demonstrated increased synthesis of class I major histocompatibility complex molecules on the surface of a murine T-cell lymphoma line after exposure to UV-A and 8-MOP. In addition, Berger and colleagues[38] used monoclonal antibodies and magnetic bead technology to demonstrate a tumor-specific cytolytic CD8+ T-cell response to distinctive class I–associated peptides on the surface of CTCL tumor cells in blood samples from 4 ECP patients with advanced CTCL. These data support the assertion that ECP exerts its immunologic effects by stimulating a tumor-specific CD8 T-cell response triggered by a population of tumor-loaded DCs after the ECP procedure.

To summarize: In patients with MF/SS and significant blood involvement, ECP treatment not only induces apoptosis of malignant Th2/Treg cells but also induces more mDCs, creates a proinflammatory environment for DCs to activate, and further stimulates Th1/cytotoxic T cells and immune responses.[35]

PHARMACOKINETICS

8-MOP or methoxsalen is a furocoumarin with photoactivating properties. Methoxsalen, on photoactivation, conjugates and forms covalent bonds with DNA, which lead to the formation of both monofunctional (addition to a single strand of DNA) and bifunctional (crosslinking of psoralen to both strands of DNA) adducts.[39] Reactions with proteins have also been described. The formation of photoadducts results in inhibition of DNA synthesis, cell division, and epidermal turnover.[39] Liquid methoxsalen (UVADEX 20 mcg/mL) is administered in a dose of 0.017 mL per 1 mL of pheresed leukocyte volume.[18] The total dose of methoxsalen delivered in UVADEX is substantially less than (approximately 200 times) that used with oral administration. More than 80% of blood samples collected 30 minutes after reinfusion of the photoactivated cells had methoxsalen levels less than the detection limits of the assay (<10 ng/mL).[40]

Just and colleagues[41] explored the trafficking of the treated leukocytes following ECP using radioactively labeled leucocytes and monitoring with whole-body scintigraphy. Comparison of distribution patterns showed that PBMCs and neutrophils have different kinetic patterns after intravenous reinjection. The most prominent difference was immediate retention of PBMCs but not of neutrophils in the lungs corresponding to a signal 3 times more intense. After 24 hours, more than 80% of both cell populations could be detected in the liver and spleen.

TYPICAL REGIMEN

For patients with MF/SS, the typical ECP regimen is one treatment on 2 consecutive days every 4 weeks. Since FDA approval of ECP in 1988, there has been minor variability in the 2-day cycle every 4 weeks in the treatment of MF/SS. Duvic and colleagues[42] found no increased response rate using an accelerated regimen of one 2-day cycle every 2 weeks to treat a small cohort of patients with MF/SS. More recently, Siakantaris and colleagues[43] from Greece published their retrospective experience (N = 18) using an accelerated treatment schedule of one cycle of ECP every week for 1 month, followed by 1 cycle of ECP every 2 weeks for 2 months, and then one cycle of ECP every month. The overall response rate of 61% compares quite favorably with previously published response rates of patients with MF/SS treated with ECP combined with other systemic therapies.

The European Dermatology Forum's guidelines on the use of ECP published in January 2014 recommends the following ECP schedule for the treatment of MF/SS: 1 cycle every 2 weeks for the first 3 months then once monthly or every 3 weeks.[44] The investigators note, however, that there is no clear optimal therapy; other published guidelines, including the UK consensus statement on the use of ECP,[45] have recommended 1 cycle every 2 to 4 weeks followed by tapering after maximum response.[44]

Each ECP procedure varies between 2 and 3 hours in length based on several factors, including venous access, blood flow, hemoglobin concentrations, and technical issues. Most centers achieve peripheral access using one 16-gauge or 18-gauge needle inserted into the antecubital vein though central venous catheters, or specialized subcutaneous ports (eg, Vortex AngioDynamics, Latham, NY) that allow for rapid reverse flow during the blood collection phase of the procedure may also be used.[46]

RESPONSE TO THERAPY

The efficacy of ECP has been reported in more than 500 patients worldwide. Most of these reports have been small to medium size case series. There are no randomized controlled clinical trials demonstrating the efficacy of photopheresis as monotherapy in the treatment of MF/SS. Despite this, several national and international organizations have listed photopheresis as first-, second-, or third-line therapy for various stages of MF/SS.

The clinical data support the use of ECP to treat patients with erythrodermic MF ($T_4N_{0-3}M0B_1$) with at least some atypical circulating lymphocytes or SS ($T_4N_{0-3}M0B_2$), which requires significant blood involvement for diagnosis. The clinical data do not support the use of ECP to treat patients with tumor stage MF. There is some clinical data to support the use of photopheresis to treat early stage patients with MF, especially those that have at least some atypical circulating lymphocytes.

EARLY STAGE MYCOSIS FUNGOIDES

After ECP was FDA approved in 1988, several reports emerged of patients with early stage MF

responding to ECP often combined with other treatment modalities.[47–50] Zic and colleagues[48,49] at Vanderbilt reported preliminary and long-term follow-up data on a cohort of 20 refractory patients with MF/SS treated with ECP and adjunctive therapies. This cohort included 14 treatment-refractory patients with early stage disease (T2). Nine of 14 (64%) achieved an objective response (OR) in the skin (greater than 50% clearing of skin lesions) with 4 complete responses (CRs). For the 7 patients who at some point in their treatment achieved a CR, the median time to clearing was 11 months. For the 7 patients weaned from ECP, the mean relapse-free interval was approximately 45 months (range, 20–64 months, 2 relapses). Another important observation was that patients who responded within 6 to 8 months after starting ECP maintained their response over time.[49]

In 2004, Child and colleagues[51] published the results of a randomized crossover study comparing PUVA and ECP in the treatment of 20 patients with plaque stage (T2) MF who had a detectable peripheral blood T-cell clone. Eight patients completed the study. Although PUVA was more effective than ECP in improving skin scores, neither treatment modality cleared malignant T cells from the peripheral blood.

In a retrospective analysis of patients treated with ECP combined with adjuvant therapies, Siakantaris and colleagues[43] from Greece reported a response rate of 40% (2 of 5) in patients with early stage MF as compared with a response rate of 62% (9 of 13) in patients with advanced MF/SS.

Recently, a prospective, open-label, single-arm, multicenter, investigator-initiated pilot study was completed to assess the response to ECP in patients with early stage MF (stages IA–IIA).[52] The UVAR XTS Photopheresis System (Therakos, Inc Raritan, NJ) was used to administer ECP for 2 consecutive days once monthly for 12 months. Patients who did not respond after 6 months of ECP were treated adjunctively with oral bexarotene (150 mg/m^2) alone or combined with interferon (IFN) alfa (1–3 million units 3 times per week). Patients with stage IA disease were only enrolled if they showed evidence of minor blood abnormality by flow cytometry assessment (B1). The primary end point was a skin involvement response assessed monthly by using the modified severity weighted assessment tool (mSWAT) assessment tool (partial response [PR] >50% improvement in mSWAT). A total of 19 patients with early stage MF (IA = 3, IB = 14, IIA = 2) were enrolled. Eight of the 12 patients who were treated with ECP monotherapy responded (67%, 2 CR), and 4 of the 7 patients who received combination therapy responded (57%, 0 CR). The overall response rate for the entire cohort (12 of 19) was 63.1%. However, if the 7 patients requiring combination therapy are considered ECP treatment failures, then the overall response rate for ECP alone was 42% (8 of 19). The median time to response was 4 months (3–8 months), and the median duration of response was 6.5 months (1–48 months). Also, quality-of-life measurements indicated an improvement in emotional scores over time.[52]

Current National Comprehensive Cancer Network (NCCN) guidelines for non-Hodgkin lymphoma (NHL) (Version 5.2014) do not recommend ECP as primary treatment in early stage MF (IA, IB, IIA). However, in patients with stage IA, IB, and IIA disease and B1 blood involvement or those with treatment refractory disease, ECP is listed as a systemic treatment option along with retinoids, IFNs, histone deacetylase inhibitors, and methotrexate.[53] The European Dermatology Forum published guidelines on the use of ECP in January 2014. The consensus decision was that ECP should only be considered in patients with early stage MF for clinical trial purposes as a variety of other safe, effective, and easily accessible treatment options are available for use at these stages.[44]

TUMOR STAGE MYCOSIS FUNGOIDES

ECP should not be considered a primary treatment option in patients with tumor stage MF (stage IIB). In 15 patients extracted from the literature with skin stage T3 (tumor stage), no patient responded to photopheresis.[49,50,54,55] One retrospective study examined the use of ECP or chemotherapy as a maintenance adjuvant treatment regimen in patients with tumor stage MF (N = 41) or erythrodermic MF/SS (N = 21) who had achieved a CR from total skin electron beam radiotherapy (TSEB).[56] The difference between overall survival for those who received ECP (100% at 3 years) versus those who received no adjuvant therapy (50% at 3 years) approached statistical significance ($P<.06$), whereas significant survival benefit from the addition of chemotherapy (75% at 3 years) for TSEB CRs was not observed. Neither adjuvant therapy provided benefit with respect to relapse-free survival after TSEB.[56]

ERYTHRODERMIC MYCOSIS FUNGOIDES AND SÉZARY SYNDROME

Erythrodermic CTCL may be divided into erythrodermic MF (stage III, $T_4N_{0-2}M_0B_{0-1}$) and SS (stage $IVA_{1\ or\ 2}$, $T_4N_{0-3}M_0B_2$). Although there is considerable variability in the presentation and prognosis of patients with erythrodermic MF/SS, photopheresis is considered the first-line treatment by most experts. The publication of the landmark article in 1987 by Edelson and colleagues[17] established the safety and efficacy of ECP in 22 of 29 erythrodermic patients with MF/SS. Since then, the responses of more than 518 ECP-treated patients with erythrodermic MF/SS have been published and summarized with a wide range of response rates from 33% to 74%.[44,57] Many of these patients were treated with photopheresis in combination with other therapies. In addition, none of the patients were part of prospective randomized controlled clinical trials.

The United States Cutaneous Lymphoma Consortium (USCLC) recently published guidelines for the treatment of SS.[58] In this review 118 patients with SS treated with ECP as monotherapy were extracted from the literature based on clearly defined criteria and an overall response rate defined as at least 50% clearing. Of these 118 patients, 28 (24%) responded to ECP monotherapy and 11 patients achieved a CR (9%). Higher response rates were seen in patients who received ECP in combination with other therapies (**Fig. 1**). ECP was recommended by the USCLC as one of the primary (category A) systemic monotherapies for the treatment of SS (II-2 evidence: ≥ 1 prospective, well-designed cohort or case-controlled study, preferably >1 center or research group). Others in this category included IFN alfa, bexarotene, low-dose methotrexate, and denileukin diftitox plus corticosteroids.[58]

Based on ECP data from 1987 to 2001, the British Photodermatology Group and United Kingdom Skin Lymphoma Group published their report in 2006 on evidence-based practice of ECP.[59] The investigators concluded that there was fair evidence of clinical benefit in erythrodermic MF/SS from ECP (B level recommendation [A to E], II-i evidence [non-randomized controlled trials]).

Based on category 2A evidence (lower-level evidence and uniform NCCN consensus that the intervention is appropriate), current NCCN guidelines for NHL (version .5.2014) do recommend ECP as one of the primary treatments for SS and erythrodermic MF with B1 blood stage but not for patients with erythrodermic MF with no evidence of blood involvement (B0).[53] In contrast, the European Dermatology Forum's guidelines recommend ECP as first-line therapy for all patients with T4 skin stage regardless of blood and lymph node involvement and patients with T1/T2 skin stage with B2 blood involvement according to the revised International Society for Cutaneous Lymphomas (ISCL)/European Organization of Research and Treatment of Cancer (EORTC)

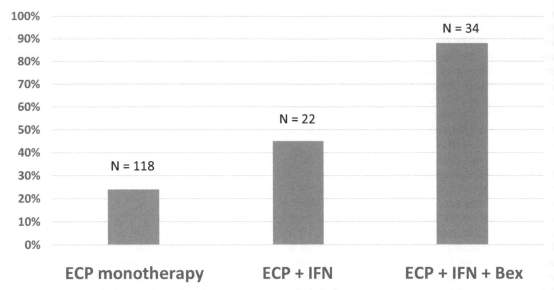

Fig. 1. Estimated pooled response rates for patients with SS to ECP monotherapy, ECP + IFN alfa or gamma, and ECP + IFN + bexarotene capsules (Bex). N = number of patients extracted from the literature with a clear definition of SS and an overall response rate defined as 50% or greater clearing of skin. (*Data from* Olsen EA, Rook AH, Zic J, et al. Sezary syndrome: immunopathogenesis, literature review of therapeutic options, and recommendations for therapy by the United States Cutaneous Lymphoma Consortium (USCLC). J Am Acad Dermatol 2011;64(2):352–404.)

staging.[60] The American Society for Apheresis also categorized ECP as an accepted first-line therapy for erythrodermic MF/SS as a primary stand-alone treatment or in conjunction with other modes of treatment.[61]

EXTRACORPOREAL PHOTOPHERESIS AND ADJUNCTIVE THERAPIES

Most patients with MF/SS treated with ECP receive adjunctive therapies, especially IFN alfa and bexarotene capsules. There is evidence to support higher response rates when ECP is combined with adjunctive therapies. In one report, ECP monotherapy showed a 40% response rate in patients with stage III/IV MF/SS in contrast to a 57% response rate in those treated with a combination of ECP plus IFN alfa, bexarotene, or GM-CSF.[62] In a retrospective review of 98 patients with SS treated with ECP (>3 months) and 1 or more systemic immunostimulatory agents (IFN gamma, IFN alfa, GM-CSF, systemic retinoids), Raphael and colleagues[63] at the University of Pennsylvania reported a significant improvement in 73 patients (75%) with 29 CRs (30%).

There are retrospective and small cohort data to support the combination of photopheresis and IFN in the treatment of erythrodermic CTCL. In the USCLC review of SS in which all patients so reported had to meet the criteria of T4B2 staging and an overall response rate defined as at least 50% clearing of disease, 10 of 22 patients treated with ECP and IFN alfa (45.4%) responded, including 4 patients who achieved a CR (18.2%) (see **Fig. 1**).[58] In the only published prospective randomized trial of IFN versus IFN and ECP, 20 patients with MF/SS stages IA to IVB were treated with IFN 3 to 18 million units (MU) daily intramuscularly versus same-dosing IFN plus ECP 2 days per month. Two of the 9 patients (22%) assigned to the combination arm had an OR versus 4 of the 11 patients (36%) assigned to the IFN alone arm, including one CR.[64] Thus there was no advantage to adding ECP to IFN alone in this small study.

The combination of ECP, IFN alfa/gamma, and bexarotene capsules may lead to the highest response rates in patients with SS. In the USCLC review of the 34 patients with SS treated with ECP, IFN, and bexarotene, 30 of 34 (88.2%) responded to the combined therapy, including 11 patients with a CR (32.4%) (see **Fig. 1**).[58] Bexarotene dosages ranged from 75 mg to 450 mg by mouth per day. IFN alfa dosages ranged from 1.5 MU to 6 MU subcutaneous injections 3 to 5 times weekly. IFN gamma dosages ranged from 40 mcg to 100 mcg subcutaneous injections 3 to 5 times weekly.[58]

In contrast to these pooled results, Polansky and colleagues[65] at the M.D. Anderson Cancer

Center recently reported the results of 18 of 217 patients with SS who had achieved long-term CR of greater than 1 year: 3 CRs were achieved with combined immunomodulatory therapy (ECP, IFN alfa, and/or retinoids), 13 CRs were achieved after allogeneic stem cell transplantation, one CR with alemtuzumab, and one CR with mogamulizumab.

PREDICTORS OF RESPONSE

In a small cohort of 21 patients with MF/SS treated with ECP as monotherapy for at least 6 months, the following baseline blood parameters were associated with a favorable clinical response: lower percentage of Sézary cells (32% vs 54% lymphocytes) and a higher absolute eosinophil count (388/mm^3 vs 87/mm^3). Comparison of cytokines, gene transcripts, and other laboratory measures of disease did not correlate with the subsequent clinical response.[66] In a more recent analysis of microRNA (miR) levels on a subset of this cohort (n = 13), McGirt and colleagues[67] discovered that an early increase of PBMC miR-191, miR-223, and miR-342 at 3 months into ECP monotherapy predicted a clinical response to ECP at 6 and 12 months.

In a large cohort of patients (n = 98) with SS treated with ECP and immunostimulatory agents, Raphael and colleagues[63] found the following baseline differences in the CR group as compared with the nonresponse group: lower CD4/CD8 ratio (13.2 vs 44.2), lower median percentage of CD4+/CD26− cells (27.4% vs 57.2%), lower median percentage of CD4+/CD7− cells (20.0% vs 41.3%), and higher median monocyte percentage (9.5% vs 7.3%). There were no differences between the group with PR when compared with the nonresponse group.

Other factors that have been reported to predict response to ECP have been recently summarized.[57,68] They include relatively low tumor load of malignant T cells in the blood, lymph nodes, and skin; peripheral blood involvement; relatively intact immune system; erythroderma; and plaques covering less than 10% to 15% of the total skin surface[68] (Table 1).

SURVIVAL

The impact of ECP alone or ECP in combination with other therapies on the survival of patients with erythrodermic MF/SS remains to be confirmed with a prospective study. A follow-up analysis of the original cohort of Edelson and colleagues[69] was published in 1992 showing that the median survival for patients who received ECP was 60 months. Gottlieb and colleagues[47] and Zic and colleagues[49] reported similar median survivals in their respective cohorts of ECP-treated patients with MF/SS. In 2012, Knobler and colleagues[70] used ISCL/EORTC criteria to reevaluate the original cohort of 39 patients in the 1987 pivotal trial by Edelson and colleagues[17] with a median follow-up of 71.6 months in this cohort; the median overall survival for a subgroup of 26 patients with erythroderma was 76.9 months from diagnosis.

Fraser-Andrews and colleagues[71] published a retrospective historical control study comparing the survival of a cohort of 44 patients with SS separated into 3 groups: ECP treated 1991 to 1996 (n = 29, median survival 39 months), no ECP treatment 1991 to 1996 (n = 8, median survival 22 months), and no ECP treatment before 1991 (n = 7, median survival 26.5 months). In contrast to the previously published survival data at that time, this study showed no statistically significant difference between the groups and did not support the contention that ECP prolongs survival in patients with SS. In a letter to the editor, Stevens and colleagues[72] argued that this study had low statistical power and an inadequate treatment regimen for proper comparison.

ADVERSE EFFECTS

ECP is well tolerated with rare grade III-IV systemic toxicities reported in the literature and no reports of immunosuppression. In a recent series of 51 patients with erythrodermic MF/SS treated with ECP, the following adverse effects were reported using the National Cancer Institute Common Toxicity Criteria system: transient grade I hypotension (12%), grade I-II anemia (6%), hypokalemia (4%), and 1 urticarial eruption interpreted as a drug reaction to either 8-MOP or heparin.[57] Discomfort and mild hematomas at venipuncture sites are not uncommon and can be relieved with pressure bandages and ice compresses.[17] To avoid catheter-related infections, intermittent peripheral venous access is preferred over indwelling catheters because of the high rate of Staphylococcus aureus colonization on the skin in patients with erythrodermic MF/SS. Transient low-grade fever and increased erythroderma have been observed in some patients within 6 to 8 hours of reinfusion of the photoactivated leukocyte-enriched blood.[18] Nausea was a common side effect to the oral formulation of 8-MOP but has now been eliminated with the introduction of the liquid formulation directly injected into the collection bag.[15] A single case of grade III anemia was reported in a patient with SS undergoing treatment with bexarotene and ECP caused by undiagnosed cold agglutinin disease, which was suspected when agglutinated blood was noted in the centrifuge bowl of the photopheresis device.[73]

Table 1
Baseline predictors of response to photopheresis

Low Tumor Load of Malignant T Cells		
Skin	Erythroderma[a]	Quaglino et al,[57] 2013; Knobler et al,[44] 2014
	Plaques <10%–15% total skin surface	Atta et al,[68] 2012; Knobler et al,[44] 2014
Blood	Lower percentage of elevated circulating Sézary cells	Heald et al,[69] 1992; Raphael et al,[63] 2011; McGirt et al,[66] 2010
	Lower CD4/CD8 ratio <10–15	Heald et al,[69] 1992; Knobler et al,[74] 2002; Raphael et al,[63] 2011; Quaglino et al,[57] 2013
	Lower % CD4+CD7− <30%	Stevens et al,[75] 2002; Raphael et al,[63] 2011
	Lower % CD4+CD26− <30%	Raphael et al,[63] 2011
	Normal LDH levels	Knobler et al,[74] 2002; Quaglino et al,[57] 2013
	B0 or B1 blood stage	Quaglino et al,[57] 2013
	Lymphocyte count <20,000/μl	Atta et al,[68] 2012
Lymph nodes	Lack of bulky adenopathy	Atta et al,[68] 2012
Visceral organs	Lack of visceral organ involvement	Atta et al,[68] 2012
Peripheral Blood Involvement	B1 blood stage >B2 blood stage[60]	Quaglino et al,[57] 2013; Evans et al,[76] 2001; Atta et al,[68] 2012
	Presence of a discrete number of Sézary cells (10%–20% mononuclear cells)	Knobler et al,[44] 2014
Relatively Intact Immune System	Higher % monocytes >9%	Raphael et al,[63] 2011
	Increased eosinophil count >300/mm³	McGirt et al,[66] 2010
	No previous intense chemotherapy	Zic,[18] 2012; Atta et al,[68] 2012
	Short disease duration before ECP (<2 y from diagnosis)	Atta et al,[68] 2012; Quaglino et al,[57] 2013
	↑ NK cell count at 6 mo into ECP therapy	Prinz et al,[77] 1995; Quaglino et al,[57] 2013
	Near-normal NK cell activity	Knobler et al,[44] 2014
	Normal CD3+CD8+ cell count >200/mm³	Quaglino et al,[57] 2013
Other Monitored Factors		
PBMC miR levels	↑ miR-191, ↑ miR-223, ↑ miR-342 at 3 mo into ECP monotherapy	McGirt et al,[67] 2014
Soluble interleukin-2 receptor	↓ sIL-2R at 6 mo into ECP	Rao et al,[78] 2006
Neopterin	↓ Neopterin at 6 mo into ECP	Rao et al,[78] 2006
Beta²-microglobulin	↓ Beta²-microglobulin at 6 mo into ECP	Rao et al,[78] 2006
Response at 5–6 mo of ECP	Predicts durable response and long-term survival	Stevens et al,[75] 2002; Zic et al,[49] 1996

Abbreviations: LDH, lactate dehydrogenase; NK, natural killer; sIL-2R, soluble interleukin-2 receptor.
[a] Patients with erythrodermic MF/SS often show fewer malignant T cells in skin biopsies than T3 and T2 skin stages.

PEARLS TO HELP THE MANAGEMENT OF PATIENTS WITH MYCOSIS FUNGOIDES/ SÉZARY SYNDROME BEING TREATED WITH EXTRACORPOREAL PHOTOPHERESIS

As with any therapy, patient selection is important. It is important to set patient expectations at the beginning of ECP treatment. Patients rarely obtain a rapid response to ECP; they should, therefore, be told that it may take at least 6 to 8 months of treatment to see a significant response. Patients who tend to respond best to ECP are those with erythrodermic variants (T4 MF or SS), including patients that one suspects are evolving into SS.

Patients who have many predictive factors for response can initiate ECP as monotherapy. If patients do not show a significant response by 6 to 8 months of ECP (stable disease), then the author recommends adding adjunctive therapies (IFN, bexarotene) or switching to an alternative therapy. If patients show progressive disease, then the author would add or switch therapies sooner. In contrast, patients with fewer predictive factors for response, especially those with SS and lymphadenopathy, should be treated up front with combination immunotherapy (ECP, IFN alfa or gamma, bexarotene). If patients do not show a significant response by 6 to 8 months of ECP, the author recommends stopping ECP and switching to an alternative systemic therapy.

Venous access can be a challenge for heavily pretreated patients and older patients. To increase the caliber of the antecubital veins, the author recommends instructing patients to squeeze rubber balls with both hands as a daily exercise.

SUMMARY

In the setting of MF/SS, photopheresis leads to an expansion of peripheral blood DC populations and an enhanced TH1 immune response. ECP is a first-line therapy for erythrodermic MF/SS based on the excellent side effect profile and moderate efficacy in the treatment of patients with T4 (erythroderma) skin stage. Patients with erythrodermic MF/SS are most likely to respond to ECP when they have a measurable but low blood tumor burden. The addition of adjunctive immunostimulatory agents seems to increase the response to ECP. There may be a role for the treatment of refractory early stage MF with ECP, though data are limited. Further studies are needed not only to clarify the mechanism of action of ECP to better optimize therapy but also to maximize the response for patients with advanced MF/SS.

REFERENCES

1. Alibert JL. Description des Maladies de la Peau: observees a l'Hospital St louis et Exposition des Meilleurs Methodes Suivies pour leur Traitement. Paris: Barrois l'aine et Fil; 1806.
2. Broome JD, Zucker-Franklin D, Weiner MS, et al. Leukemic cells with membrane properties of thymus-derived (T) lymphocytes in a case of Sezary's syndrome: morphologic and immunologic studies. Clin Immunol Immunopathol 1973;1(3):319–29.
3. Heymans JF. Iso, hyper et hypothermisation des mammiferes par calorification et frigorification du sang de la circulation carotid-jugulaire anastomosee. Arch Int Pharmacodyn 1921;25:1–5.
4. Cronkite EP. Extracorporeal irradiation of the blood and lymph in the treatment of leukemia and for immunosuppression. Ann Intern Med 1967;67(2):415–23.
5. Cronkite EP, Jansen CR, Mather GC, et al. Studies on lymphocytes. I. Lymphopenia produced by prolonged extracorporeal irradiation of the circulation of the blood. Blood 1962;20:203–8.
6. Schiffer LM, Chanana AD, Cronkite EP, et al. Extracorporeal irradiation of the blood. Semin Hematol 1966;3(2):154–67.
7. Schiffer LM, Chanana AD, Cronkite EP, et al. Lymphocyte kinetics in chronic lymphocytic leukaemia (CLL) studied by ECIB. Br J Haematol 1969;17(4):408.
8. Binet JL, Villeneuve B, Rapenbusch RV, et al. [Extracorporeal radiation of the blood by ultraviolet rays]. Nouv Rev Fr Hematol 1968;8(5):733–44 [in French].
9. Binet JL, Villeneuve B, Vaugier G, et al. Extracorporeal irradiation of blood by ultra-violet light in four cases of chronic lymphocytic leukaemia. Br J Haematol 1969;17(4):406.
10. Gilchrest BA. Methoxsalen photochemotherapy for mycosis fungoides. Cancer Treat Rep 1979;63(4):663–7.
11. Gilchrest BA, Parrish JA, Tanenbaum L, et al. Oral methoxsalen photochemotherapy of mycosis fungoides. Cancer 1976;38(2):683–9.
12. Edelson RL. Recent advances in the cutaneous T cell lymphomas. Bull Cancer 1977;64(2):209–24.
13. Ben-Nun A, Wekerle H, Cohen IR. Vaccination against autoimmune encephalomyelitis with T-lymphocyte line cells reactive against myelin basic protein. Nature 1981;292(5818):60–1.
14. Perez MI, Edelson RL, John L, et al. Inhibition of anti-skin allograft immunity induced by infusions with photoinactivated effector T lymphocytes (PET cells). Yale J Biol Med 1989;62(6):595–609.
15. Trautinger F, Just U, Knobler R. Photopheresis (extracorporeal photochemotherapy). Photochem Photobiol Sci 2013;12(1):22–8.
16. Edelson RL. Mechanistic insights into extracorporeal photochemotherapy: efficient induction of monocyte-to-dendritic cell maturation. Transfus Apher Sci 2014;50(3):322–9.
17. Edelson R, Berger C, Gasparro F, et al. Treatment of cutaneous T-cell lymphoma by extracorporeal photochemotherapy. Preliminary results. N Engl J Med 1987;316(6):297–303.
18. Zic JA. Photopheresis in the treatment of cutaneous T-cell lymphoma: current status. Curr Opin Oncol 2012;24(Suppl 1):S1–10.
19. Edelson RL. Photopheresis: a new therapeutic concept. Yale J Biol Med 1989;62(6):565–77.
20. Heylmann D, Rodel F, Kindler T, et al. Radiation sensitivity of human and murine peripheral blood lymphocytes, stem and progenitor cells. Biochim Biophys Acta 2014;1846(1):121–9.

21. Nichols WS, Troup GM, Anderson RE. Radiosensitivity of sensitized and nonsensitized human lymphocytes evaluated in vitro. Am J Pathol 1975; 79(3):499–508.

22. Spary LK, Al-Taei S, Salimu J, et al. Enhancement of T cell responses as a result of synergy between lower doses of radiation and T cell stimulation. J Immunol 2014;192(7):3101–10.

23. Bladon J, Taylor PC. Extracorporeal photopheresis induces apoptosis in the lymphocytes of cutaneous T-cell lymphoma and graft-versus-host disease patients. Br J Haematol 1999;107(4):707–11.

24. Bladon J, Taylor PC. Lymphocytes treated by extracorporeal photopheresis demonstrate a drop in the Bcl-2/Bax ratio: a possible mechanism involved in extracorporeal-photopheresis-induced apoptosis. Dermatology 2002;204(2):104–7.

25. Bladon J, Taylor PC. Extracorporeal photopheresis in cutaneous T-cell lymphoma and graft-versus-host disease induces both immediate and progressive apoptotic processes. Br J Dermatol 2002; 146(1):59–68.

26. Enomoto DN, Schellekens PT, Yong SL, et al. Extracorporeal photochemotherapy (photopheresis) induces apoptosis in lymphocytes: a possible mechanism of action of PUVA therapy. Photochem Photobiol 1997;65(1):177–80.

27. Gameiro SR, Jammeh ML, Wattenberg MM, et al. Radiation-induced immunogenic modulation of tumor enhances antigen processing and calreticulin exposure, resulting in enhanced T-cell killing. Oncotarget 2014;5(2):403–16.

28. Santini SM, Lapenta C, Logozzi M, et al. Type I interferon as a powerful adjuvant for monocyte-derived dendritic cell development and activity in vitro and in Hu-PBL-SCID mice. J Exp Med 2000;191(10): 1777–88.

29. Berger CL, Xu AL, Hanlon D, et al. Induction of human tumor-loaded dendritic cells. Int J Cancer 2001;91(4):438–47.

30. Edelson RL. Cutaneous T cell lymphoma: the helping hand of dendritic cells. Ann N Y Acad Sci 2001;941:1–11.

31. Gonzalez AL, Berger CL, Remington J, et al. Integrin-driven monocyte to dendritic cell conversion in modified extracorporeal photochemotherapy. Clin Exp Immunol 2014;175(3):449–57.

32. Berger C, Hoffmann K, Vasquez JG, et al. Rapid generation of maturationally synchronized human dendritic cells: contribution to the clinical efficacy of extracorporeal photochemotherapy. Blood 2010; 116(23):4838–47.

33. Ni X, Duvic M. Dendritic cells and cutaneous T-cell lymphomas. G Ital Dermatol Venereol 2011;146(2): 103–13.

34. Kadowaki N. Dendritic cells: a conductor of T cell differentiation. Allergol Int 2007;56(3):193–9.

35. Shiue LH, Alousi AM, Wei C, et al. Augmentation of blood dendritic cells by extracorporeal photopheresis in patients with leukemic cutaneous T-cell lymphoma and graft-versus-host disease. J Invest Dermatol 2013;133(8):2098–100.

36. Di Renzo M, Rubegni P, De Aloe G, et al. Extracorporeal photochemotherapy restores Th1/Th2 imbalance in patients with early stage cutaneous T-cell lymphoma. Immunology 1997;92(1):99–103.

37. Moor AC, Schmitt IM. Beijersbergen van Henegouwen GM, Chimenti S, Edelson RL, Gasparro FP. Treatment with 8-MOP and UVA enhances MHC class I synthesis in RMA cells: preliminary results. J Photochem Photobiol B 1995;29(2–3):193–8.

38. Berger CL, Wang N, Christensen I, et al. The immune response to class I-associated tumor-specific cutaneous T-cell lymphoma antigens. J Invest Dermatol 1996;107(3):392–7.

39. Gasparro FP, Chan G, Edelson RL. Phototherapy and photopharmacology. Yale J Biol Med 1985; 58(6):519–34.

40. Balogh A, Merkel U, Looks A, et al. Plasma and buffy coat concentration of 8-methoxypsoralen in patients treated with extracorporeal photopheresis. Exp Toxicol Pathol 1998;50(4–6):397–401.

41. Just U, Dimou E, Knobler R, et al. Leucocyte scintigraphy with 111In-oxine for assessment of cell trafficking after extracorporeal photopheresis. Exp Dermatol 2012;21(6):443–7.

42. Duvic M, Hagemeister F, Hester J. Accelerated delivery of extracorporeal photopheresis in patients with cutaneous T-cell lymphoma. J Invest Dermatol 1989;92:423.

43. Siakantaris MP, Tsirigotis P, Stavroyianni N, et al. Management of cutaneous T-cell lymphoma patients with extracorporeal photopheresis. The Hellenic experience. Transfus Apher Sci 2012;46(2):189–93.

44. Knobler R, Berlin G, Calzavara-Pinton P, et al. Guidelines on the use of extracorporeal photopheresis. J Eur Acad Dermatol Venereol 2014;28(Suppl 1): 1–37.

45. Scarisbrick JJ, Taylor P, Holtick U, et al. U.K. consensus statement on the use of extracorporeal photopheresis for treatment of cutaneous T-cell lymphoma and chronic graft-versus-host disease. Br J Dermatol 2008;158(4):659–78.

46. Marques MB, Adamski J. Extracorporeal photopheresis: technique, established and novel indications. J Clin Apher 2014;29(4):228–34.

47. Gottlieb SL, Wolfe JT, Fox FE, et al. Treatment of cutaneous T-cell lymphoma with extracorporeal photopheresis monotherapy and in combination with recombinant interferon alfa: a 10-year experience at a single institution. J Am Acad Dermatol 1996;35(6): 946–57.

48. Zic J, Arzubiaga C, Salhany KE, et al. Extracorporeal photopheresis for the treatment of cutaneous T-cell

lymphoma [see comments]. J Am Acad Dermatol 1992;27(5 Pt 1):729–36.

49. Zic JA, Stricklin GP, Greer JP, et al. Long-term follow-up of patients with cutaneous T-cell lymphoma treated with extracorporeal photochemotherapy. J Am Acad Dermatol 1996;35(6):935–45.

50. Vonderheid EC, Zhang Q, Lessin SR, et al. Use of serum soluble interleukin-2 receptor levels to monitor the progression of cutaneous T-cell lymphoma. J Am Acad Dermatol 1998;38(2 Pt 1):207–20.

51. Child FJ, Mitchell TJ, Whittaker SJ, et al. A randomized cross-over study to compare PUVA and extracorporeal photopheresis in the treatment of plaque stage (T2) mycosis fungoides. Clin Exp Dermatol 2004;29(3):231–6.

52. Talpur R, Demierre MF, Geskin L, et al. Multicenter photopheresis intervention trial in early-stage mycosis fungoides. Clin Lymphoma Myeloma Leuk 2011;11(2):219–27.

53. NCCN clinical practice guidelines: non-Hodgkins lymphoma. 2014. Available at: http://www.nccn.org/professionals/physician_gls/f_guidelines.asp#site. Accessed December 12, 2014.

54. Heald PW, Perez MI, Christensen I, et al. Photopheresis therapy of cutaneous T-cell lymphoma: the Yale-New Haven Hospital experience. Yale J Biol Med 1989;62(6):629–38.

55. Zic JA, Miller JL, Stricklin GP, et al. The North American experience with photopheresis. Ther Apher 1999;3(1):50–62.

56. Wilson LD, Licata AL, Braverman IM, et al. Systemic chemotherapy and extracorporeal photochemotherapy for T3 and T4 cutaneous T-cell lymphoma patients who have achieved a complete response to total skin electron beam therapy. Int J Radiat Oncol Biol Phys 1995;32(4):987–95.

57. Quaglino P, Knobler R, Fierro MT, et al. Extracorporeal photopheresis for the treatment of erythrodermic cutaneous T-cell lymphoma: a single center clinical experience with long-term follow-up data and a brief overview of the literature. Int J Dermatol 2013;52(11):1308–18.

58. Olsen EA, Rook AH, Zic J, et al. Sezary syndrome: immunopathogenesis, literature review of therapeutic options, and recommendations for therapy by the United States Cutaneous Lymphoma Consortium (USCLC). J Am Acad Dermatol 2011;64(2):352–404.

59. McKenna KE, Whittaker S, Rhodes LE, et al. Evidence-based practice of photopheresis 1987–2001: a report of a workshop of the British Photodermatology Group and the U.K. Skin Lymphoma Group. Br J Dermatol 2006;154(1):7–20.

60. Olsen E, Vonderheid E, Pimpinelli N, et al. Revisions to the staging and classification of mycosis fungoides and Sezary syndrome: a proposal of the International Society for Cutaneous Lymphomas (ISCL) and the cutaneous lymphoma task force of the European Organization of Research and Treatment of Cancer (EORTC). Blood 2007;110(6):1713–22.

61. Ratcliffe N, Dunbar NM, Adamski J, et al. National Institutes of Health state of the science symposium in therapeutic apheresis: scientific opportunities in extracorporeal photopheresis. Transfus Med Rev 2015;29(1):62–70.

62. Duvic M, Chiao N, Talpur R. Extracorporeal photopheresis for the treatment of cutaneous T-cell lymphoma. J Cutan Med Surg 2003;7(4 Suppl):3–7.

63. Raphael BA, Shin DB, Suchin KR, et al. High clinical response rate of Sezary syndrome to immunomodulatory therapies: prognostic markers of response. Arch Dermatol 2011;147(12):1410–5.

64. Olsen EA, Bunn PA. Interferon in the treatment of cutaneous T-cell lymphoma. Hematol Oncol Clin North Am 1995;9(5):1089–107.

65. Polansky M, Talpur R, Daulat S, et al. Long-term complete responses to combination therapies and allogeneic stem cell transplants in patients with Sézary syndrome. Clin Lymphoma Myeloma Leuk 2015;15(5):e83–93.

66. McGirt LY, Thoburn C, Hess A, et al. Predictors of response to extracorporeal photopheresis in advanced mycosis fungoides and Sézary syndrome. Photodermatol Photoimmunol Photomed 2010;26(4):182–91.

67. McGirt LY, Baerenwald DA, Vonderheid EC, et al. Early changes in miRNA expression are predictive of response to extracorporeal photopheresis in cutaneous T-cell lymphoma. J Eur Acad Dermatol Venereol 2014. [Epub ahead of print].

68. Atta M, Papanicolaou N, Tsirigotis P. The role of extracorporeal photopheresis in the treatment of cutaneous T-cell lymphomas. Transfus Apher Sci 2012;46(2):195–202.

69. Heald P, Rook A, Perez M, et al. Treatment of erythrodermic cutaneous T-cell lymphoma with extracorporeal photochemotherapy [see comments]. J Am Acad Dermatol 1992;27(3):427–33.

70. Knobler R, Duvic M, Querfeld C, et al. Long-term follow-up and survival of cutaneous T-cell lymphoma patients treated with extracorporeal photopheresis. Photodermatol Photoimmunol Photomed 2012;28(5):250–7.

71. Fraser-Andrews E, Seed P, Whittaker S, et al. Extracorporeal photopheresis in Sezary syndrome. No significant effect in the survival of 44 patients with a peripheral blood T-cell clone. Arch Dermatol 1998;134(8):1001–5.

72. Stevens SR, Bowen GM, Duvic M, et al. Effectiveness of photopheresis in Sezary syndrome. Arch Dermatol 1999;135(8):995–7.

73. Mask-Bull L, Likhari SB, Zic JA, et al. Hemagglutination during photopheresis. J Am Acad Dermatol 2014;70(3):e61–2.

74. Knobler E, Warmuth I, Cocco C, et al. Extracorporeal photochemotherapy–the Columbia experience. Photodermatol Photoimmunol Photomed 2002;18(5):232–7.

75. Stevens SR, Baron ED, Masten S, et al. Circulating CD4+CD7- lymphocyte burden and rapidity of response predictors of outcome in the treatment of Sezary syndrome and erythrodermic mycosis fungoides with extracorporeal photopheresis. Arch Dermatol 2002;138(10):1347–50.

76. Evans AV, Wood BP, Scarisbrick JJ, et al. Extracorporeal photopheresis in Sezary syndrome: hematologic parameters as predictors of response. Blood 2001;98(5):1298–301.

77. Prinz B, Behrens W, Holzle E, et al. Extracorporeal photopheresis for the treatment of cutaneous T-cell lymphoma- the Dusseldorf and Munich experience. Arch Dermatol Res 1995;287(7):621–6.

78. Rao V, Ryggen K, Aahaug M, et al. Extracorporeal photochemotherapy in patients with cutaneous T-cell lymphoma: is clinical response predictable? J Eur Acad Dermatol Venereol 2006;20(9):1100–7.

Monoclonal Antibodies

Larisa J. Geskin, MD

KEYWORDS

- Cutaneous lymphoma • Antibody therapy • Antibody conjugates • Clinical trials

KEY POINTS

- Monoclonal antibodies (mAbs) have been proved to be successful in hematologic malignancies, including cutaneous lymphomas.
- Some mAbs demonstrated high response rates (RRs) and a favorable toxicity profile in clinical trials.
- Safe and effective mAbs can be used as combinational agents and for sequential therapies in a rational stepwise therapy for cutaneous lymphomas.

INTRODUCTION

Since the initial description of the production of mAbs using hybridoma technology by Köhler and Milstein in 1975,[1] significant advances have been made in the use of mAbs and their derivatives in clinical practice. The technology has enjoyed many advances. Antibody immunogenicity progressively decreased from mouse to chimeric humanized to fully human mAbs. Various structural modifications to improve led to improvement of specificity of the antibodies and their targeted and selective cytotoxicity. Targeting specific cellular targets has been successful in hematologic malignancies and solid tumors, demonstrating significantly improved patient survival. Cutaneous lymphomas have also been successfully targeted with specific mAbs for B-cell or T-cell lymphomas and through nonspecific broad antitumor activity.

mAbs and their derivatives can be grouped using various classifications. mAbs can be classified based on their respective targets or functions, such as direct tumor cell killers, checkpoint blockade inhibitors, tumor microenvironment modifiers, or immune primers,[2] among others (**Table 1**). Currently available mAbs also can be classified by their alteration in immunoglobulin scaffold and/or addition of a conjugate designed to enhance immune activation or trigger direct cell death. Agents conjugated to mAbs include immunotoxins (ITs),

such as the diphtheria toxin (DT), radioisotopes (radioimmunoconjugates, such as yttrium 90), or cytotoxic drugs (antibody-drug conjugates [ADC] such as auristatins). Most approved mAbs in clinical practice are unconjugated antibodies that exert antitumor effects through complement- or antibody-dependent cell-mediated cytotoxicity (ADCC).

Progress in biotechnology and improved understanding in cancer biology have sparked a flurry of inventions leading to improving effective mAb-based therapies while limiting overall drug toxicity.[3] Most of these antibodies are undergoing clinical investigation, and many show promise in clinical trials (see below). Engineering of new second- and third-generation mAbs and immunoconjugates with improved clinical efficacy and safety profile offers the potential of going further than optimization of naturally occurring antibodies. For example, defucosylation of the residues in the carbohydrate backbone of the antibody is thought to increase affinity for FcγRIIIa/b and other receptors, improving ADCC.[4] Certain modifications are capable of creating entirely new mAbs not found in nature, designed specifically to match desired characteristics, with nearly limitless possibilities.

The next generation of targeted biologics for cancer therapy in clinical development represents a wide variety of manmade rationally designed modifications of the antibodies directed toward

Comprehensive Cutaneous Oncology Center, Department of Dermatology, Columbia University, 161 Fort Washington Avenue, 12th floor, New York, NY 10032, USA
E-mail address: geskinlj@gmail.com

Dermatol Clin 33 (2015) 777–786
http://dx.doi.org/10.1016/j.det.2015.05.015

Table 1
Classification of therapeutic antibodies based on their function

Action	Antibody Target
Tumor cell killing	CD2, CD3[a], CD4, CD25[a], CD30[a], CD52[a], CCR4[a], KIR3DL2
T-cell activation	PD-1[a], PD-L1[a], CTLA-4[a], CD137, OX40
Tumor microenvironment	CD25[a], PD-1[a], PD-L1[a], CD137, OX40, STAT3
Immune priming	CD40, CD137

Abbreviations: CTLA-4, cytotoxic T-lymphocyte antigen; KIR3DL2, killer cell immunoglobulin-like receptor 3DL2; PD-1, programmed death-1.
[a] In clinical practice.
Data from Martinez Forero I, Okada H, Topalian SL, et al. Workshop on immunotherapy combinations. Society for Immunotherapy of Cancer annual meeting Bethesda, November 3, 2011. J Transl Med 2012;10:108.

improved tissue penetration, efficacy, and safety. Antibody fragments,[5] dimers (diabodies),[6] bispecific and multispecific antibody derivatives,[7] and many other antibody alterations, including ADCs, possess novel characteristics, not normally observed in nature. Such novel molecules are capable of synergistically affecting many complementing pathways resulting in more effective blocking of malignant cell proliferation, angiogenesis, and tumor escape.[7] While this is an exciting area of investigation that will undoubtedly yield positive clinical results applicable to cutaneous lymphomas, it is beyond the scope of this discussion.

The US Food and Drug Administration (FDA) has now approved more than 20 mAbs for clinical use in various malignancies, and over 350 other mAbs are currently in the pipeline, including clinical trials in lymphomas. mAbs are now established as targeted therapies for malignancies, transplant rejection, autoimmune and infectious diseases, as well as a range of new indications. This article discusses FDA-approved mAb-based therapies for cutaneous lymphomas, mAbs used off-label for therapy for cutaneous lymphomas, and clinical trials of other mAbs that have the potential to be of benefit to patients with skin lymphomas.

ANTIBODIES CURRENTLY IN CLINICAL PRACTICE
Anti-CD52

The Campath series of mAbs was originally produced at the Cambridge University Pathology Department in the 1980s. Alemtuzumab (Campath) is a humanized IgG1 mAb directed against the CD52 antigen. CD52 is a nonmodulating glycoprotein expressed on lymphocytes, monocytes, and macrophages but not on stem cells or bone marrow progenitor cells. As CD52 is expressed by both B and T lymphocytes, alemtuzumab is immunosuppressive. This mAb causes lymphocyte lysis via ADCC and complement fixation and may also induce apoptosis. Alemtuzumab is approved by the FDA for patients with chronic lymphocytic leukemia (CLL) who have been treated with alkylating agents and have failed fludarabine therapy and for patients with relapsing multiple sclerosis. This mAb is used for CTCL off-label. Per package insert, alemtuzumab is administered as an infusion over 2 hours thrice a week in a dose-escalating manner starting at 3 mg, then increasing to 10 mg, and then up to 30 mg for a total of 12 weeks depending on tolerability. Because of marked immunosuppression due to the drug, careful monitoring for cytomegalovirus (CMV) reactivation and appropriate prophylaxis for PCP/ herpes simplex virus/varicella zoster virus are recommended. Responses are generally evaluated at the end of the 12 weeks. However, alemtuzumab administration in CTCL differs from that recommended for CLL (see below).

In 2003, a phase 2 study conducted by Lundin and colleagues[8] reported on 22 patients with refractory, advanced, CD52-positive CTCL (7 patients with Sézary syndrome [SS] and 15 with advanced mycosis fungoides [MF]) successfully treated with alemtuzumab with an overall RR of 55% (32% complete response [CR], 23% partial response [PR]). The investigators reported better responses in erythrodermic patients with SS than in those with plaques or skin tumors and clearing of Sézary cells in 6 of 7 patients. After 10 years, this early observation was explained by Clark and colleagues[9] when they determined that in leukemic SS, alemtuzumab depleted recirculating benign and malignant central memory T cells in blood and skin of patients with SS, but did not affect a diverse population of sessile skin-resident effector memory T cells found in MF. Low-dose alemtuzumab (10 mg) was also associated with lack of infections in alemtuzumab-treated patients with SS despite the complete absence of T cells in the blood, suggesting that sessile skin-resident effector memory T cells can protect the skin from pathogens even in the absence of T-cell recruitment from the circulation.

Because high-dose alemtuzumab is associated with profound immunosuppression and infectious complications including bacterial sepsis and CMV reactivation in two-thirds of patients treated with alemtuzumab, alternative administration routes and dosages were explored. The efficacy of intermittent low-dose subcutaneous (SQ) alemtuzumab was tested in 14 patients with SS (11 with relapse and 3 untreated).[10] Most patients in this study received a reduced dose of 3 mg on day 1 and then 10 mg on alternating days SQ. Overall, 12 (85.7%) of the 14 patients achieved a clinical response, with 3 CRs (21.4%) at a median follow-up of 16 months with time to treatment failure of 12 months. Importantly, there was no hematologic toxicity or infection observed at the 10-mg dose level, whereas almost a third of the patients receiving 15 mg or more experienced infectious complications. The study showed that low-dose intermittent SQ alemtuzumab therapy resulted in durable clinical responses and reduced risk of infections.

To summarize, alemtuzumab is successfully used for symptomatic relief and palliation in patients with SS and MF. Alemtuzumab is safe and effective even when used in low doses SQ in short courses; it is considered to be safe even in patients with a very poor performance status and in the very elderly.[11] All patients treated with alemtuzumab inevitably show relapse of the condition. However, re-treatment with the same regimen is acceptable and may result in clinical responses.

Anti-CD30

CD30 (Ki-1 antigen) is a cell surface leukocyte activation transmembrane protein of 120 kDa belonging to the tumor necrosis factor receptor superfamily that is expressed on activated B and T lymphocytes and on malignant hematopoietic cells including Hodgkin lymphoma (HL), anaplastic large cell lymphoma (ALCL), primary cutaneous ALCL (PCALCL), lymphomatoid papulosis (LyP), and MF with large cell transformation (LCT) and can also be expressed at low levels in nontransformed MF. In fact, it may carry a prognostic significance in nontransformed disease[12] even when observed in low levels. Consequently, CD30 represents an attractive therapeutic target in these pathologic entities. Numerous unsuccessful clinical trials targeting CD30 were attempted until the recently developed ADC brentuximab vedotin (CD30-monomethyl auristatin E [MMAE], SGN-35) was shown to be safe and effective in lymphoid malignancies expressing CD30.[13-17]

Historically, CD30 antigen was evaluated as a therapeutic target in various CD30-expressing malignancies, including HL, systemic ALCL and PCALCL, as well as MF. Initial clinical trials using the chimeric unconjugated anti-CD30 antibody SGN-30 and the fully human anti-CD30 antibody MDX-060 conducted in HL did not reveal satisfactory clinical responses.[18,19] The second-generation anti-CD30 antibodies, the defucosylated fully human MDX-1401 and XmAb2513, were evaluated in clinical trials, but responses were also limited.[20,21] In the 1990s, attempts to increase the cytotoxic potential of the CD30-targeting antibody led to development of the bispecific mouse antibodies targeting CD30 and CD16 with the goal of recruiting natural killer (NK) cells. There was 1 CR in a patient with heavily pretreated HL in this clinical trial, but significant immunogenicity was observed,[22] and although the molecule was abandoned, the approach was considered to be promising. At present, AFM13, a tetravalent bispecific (antihuman CD30 and anti-human CD16A) recombinant antibody construct is being investigated for the treatment of HL; the results of this clinical trial are pending.

In CTCL, the efficacy of naked chimeric mAb brentuximab (anti-CD30) was tested in patients with PCALCL, LyP, MF with LCT, as well as multiple simultaneous subtypes of CTCL.[17] The overall RR was 70% (16 of 23 patients) with 10 patients achieving a CR and another 6 patients achieving a PR; 9 of the 10 patients who achieved a CR and 5 of the 6 patients who achieved a PR were in remission at their follow-up evaluation (median duration, 84 days). The adverse events during the study were mild or moderate.

To increase antitumor activity, the chimeric mAb brentuximab (anti-CD30) was conjugated with the antitubulin agent MMAE (or vedotin). After binding CD30, the conjugate is rapidly internalized inside the cell by endocytosis. Once inside the lysosome, cathepsin B and other proteolytic enzymes cleave MMAE off the conjugate. Once released, it binds to tubulin and causes cell cycle arrest. In 2003, the successful use of CD30-MMAE ADC named brentuximab vedotin was first reported in cell lines and mouse models[23,24] leading to the launch of phase 1 clinical trials in HL and ALCL. After unprecedented results in phase 1 clinical trials with overall responses of nearly 50% and reduction in tumor size in most patients,[14,15] several phase 2 clinical trials were launched.[13,16,25] The overall RR in patients with heavily pretreated HL and ALCL ranged from 75% to 86% with CRs of 34% to 53%, leading to accelerated FDA approval of this drug for the treatment of relapsed and refractory HL and ALCL. The recommended dose was 1.8 mg/kg every 3 weeks for up to 16 cycles. In CTCL, brentuximab vedotin also demonstrated significant activity. However, the expression of CD30 in MF is highly variable. Phase 2 clinical trials of patients with MF and SS with various degrees of CD30+ expression on skin biopsies is ongoing.

Adverse events of brentuximab vedotin are usually manageable, but include potentially serious neutropenia and hyperkalemia. Fatigue, nausea, anemia, upper respiratory tract infection, diarrhea, fever, rash, thrombocytopenia, cough, and vomiting have also been reported. Progressive, and often irreversible peripheral neuropathy with intense pain and hypersensitivity to cold, beginning in the hands and feet and sometimes involving the arms and legs, is cumulative and constitutes an important clinical consideration because it may limit prolonged administration of the drug. The mechanism of this toxicity is not entirely clear, but diffusion of MMAE in the tumor microenvironment and cytotoxicity of bystander cells may in part explain its activity. Progressive multifocal leukoencephalopathy associated with brentuximab vedotin therapy, which led to death, has been reported[26] and resulted in the FDA issuing a black box warning. Owing to potentially irreversible and serious side effects when the drug is used for long term, its use probably should be limited to the current approved duration, which can be broken down to several shorter courses with periods of drug holiday. The loss of CD30 expression after brentuximab vedotin has not been reported.[27]

Anti-CD25

CD25 is the α-subunit of interleukin-2 receptor (IL-2R). CD25 is a transmembrane protein present on activated B and T cells and NK cells; it is also a marker for CD4+FoxP3+ regulatory T cells (Tregs) and is constitutively expressed on a small proportion of resting memory T cells and a significant proportion of malignant CD4+ cells in CTCL,[28] most B-cell neoplasms, and some leukemias. Thus, CD25 was historically considered to be an attractive target for targeting CTCL cells. The levels of the soluble form of CD25, sIL-2R, may be elevated in these diseases and is occasionally used to track disease progression and prognosis.[29]

IL-2R is composed of 3 subunits: α (CD25, p55), β (CD122, p75), and γ (CD132, p64). The β and γ (CD122, CD132) subunits are essential for the molecule targeting CD25 to be effective because only interleukin (IL)-2 binding to the intermediate- and high-affinity receptors (IL-2R-β/γ, CD122, CD132 or IL-2R-α/β/γ, CD25, CD122, and CD133) results in signal transduction.[30] Denileukin diftitox (DD, DAB389IL-2, Ontak) is a fusion protein in which the receptor-binding domain of DT has been replaced by the IL-2 molecule, making it capable of binding the IL-2R. After DD binds to the high-affinity IL-2 receptor, it is internalized by receptor-mediated endocytosis, the molecule is proteolytically cleaved within the lysosomal compartment, and the DT portion translocates into the cytoplasm where it inhibits messenger RNA prolongation and ultimately, protein synthesis.[31]

Initial phase 1 studies using original DD molecules indicated minimal activity in CTCL.[32,33] In these early studies, the heterogeneity of CD25 expression was extremely variable and ranged from 40% to less than 5% in the analyzed samples; they also demonstrated generation of neutralizing antibodies. The presence of antitoxin antibodies did not preclude response to treatment, and the presence of CD25 did not differentiate between responders and nonresponders.[34] Of note, all clinical studies using DD did not use rigorous end point criteria, which are now standard for the assessment of patients with MF and SS.[35]

The original DAB486-IL-2 molecule was later modified (in-frame deletion of 97 amino acids from the receptor-binding domain) to produce a fusion protein with a 5-fold greater affinity for target cells, resulting in an overall increase in its half-life and a 10-fold increase in potency.[36] This new DD showed improved RRs in the mid-30s percentages.[36,37] There was no correlation between the expression of the CD25 or CD122 subunits and a clinical response, but expression of CD132, which is necessary for a response, was not assayed.[30]

The pivotal phase 3 trial, a randomized, blinded, multicenter study for stage IB to IVA MF/SS, required greater than 20% of lymphocytes within the skin biopsy to stain positive for CD25. A total of 71 patients were randomly assigned to receive either a 9 or 18 μg/kg/d dose intravenously (IV) for 5 consecutive days; treatment was repeated every 21 days for up to 8 cycles. There was further randomization of the population into those with disease of stage IIA or less and IIB or more (68% with stages > IIB). The overall RR was about 30% with 10% of patients exhibiting a CR. The overall RR between the 2 dosage groups did not reach statistical difference; however, there was a trend to superiority in efficacy of the higher dose in patients with greater than stage IIB disease. The median duration of response for those with an objective result was almost 7 months (from 2.7 to >46 months). Approximately 68% of patients had a significant clinical improvement of their pruritus.[38] Based on these results, the FDA approved the use of DD in patients with CTCL relapse and positive test result for CD25.

Adverse effects (AEs) include hypersensitivity reactions, mild to moderate flulike symptoms, fever, chills, asthenia, arthralgia, headache, myalgia, gastrointestinal symptoms, rash, transient lymphopenia, and infections. Because premedication with steroids and antihistamines were not permitted with this clinical trial, the observed toxicities were more severe than those experienced by patients receiving effective premedication in clinical practice.[39] A capillary leak syndrome (defined as edema, hypoalbuminemia, and hypotension) occurred in up to 25% of the patients and was usually seen in the first 14 days. Premedication with dexamethasone, diphenhydramine, and acetaminophen is recommended, and adequate saline hydration should continue because this has also shown to diminish the incidence of vascular leak syndrome.[40] Since FDA approval, there have been case reports of other AEs, including thyrotoxicosis, retinopathy, and vision loss.[41–43] To improve DD efficacy, combination therapies were investigated in small clinical trials, including with HDAC inhibitors, bexarotene (Targretin), and systemic steroids. The combination studies all demonstrated improved RRs, but it has not been confirmed in larger clinical trials.[44,45]

Recently, several meta-analyses have been performed of all combined DD phase 3 clinical trials analyzing the efficacy, response duration, and safety of DD in CTCL.[46,47] The data indicate that DD showed a significant overall RR, progression-free survival (PFS), and failure of progression of disease when compared with placebo. The significant toxicity observed in clinical trials can be reduced using a premedication regimen[40] and resolved to placebo levels after the second or third course of treatment. Recently, as a part of a postmarketing commitment, the pharmaceutical company Eisai has conducted a clinical trial to assess the efficacy and safety of E7777 (improved purity DD) in patients with persistent and recurrent CTCL: the results of this clinical trial are pending.

MONOCLONAL ANTIBODIES IN CLINICAL TRIALS
Anti-CD4 (Zanolimumab)

Most cases of MF and SS express the CD4 molecule highly and constitutively on the malignant lymphocytes, making it an attractive candidate for therapeutic targeting. CD4 is a coreceptor of the T-cell receptor (TCR), normally expressed on T cells (helper T cells [T_H] and Tregs), macrophages, monocytes, and dendritic cells. Development of effective anti-CD4 therapy early on was hampered by the development of antichimeric antibodies.[48,49] The anti-CD4 antibodies were well tolerated and demonstrated some clinical efficacy.

Recently, a novel anti-CD4 fully human mAb called zanolimumab that reacts with CD4-positive T cells and tumor cells and to a lesser degree with monocytes and macrophages[50] has been developed. Zanolimumab has been shown to induce a dose-dependent decrease in T-cell activation by interference with interaction between the CD4 antigen and the major histocompatibility complex class II molecule and by inhibiting signal transduction through the TCR. It has also been shown to delete CD4$^+$ cells by Fc-mediated ADCC.[50]

In 2 prospective, multicenter phase 2 clinical trials (Hx-CD4-007 and Hx-CD4-008) with patients with relapsed/refractory MF or SS, 47 patients (38 with MF and 9 with SS; 25 patients with early-stage and 22 with advanced-stage disease), were treated with 17 weekly infusions of zanolimumab. Doses ranged from 280 to 580 mg for patients with early-stage disease and from 280 to 980 mg for patients with advanced-stage disease with assessment of response by Composite Assessment of Index Lesion Disease Severity.[51] The RR was dose dependent with the highest response of 56% noted in the high-dose group with a median response duration of 81 weeks. The most common treatment-related AEs included inflammatory skin reactions and infections of the skin and upper respiratory tract. The infections were thought to be related to profound and long-term depletion of CD4$^+$ lymphocytes from the peripheral blood. A phase 3 clinical trial in CTCL was suspended by the company. At the moment, zanolimumab is being tested in other noncutaneous lymphomas and is showing clinical activity.[52,53]

Anti–CC Chemokine Receptor 4 (Mogamulizumab)

Mogamulizumab is the first approved glycoengineered therapeutic humanized IgG1 mAb and first approved mAb to target the CC chemokine receptor 4 (CCR4). It is has a defucosylated Fc region that leads to enhanced ADCC without a complement effect.[54] CCR4 is principally expressed on Tregs and T_H, including malignant CD4$^+$ CTCL cells, where it functions to induce homing of these leukocytes to sites of inflammation. Tregs impair host antitumor immunity and provide a favorable environment for tumors to grow. CCR4 is highly expressed by aggressive peripheral T-cell lymphomas (PTCLs), particularly adult T-cell leukemia/lymphoma (ATLL) and CTCL. In addition to targeting malignant cells, mogamulizumab depletes CCR4+ Tregs, potentially evoking antitumor immune responses by autologous effector cells.[55] This mode of action is especially important in CTCL, where the malignant cells were shown to have Treg phenotype and function.[55] In addition, CCR4+ T cells are the main source of IL-31 in CTCL, an antibody associated with intractable pruritus. Neutralizing the IL-31 pathway through targeting of the CCR4-expressing T cells may represent a promising therapeutic strategy for symptomatic relief in CTCL.[56]

Mogamulizumab is approved for use in Japan, based on the phase 2 clinical trial demonstrating an overall RR of 35%, including 5 patients (14%) with a CR. The median PFS was 3.0 months.

In a phase 1/2 trial in the United States evaluating the efficacy of mogamulizumab in 41 pretreated patients with CTCL, no dose-limiting toxicity was observed and the maximum tolerated dose was not reached in phase 1 after IV infusion of mogamulizumab (0.1, 0.3, and 1.0 mg/kg) once weekly for 4 weeks followed by a 2-week observation period.[57] In phase 2, patients were dosed with 1.0 mg/kg mogamulizumab according to the same schedule for the first course followed by infusion every 2 weeks during subsequent courses until disease progression. The overall RR was 36.8%: 47.1% in SS and 28.6% in MF. Of the19 (94.7%) patients with greater than or equal to B1 blood involvement, 18 had a response in blood, including 11 CRs. Adverse events were nausea (31.0%), chills (23.8%), headache (21.4%), and infusion-related reaction (21.4%); most events were grade 1/2. There were no significant hematologic effects.

Based on the reported safety and efficacy of mogamulizumab, phase 3 investigation of mogamulizumab in patients with CTCL is ongoing.

Anti–Killer Cell Immunoglobulin-Like Receptor 3DL2 (IPH4102)

Since the discovery of high expression of killer cell immunoglobulin-like receptor (KIR) 3DL2 (KIR3DL2) on malignant SS cells, it has become an established marker for malignant cells in SS,[58] but it has also been shown to be expressed in MF.[59] Thus it may be a universal marker for CTCL. KIRs are transmembrane glycoproteins normally expressed by NK cells and a small subset of T cells, but they are highly and constitutively expressed in CTCL.[60]

A recent study reported the development of IPH4102, a humanized mAb that targets the immune receptor KIR3DL2.[61] Potent antitumor properties of IPH4102 were documented in allogeneic human CTCL cells and a mouse model of KIR3DL2(+) disease. IPH4102 antitumor activity was mediated by ADCC and phagocytosis.[61] IPH4102 improved survival and reduced tumor growth in mice inoculated with KIR3DL2(+) tumors. Ex vivo IPH4102 selectively and efficiently killed primary Sézary cells.[61] These results present a preclinical proof of concept for the clinical development of IPH4102 to treat patients with advanced CTCL. The clinical trials with IPH4102 will be opening in the summer of 2015.

MONOCLONAL ANTIBODIES WITH POTENTIAL UTILITY IN CUTANEOUS LYMPHOMAS
LMB-2

LMB-2 is a recombinant IT with mAb to IL-2 (anti-CD25) fused to the truncated form of the pseudomonas exotoxin. LMB-2 binds to CD25 for internalization and processing of toxin and causes apoptosis and cell death similar to DD.[62] In a phase 1 dose escalation clinical trial in 35 patients, including 1 patient with CTCL and 2 with PTCL (others had HL, non-HL, CLL, hairy cell leukemia, ATLL), an overall response was observed in 8 of 35 (23%), including 1 CR and 7 PRs at 30 to 50 μg/kg. Patients with stage IVB SS had significant PRs with rapid reduction of circulating malignant cells and maintenance of 80% to 95% improvement in erythroderma. The most common adverse events were elevated results of liver function tests, but no cumulative toxicity was observed.

Checkpoint Blockade Inhibitors

Anti–cytotoxic T-lymphocyte antigen 4 (ipilimumab)
Cytotoxic T-lymphocyte antigen (CTLA-4, Ipilimumab) is the first mAb, a checkpoint blockade inhibitor, approved by the FDA for the treatment of melanoma. However, CTCL may be an attractive target for this antibody not only because of the removal of immune tolerance[63,64] but also because it can directly target the malignant T cells expressing CTLA-4.[65,66] Ipilimumab is a fully human IgG1κ mAb against CTLA-4, which inhibits the function of a cell surface receptor on activated CD4 and CD8 cells and Tregs. Anti-CTLA-4 competes for binding of the CD80 costimulatory molecule on antigen-presenting cells, which leads to inhibition of IL-2 production and kinase cascades and downregulates key components of the cell cycle machinery.[67] Anti-CTLA-4 is being tested in

clinical trials in patients with other lymphoproliferative disorders.[68]

Programmed death-1 (nivolumab, pembrolizumab)

One of the most critical checkpoint pathways responsible for mediating tumor-induced immune suppression is the programmed death-1 (PD-1) pathway. This pathway is normally involved in promoting tolerance and preventing tissue damage in settings of chronic inflammation. CTCL cells were shown to be highly positive for PD-1 and PD-L1.[69–72] Two anti–PD-1 antibodies have been recently approved by the FDA for the therapy for melanoma because of their unprecedented improvement in patient survival.[73–77] Clinical trials investigating the therapeutic potential of PD-1 pathway–targeted antibodies in CTCL are underway, and the results are eagerly awaited.

SUMMARY

Antibody-based therapies are an integral part of the therapeutic armamentarium in CTCL management. Clinical responses have been clearly demonstrated with many available drugs in clinical practice. Scientific progress and understanding of the disease pathogenesis is uncovering new potential targets for more effective and safe therapy. An approach to cancer and, specifically, CTCL as a disease of immune dysregulation, shifts the paradigm toward immunomodulatory regimens not only to reduce the need for cytotoxic therapies but also to deliver such cytotoxic therapies in an exceptionally precise manner to minimize overall toxicity. Heterogeneity of the disease pathogenesis underscores the need for an individualized approach to each patient and stresses the need for precise molecular testing, which will be available in the near future. Such testing will help to guide patient-specific therapies. Although a common notion is that no current therapy has improved survival in MF or SS, retrospective studies have in fact shown improved survival of patients with CTCL currently over historic controls.[78,79] This improvement may be due to novel therapies, including immunomodulators, which were not available previously. Antibody-based therapies frequently offer safe therapies, which improve quality of life and treat or palliate the disease in a very effective manner.

REFERENCES

1. Köhler G, Milstein C. Continuous cultures of fused cells secreting antibody of predefined specificity. Nature 1975;256(5517):495–7.

2. Martinez Forero I, Okada H, Topalian SL, et al. Workshop on immunotherapy combinations. Society for Immunotherapy of Cancer annual meeting Bethesda, November 3, 2011. J Transl Med 2012;10:108.

3. Chames P, Van Regenmortel M, Weiss E, et al. Therapeutic antibodies: successes, limitations and hopes for the future. Br J Pharmacol 2009;157(2):220–33.

4. Natsume A, Niwa R, Satoh M. Improving effector functions of antibodies for cancer treatment: enhancing ADCC and CDC. Drug Des Devel Ther 2009;3:7–16.

5. Holliger P, Hudson PJ. Engineered antibody fragments and the rise of single domains. Nat Biotechnol 2005;23(9):1126–36.

6. Holliger P, Prospero T, Winter G. "Diabodies": small bivalent and bispecific antibody fragments. Proc Natl Acad Sci U S A 1993;90(14):6444–8.

7. Weidle UH, Kontermann RE, Brinkmann U. Tumor-antigen-binding bispecific antibodies for cancer treatment. Semin Oncol 2014;41(5):653–60.

8. Lundin J, Hagberg H, Repp R, et al. Phase 2 study of alemtuzumab (anti-CD52 monoclonal antibody) in patients with advanced mycosis fungoides/Sezary syndrome. Blood 2003;101(11):4267–72.

9. Clark RA, Watanabe R, Teague JE, et al. Skin effector memory T cells do not recirculate and provide immune protection in alemtuzumab-treated CTCL patients. Sci Transl Med 2012;4(117):117ra117.

10. Bernengo MG, Quaglino P, Comessatti A, et al. Low-dose intermittent alemtuzumab in the treatment of Sezary syndrome: clinical and immunologic findings in 14 patients. Haematologica 2007;92(6):784–94.

11. Alinari L, Geskin L, Grady T, et al. Subcutaneous alemtuzumab for Sezary Syndrome in the very elderly. Leuk Res 2008;32(8):1299–303.

12. Edinger JT, Clark BZ, Pucevich BE, et al. CD30 expression and proliferative fraction in nontransformed mycosis fungoides. Am J Surg Pathol 2009;33(12):1860–8.

13. Younes A, Gopal AK, Smith SE, et al. Results of a pivotal phase II study of brentuximab vedotin for patients with relapsed or refractory Hodgkin's lymphoma. J Clin Oncol 2012;30(18):2183–9.

14. Fanale MA, Forero-Torres A, Rosenblatt JD, et al. A phase I weekly dosing study of brentuximab vedotin in patients with relapsed/refractory CD30-positive hematologic malignancies. Clin Cancer Res 2012;18(1):248–55.

15. Younes A, Bartlett NL, Leonard JP, et al. Brentuximab vedotin (SGN-35) for relapsed CD30-positive lymphomas. N Engl J Med 2010;363(19):1812–21.

16. Phase II trial of brentuximab vedotin for CD30+ cutaneous T-cell lymphomas and lymphoproliferative disorders. Clin Adv Hematol Oncol 2014;12(2 Suppl 5):12–4.

17. Duvic M, Reddy SA, Pinter-Brown L, et al. A phase II study of SGN-30 in cutaneous anaplastic large cell lymphoma and related lymphoproliferative disorders. Clin Cancer Res 2009;15(19):6217–24.

18. Bartlett NL, Younes A, Carabasi MH, et al. A phase 1 multidose study of SGN-30 immunotherapy in patients with refractory or recurrent CD30+ hematologic malignancies. Blood 2008;111(4):1848–54.

19. Ansell SM, Horwitz SM, Engert A, et al. Phase I/II study of an anti-CD30 monoclonal antibody (MDX-060) in Hodgkin's lymphoma and anaplastic large-cell lymphoma. J Clin Oncol 2007;25(19):2764–9.

20. Cardarelli PM, Moldovan-Loomis MC, Preston B, et al. In vitro and in vivo characterization of MDX-1401 for therapy of malignant lymphoma. Clin Cancer Res 2009;15(10):3376–83.

21. Kumar A, Blum KA, Fung HC, et al. A phase 1 dose-escalation study of XmAb((R)) 2513 in patients with relapsed or refractory Hodgkin lymphoma. Br J Haematol 2015;168(6):902–4.

22. Hartmann F, Renner C, Jung W, et al. Treatment of refractory Hodgkin's disease with an anti-CD16/CD30 bispecific antibody. Blood 1997;89(6):2042–7.

23. Doronina SO, Toki BE, Torgov MY, et al. Development of potent monoclonal antibody auristatin conjugates for cancer therapy. Nat Biotechnol 2003;21(7):778–84.

24. Francisco JA, Cerveny CG, Meyer DL, et al. cAC10-vcMMAE, an anti-CD30-monomethyl auristatin E conjugate with potent and selective antitumor activity. Blood 2003;102(4):1458–65.

25. Pro B, Advani R, Brice P, et al. Brentuximab vedotin (SGN-35) in patients with relapsed or refractory systemic anaplastic large-cell lymphoma: results of a phase II study. J Clin Oncol 2012;30(18):2190–6.

26. Carson KR, Newsome SD, Kim EJ, et al. Progressive multifocal leukoencephalopathy associated with brentuximab vedotin therapy: a report of 5 cases from the Southern Network on Adverse Reactions (SONAR) project. Cancer 2014;120(16):2464–71.

27. Nathwani N, Krishnan AY, Huang Q, et al. Persistence of CD30 expression in Hodgkin lymphoma following brentuximab vedotin (SGN-35) treatment failure. Leuk Lymphoma 2012;53(10):2051–3.

28. Nichols J, Foss F, Kuzel TM, et al. Interleukin-2 fusion protein: an investigational therapy for interleukin-2 receptor expressing malignancies. Eur J Cancer 1997;33(Suppl 1):S34–6.

29. Wasik MA, Vonderheid EC, Bigler RD, et al. Increased serum concentration of the soluble interleukin-2 receptor in cutaneous T-cell lymphoma. Clinical and prognostic implications. Arch Dermatol 1996;132(1):42–7.

30. Re GG, Waters C, Poisson L, et al. Interleukin 2 (IL-2) receptor expression and sensitivity to diphtheria fusion toxin DAB389IL-2 in cultured hematopoietic cells. Cancer Res 1996;56(11):2590–5.

31. Bacha P, Williams DP, Waters C, et al. Interleukin 2 receptor-targeted cytotoxicity. Interleukin 2 receptor-mediated action of a diphtheria toxin-related interleukin 2 fusion protein. J Exp Med 1988;167(2):612–22.

32. LeMaistre CF, Meneghetti C, Rosenblum M, et al. Phase I trial of an interleukin-2 (IL-2) fusion toxin (DAB486IL-2) in hematologic malignancies expressing the IL-2 receptor. Blood 1992;79(10):2547–54.

33. Hesketh P, Caguioa P, Koh H, et al. Clinical activity of a cytotoxic fusion protein in the treatment of cutaneous T-cell lymphoma. J Clin Oncol 1993;11(9):1682–90.

34. Kuzel TM, Rosen ST, Gordon LI, et al. Phase I trial of the diphtheria toxin/interleukin-2 fusion protein DAB486IL-2: efficacy in mycosis fungoides and other non-Hodgkin's lymphomas. Leuk Lymphoma 1993;11(5–6):369–77.

35. Olsen EA, Whittaker S, Kim YH, et al. Clinical end points and response criteria in mycosis fungoides and Sezary syndrome: a consensus statement of the International Society for Cutaneous Lymphomas, the United States Cutaneous Lymphoma Consortium, and the Cutaneous Lymphoma Task Force of the European Organisation for Research and Treatment of Cancer. J Clin Oncol 2011;29(18):2598–607.

36. LeMaistre CF, Saleh MN, Kuzel TM, et al. Phase I trial of a ligand fusion-protein (DAB389IL-2) in lymphomas expressing the receptor for interleukin-2. Blood 1998;91(2):399–405.

37. Duvic M, Cather J, Maize J, et al. DAB389IL2 diphtheria fusion toxin produces clinical responses in tumor stage cutaneous T cell lymphoma. Am J Hematol 1998;58(1):87–90.

38. Olsen E, Duvic M, Frankel A, et al. Pivotal phase III trial of two dose levels of denileukin diftitox for the treatment of cutaneous T-cell lymphoma. J Clin Oncol 2001;19(2):376–88.

39. Foss FM, Bacha P, Osann KE, et al. Biological correlates of acute hypersensitivity events with DAB(389) IL-2 (denileukin diftitox, ONTAK) in cutaneous T-cell lymphoma: decreased frequency and severity with steroid premedication. Clin Lymphoma 2001;1(4):298–302.

40. McCann S, Akilov OE, Geskin L. Adverse effects of denileukin diftitox and their management in patients with cutaneous T-cell lymphoma. Clin J Oncol Nurs 2012;16(5):E164–172.

41. Ghori F, Polder KD, Pinter-Brown LC, et al. Thyrotoxicosis after denileukin diftitox therapy in patients with mycosis fungoides. J Clin Endocrinol Metab 2006;91(6):2205–8.

42. Ruddle JB, Harper CA, Honemann D, et al. A denileukin diftitox (Ontak) associated retinopathy? Br J Ophthalmol 2006;90(8):1070–1.

43. Lubow M, Grzybowski DM, Awad H. Denileukin diftitox vision loss is not posterior ischemic optic

neuropathy. Leuk Lymphoma 2008;49(2):370–1 [author reply: 372].

44. Shao RH, Tian X, Gorgun G, et al. Arginine butyrate increases the cytotoxicity of DAB(389)IL-2 in leukemia and lymphoma cells by upregulation of IL-2Rbeta gene. Leuk Res 2002;26(12):1077–83.

45. Gorgun G, Foss F. Immunomodulatory effects of RXR rexinoids: modulation of high-affinity IL-2R expression enhances susceptibility to denileukin diftitox. Blood 2002;100(4):1399–403.

46. Weberschock T, Strametz R, Lorenz M, et al. Interventions for mycosis fungoides. Cochrane Database Syst Rev 2012;(9):CD008946.

47. Duvic M, Geskin L, Prince HM. Duration of response in cutaneous T-cell lymphoma patients treated with denileukin diftitox: results from 3 phase III studies. Clin Lymphoma Myeloma Leuk 2013;13(4):377–84.

48. Knox SJ, Levy R, Hodgkinson S, et al. Observations on the effect of chimeric anti-CD4 monoclonal antibody in patients with mycosis fungoides. Blood 1991;77(1):20–30.

49. Knox S, Hoppe RT, Maloney D, et al. Treatment of cutaneous T-cell lymphoma with chimeric anti-CD4 monoclonal antibody. Blood 1996;87(3):893–9.

50. Mestel DS, Beyer M, Mobs M, et al. Zanolimumab, a human monoclonal antibody targeting CD4 in the treatment of mycosis fungoides and Sezary syndrome. Expert Opin Biol Ther 2008;8(12):1929–39.

51. Kim YH, Duvic M, Obitz E, et al. Clinical efficacy of zanolimumab (HuMax-CD4): two phase 2 studies in refractory cutaneous T-cell lymphoma. Blood 2007;109(11):4655–62.

52. Alexandroff AB, Shpadaruk V, Bamford WM, et al. Alemtuzumab-resistant Sezary syndrome responding to zanolimumab. Br J Haematol 2011;154(3):419–21.

53. d'Amore F, Radford J, Relander T, et al. Phase II trial of zanolimumab (HuMax-CD4) in relapsed or refractory non-cutaneous peripheral T cell lymphoma. Br J Haematol 2010;150(5):565–73.

54. Ito A, Ishida T, Yano H, et al. Defucosylated anti-CCR4 monoclonal antibody exercises potent ADCC-mediated antitumor effect in the novel tumor-bearing humanized NOD/Shi-scid, IL-2Rgamma(null) mouse model. Cancer Immunol Immunother 2009;58(8):1195–206.

55. Ni X, Jorgensen JL, Goswami M, et al. Reduction of regulatory T cells by Mogamulizumab, a defucosylated anti-CC chemokine receptor 4 antibody, in patients with aggressive/refractory mycosis fungoides and Sezary syndrome. Clin Cancer Res 2015;21(2):274–85.

56. Cedeno-Laurent F, Singer EM, Wysocka M, et al. Improved pruritus correlates with lower levels of IL-31 in CTCL patients under different therapeutic modalities. Clin Immunol 2015;158(1):1–7.

57. Duvic M, Pinter-Brown LC, Foss FM, et al. Phase 1/2 study of mogamulizumab, a defucosylated anti-CCR4 antibody, in previously treated patients with cutaneous T-cell lymphoma. Blood 2015;125(12):1883–9.

58. Moins-Teisserenc H, Daubord M, Clave E, et al. CD158k is a reliable marker for diagnosis of Sezary syndrome and reveals an unprecedented heterogeneity of circulating malignant cells. J Invest Dermatol 2015;135(1):247–57.

59. Dulmage BO, Geskin LJ. Lessons learned from gene expression profiling of cutaneous T-cell lymphoma. Br J Dermatol 2013;169(6):1188–97.

60. Sako N, Schiavon V, Bounfour T, et al. Membrane expression of NK receptors CD160 and CD158k contributes to delineate a unique CD4+ T-lymphocyte subset in normal and mycosis fungoides skin. Cytometry A 2014;85(10):869–82.

61. Marie-Cardine A, Viaud N, Thonnart N, et al. IPH4102, a humanized KIR3DL2 antibody with potent activity against cutaneous T-cell lymphoma. Cancer Res 2014;74(21):6060–70.

62. Kreitman RJ, Wilson WH, White JD, et al. Phase I trial of recombinant immunotoxin anti-Tac(Fv)-PE38 (LMB-2) in patients with hematologic malignancies. J Clin Oncol 2000;18(8):1622–36.

63. Walunas TL, Lenschow DJ, Bakker CY, et al. CTLA-4 can function as a negative regulator of T cell activation. Immunity 1994;1(5):405–13.

64. Wing K, Onishi Y, Prieto-Martin P, et al. CTLA-4 control over Foxp3+ regulatory T cell function. Science 2008;322(5899):271–5.

65. Krejsgaard T, Odum N, Geisler C, et al. Regulatory T cells and immunodeficiency in mycosis fungoides and Sezary syndrome. Leukemia 2012;26(3):424–32.

66. Wong HK, Wilson AJ, Gibson HM, et al. Increased expression of CTLA-4 in malignant T-cells from patients with mycosis fungoides – cutaneous T cell lymphoma. J Invest Dermatol 2006;126(1):212–9.

67. Weber JS, O'Day S, Urba W, et al. Phase I/II study of ipilimumab for patients with metastatic melanoma. J Clin Oncol 2008;26(36):5950–6.

68. Ansell SM, Hurvitz SA, Koenig PA, et al. Phase I study of ipilimumab, an anti-CTLA-4 monoclonal antibody, in patients with relapsed and refractory B-cell non-Hodgkin lymphoma. Clin Cancer Res 2009;15(20):6446–53.

69. Cetinozman F, Jansen PM, Vermeer MH, et al. Differential expression of programmed death-1 (PD-1) in Sezary syndrome and mycosis fungoides. Arch Dermatol 2012;148(12):1379–85.

70. Kantekure K, Yang Y, Raghunath P, et al. Expression patterns of the immunosuppressive proteins PD-1/CD279 and PD-L1/CD274 at different stages of cutaneous T-cell lymphoma/mycosis fungoides. Am J Dermatopathol 2012;34(1):126–8.

71. Cetinozman F, Jansen PM, Willemze R. Expression of programmed death-1 in primary cutaneous CD4-positive small/medium-sized pleomorphic T-cell lymphoma, cutaneous pseudo-T-cell lymphoma, and other types of cutaneous T-cell lymphoma. Am J Surg Pathol 2012;36(1):109–16.

72. Samimi S, Benoit B, Evans K, et al. Increased programmed death-1 expression on CD4+ T cells in cutaneous T-cell lymphoma: implications for immune suppression. Arch Dermatol 2010;146(12):1382–8.

73. Brahmer JR, Drake CG, Wollner I, et al. Phase I study of single-agent anti-programmed death-1 (MDX-1106) in refractory solid tumors: safety, clinical activity, pharmacodynamics, and immunologic correlates. J Clin Oncol 2010;28(19):3167–75.

74. Robert C, Ribas A, Wolchok JD, et al. Anti-programmed-death-receptor-1 treatment with pembrolizumab in ipilimumab-refractory advanced melanoma: a randomised dose-comparison cohort of a phase 1 trial. Lancet 2014;384(9948):1109–17.

75. Brahmer JR, Tykodi SS, Chow LQ, et al. Safety and activity of anti-PD-L1 antibody in patients with advanced cancer. N Engl J Med 2012;366(26): 2455–65.

76. Topalian SL, Hodi FS, Brahmer JR, et al. Safety, activity, and immune correlates of anti-PD-1 antibody in cancer. N Engl J Med 2012;366(26):2443–54.

77. Wolchok JD, Kluger H, Callahan MK, et al. Nivolumab plus ipilimumab in advanced melanoma. N Engl J Med 2013;369(2):122–33.

78. Kim YH, Liu HL, Mraz-Gernhard S, et al. Long-term outcome of 525 patients with mycosis fungoides and Sezary syndrome: clinical prognostic factors and risk for disease progression. Arch Dermatol 2003;139(7):857–66.

79. Vidulich KA, Talpur R, Bassett RL, et al. Overall survival in erythrodermic cutaneous T-cell lymphoma: an analysis of prognostic factors in a cohort of patients with erythrodermic cutaneous T-cell lymphoma. Int J Dermatol 2009;48(3):243–52.

Other Chemotherapeutic Agents in Cutaneous T-Cell Lymphoma

Catherine G. Chung, MD[a], Brian Poligone, MD, PhD[b],*

KEYWORDS

- Chemotherapy • Response rate • Clinical trial

KEY POINTS

- Traditional chemotherapies are used throughout the world in the treatment of cutaneous T-cell lymphoma (CTCL).
- Both single and multiagent chemotherapies can benefit patients with CTCL.
- There currently are no data to support the use of traditional chemotherapies over other therapies for CTCL. Therefore, in patients with less advanced disease, alternative therapies should be considered.

INTRODUCTION

Currently, no traditional chemotherapy agents are Food and Drug Administration (FDA) approved for the treatment of mycosis fungoides (MF) or Sézary syndrome (SS). Multiple chemotherapeutic treatments for MF and SS, such as systemic nitrogen mustard and multiagent chemotherapy regimens (eg, cyclophosphamide, adriamycin, vincristine, and prednisone [CHOP]), were initially used because of established activity in other non-Hodgkin lymphomas (NHLs) or Hodgkin lymphomas. Over time, specific treatments were reported by astute physicians to be particularly effective in MF/SS, such as the Winkelmann chlorambucil regimen. More recently, however, it has been recognized that some of these regimens, which are often characterized by significant immunosuppression and toxicity, are not more effective than agents described elsewhere in this issue (eg, interferons [IFNs]).[1] Nevertheless, these other "chemotherapeutic" agents remain an important therapy option for some patients with MF/SS. This article describes those chemotherapeutic agents not discussed elsewhere in this issue with a review of the data supporting their use. **Table 1** summarizes single-agent therapies in MF/SS and **Table 2** summarizes multiagent chemotherapies. Readers are further referred to a comprehensive review on the treatments used for SS and MF by Olsen and colleagues[2] for additional in-depth discussion of many of the agents discussed later.

ANTIMETABOLITES

Antimetabolites are typically low-molecular-weight molecules with structures resembling normal cellular constituents that act by disrupting normal metabolic pathways. There are 3 common subgroups: (1) purine analogs, (2) pyrimidine analogs, and (3) folates.

Purine Analogs/Antagonists

Purine analogs are antimetabolites with a chemical structure that mimics the purine bases (adenine and guanine) and interferes with DNA polymerase

Disclosure: The authors declare no conflicts of interest associated with this work.
[a] Departments of Dermatology and Pathology, Penn State Hershey Medical Center, 500 University Drive, Hershey, PA 17033, USA; [b] James P. Wilmot Cancer Center, University of Rochester School of Medicine, 601 Elmwood Avenue, Rochester, NY 14642, USA
* Corresponding author.
E-mail address: bpoligone@gmail.com

Dermatol Clin 33 (2015) 787–805
http://dx.doi.org/10.1016/j.det.2015.05.012
0733-8635/15/$ – see front matter © 2015 Elsevier Inc. All rights reserved.

Table 1
Summary of single-agent and combination chemotherapy studies in the treatment of mycosis fungoides or Sézary syndrome

Agent(s)	Response Rate (Responders/Total)	Dosing	Study
Fludarabine	2/5	25 mg/m² × 5 d, q3–4 wk	Redman et al,[4] 1992
	6/31	18–25 mg/m² × 5 d, q4 wk	Von Hoff et al,[5] 1990
Fludarabine + ECP	7/27 MF; 6/17 SS	25 mg/m² × 5 d, q4 wk	Quaglino et al,[6] 2000
Fludarabine + IFN	18/35	25 mg/m² × 5 d q4 wk; 5 million units, TIW	Foss et al,[7] 1994
Fludarabine + cyclophosphamide	5/6	18 mg/m² × 3 d, q4wk; 250 mg/m² × 3 d, q4wk	Scarisbrick et al,[8] 2011
Cladribine	2/2	0.1 mg/kg × 7 d, q4wk	Betticher et al,[9] 1994
	2/9	4 mg/m² × 7 d, q4wk	O'Brien et al,[10] 1994
	9/22	0.1 mg/kg × 5–7 d, q4wk	Kuzel et al,[11] 1996
	2/8	0.06 mg/kg × 5 d, q4wk	Trautinger et al,[12] 1999
Pentostatin	10/32	3.75–5 mg/m² × 3 d, q3wk	Tsimberidou et al,[14] 2004
	4/8	5 mg/m² × 3 d, q3wk	Cummings et al,[15] 1991
	7/18	Varied	Greiner et al,[17] 1997
	5/22 MF; 7/21 SS	4 mg/m² q1–4wk	Ho et al,[18] 1999
	4/6 MF; 10/14 SS	5 mg/m² × 3 d, q3wk ± 1.25 mg/m² on subsequent cycles	Kurzrock et al,[19] 1999
Pentostatin, cyclophosphamide, and bexarotene	5/5 MF; 2/3 SS	4 mg/m² q2wk; 600 mg/m² q2wk; 300 mg/m² qd × 8 mo	Calderon Cabrera et al,[21] 2013
Pentostatin + IFN	17/41	4 mg/m² × 3 d	Foss et al,[20] 1992
Gemcitabine	9/19	1200 mg/m² d 1, 8, 15, and 28	Zinzani et al,[144] 2010
	19/26 MF; 0/1 SS	1200 mg/m² d 1, 8, 15, and 28	Marchi et al,[29] 2005
	21/30	1000 mg/m² d 1, 8, and 15	Duvic et al,[30] 2006
	3/3	1000 mg/m² d 1, 8, and 15 then 250 mg/m² weekly	Buhl et al,[32] 2009
	7/9 MF; 2/4 SS	1000 mg/m² d 1 and 8 of a 21-d cycle or d 1, 8, ± 15 of a 28-d cycle	Jidar et al,[31] 2009
Mechlorethamine	34/41	Varied	Van Scott et al,[37] 1975
Chlorambucil + prednisone	23/26 (all SS)	2–6 mg/d; 20 mg/d	Winkelmann et al,[44] 1984
	6/6	2–6 mg/d; 5–20 mg/d	Hamminga et al,[42] 1979
Chlorambucil + fluocortolone	13/13	Clorambucil 10–12 mg/d × 3 d; fluocortolone 75 mg d 1, 50 mg d 2, 25 mg d 3	Coors & von den Driesch,[43] 2000

Agent	Response	Dose/Regimen	Reference
Chlorambucil + prednisone + leukapheresis	11/11	4 mg/d; 20 mg/d; Leukapheresis 2–3 × per wk	Winkelmann et al,[44] 1984
Bendamustine	2/3	60–100 mg/m²	Zaja et al,[59] 2013
Cyclophsphamide	4/4	Varied: 200–700 mg/d	Abele & Dobson,[61] 1960
	5/11	Varied: 50–300 mg/d	Van Scott et al,[66] 1962
TMZ	3/9	150 mg/m²/d × 5 d, q4wk, Then 200 mg/m²/d × 5 d q4wk	Tani et al,[75] 2005
	7/26	200 mg/m²/d PO × 5 d q4wk	Querfeld et al,[76] 2011
Liposomal daunorubicin	3/3	20–40 mg/m² q3–4wk	Wollina et al,[92] 2003
Doxorubicin	7/13	60 mg/m² q3wk	Levi et al,[84] 1977
	26/30 MF; 1/1 SS	20–40 mg/m² q2–4wk	Wollina et al,[85] 2003
	3/10	20 mg/m² q4wk	Di Lorenzo et al,[86] 2005
	12/13 MF; 1/3 SS;	20 mg/m² q4wk	Pulini et al,[87] 2007
	6/10 MF; 3/5 SS	40 mg/m² q4wk	Quereux et al,[88] 2008
	20/49	20 mg/m² q2wk	Dummer et al,[89] 2012
Doxorubicin + bexarotene	14/34 (Doxorubicin only); 7/15 (doxorubicin + bexarotene)	Doxil 20 mg/m² q2wk; bexarotene 300 mg/m²/d	Straus et al,[90] 2014
Etoposide ± cyclophosphamide	2/5 (Etoposide only); 3/4 (etoposide + cyclophosphamide)	100 mg/m² IV × 5 d, q2–3wk ± cyclophosphamide	Molin et al,[99] 1979
IL-2	3/3 MF; 1/3 SS	20 million units/m² on d 1–5, 14–17, and 28–30 (induction) followed by 2 d/mo for 5 mo (consolidation)	Baccard et al,[111] 1997
	5/7	20 million units/m²/d for 5, 4, and 3 d (wk 1, 3, and 5) followed by optional monthly maintenance × 5 d	Gisselbrecht et al,[112] 1994
	4/22	20 million units/m²/d on d 1–4 × 6 wk in an 8-wk cycle	Querfeld et al,[107] 2007
IL-12	5/10	50, 100, or 300 ng/kg twice weekly, up to 24 wk	Rook et al,[117] 1999
	10/23	100 ng/kg twice weekly × 2 wk then 300 mg/kg twice weekly through 24 wk	Rook et al,[118] 2001
Forodesine	9/13	40–320 mg/m² BID × 4 d in a 16-d cycle	Lansigan & Foss,[127] 2010
	10/37 (MF/SS + other T-cell lymphomas)	40–320 mg/m²/d × 4 wk	Duvic et al,[128] 2006
	11/101	200 mg daily (approximately 80 mg/m²)	Dummer et al,[129] 2014
Bortezomib	7/10	1.3 mg/m² twice weekly × 2 wk in a 3-wk cycle	Zinzani et al,[133] 2007

Abbreviation: TIW, three times weekly.

Table 2
Combination chemotherapy used in the treatment of mycosis fungoides/Sézary syndrome

Therapy Regimen	No. of Patients	Complete Response + Partial Response, n (%)	Complete Response, n (%)	Median Duration of Response (mo)	Stage	Reference
MOPP/COPP + TSEB	21	19 (70)	11 (52)	14	I-III	Hallahan et al,[145] 1988; Bunn et al,[146] 1994
BLM + MTX	10	9 (90)	1 (10)	6	T3	Groth et al,[147] 1979
CHOP/HOP	12	10 (83)	5 (42)	5	II-IV	Grozea et al,[148] 1979; Lamberg et al,[149] 1979
CHOP/COP	30	9 (30)	3 (10)	6	Not reported	Fierro et al,[150] 1998
CHOP	1	0	0	—	T3	Molin et al,[151] 1980; Raafat & Oster,[152] 1980
CVP	4	3 (75)	1 (25)	Not reported	IV	Lutzner et al,[153] 1975
CVP	3	2 (67)	0 (0)	Not reported	T3	Molin et al,[151] 1980; Raafat & Oster,[152] 1980
CVP	16	8 (50)	4 (25)	12	IIB (4), III (1), IV (11)	Tirelli et al,[154] 1986
CVP ± TSEB	12	6 (50)	4 (33)	Not reported	III	Hamminga et al,[155] 1982
CBP	8	5 (63)	2 (25)	Not reported	Not reported	Molin et al,[156] 1987
CBP + retinoid	12	7 (58)	3 (25)	Not reported	Not reported	Molin et al,[156] 1987
CBP + retinoid	20	18 (90)	16 (80)	8	—	Zachariae & Thestrup-Pedersen,[157] 1987
CBP + retinoid + TF	10	8 (80)	8 (80)	Not reported	—	Zachariae et al,[158] 1987
CAVOP	5	4 (80)	1 (20)	Not reported	T3	Molin et al,[151] 1980; Raafat & Oster,[152] 1980
COP + BLM	12	11 (92)	2 (17)	11.5	II-IV	Grozea et al,[148] 1979; Lamberg et al,[149] 1979
VICOP-B	25[a]	(84)	(36)[a]	8.7	IIB and IV	Fierro et al,[96] 1997
EPOCH	15	12 (80)	4 (27)	8	IIB-IVB	Akpek et al,[159] 1999
Cyclophosphamide + VP-16	4	3 (75)	1 (25)	6	Various, majority T3	Molin et al,[99] 1979
MBPE	11	8 (73)	1 (9)	6	II-IV	Doberauer & Ohl,[160] 1989
CAVE	52	47 (90)	20 (38)	Not reported	II-IV	Kaye et al,[161] 1989
TSEB + doxorubicin + cyclophosphamide	50	49 (98)	44 (88)	Range 2-75	I (20); II (20); III (7); IV (3)	Braverman et al,[162] 1987
BAM	10	8 (80)	7 (70)	41	IIB-IVB	Zakem et al,[163] 1986

Abbreviations: BAM, bleomycin, adriamycin, and MTX; BLM, bleomycin; BVP, bleomycin, vinblastine, and prednisone; CAVE, cyclophosphamide, adriamycin, vincristine, and etoposide; CAVOP, cyclophosphamide, adriamycin, vincristine, VP-16, and prednisone; CBP, cyclophosphamide, bleomycin, and prednisone; COMP, cyclophosphamide, vincristine, MTX, and prednisone; COP/CVP, cyclophosphamide, vincristine, and prednisone; COPP, cyclophosphamide, vincristine, procarbazine, and prednisone; MBPE, MTX, bleomycin, prednisone, and etoposide; MOPP, meclorethamine, vincristine, procarbazine, and prednisone; TF, transfer factor; TSEB, total skin electron beam therapy.

[a] Includes a cohort of patients with pleomorphic lymphoma.

and ribonucleotide reductase, thus inhibiting both DNA and RNA synthesis. It is unclear which of these play a more important role in cytotoxicity, or if both do.

6-Mercaptopurine

6-Mercaptopurine (6-MP or Purinethol) is an oral thiopurine used in acute lymphocytic leukemia. It has not been studied in MF/SS and is not recommended in the National Comprehensive Cancer Network (NCCN) guidelines for NHL.[3]

Fludarabine

Fludarabine (Fludara) is an adenosine analog that inhibits adenosine deaminase, leading to an accumulation of deoxyadenosine triphosphate, which in turn inhibits DNA polymerase and ribonucleotide reductase. It can be given both orally (available in Canada but not in the United States) and intravenously (IV). It is FDA approved for use in chronic lymphocytic leukemia (CLL) and is also used as a component of multiagent chemotherapy for NHL. As a single agent, fludarabine at 18 to 25 mg/m^2 for 5 days every 3 to 4 weeks was modestly effective in advanced-staged MF with an overall response rate (ORR) of 26% (21/80 patients) between three trials [2/5 (40%)] of patients with MF (Redman and colleagues[4]), stage not otherwise reported; 6/31 (19%) evaluable patients with stage IB–IVB MF (Von Hoff and colleagues[5]); and 13/44 (29.5%) patients with stage IIB–IV MF (Quaglino and colleagues).[6] Fludarabine has been used in combination with IFN (5–7.5 million units/m^2 3 times a week)[7] in 35 patients with MF, 31 who had stage IV disease, with an ORR of 51%. Fludarabine has also been used in combination with cyclophosphamide (250 mg/m^2 × 3 days every 4 weeks × 3–6 months)[8] in 12 patients with stage III–IVA MF/SS, with an ORR of 42%. The duration of response was low.

Given its modest benefit and significant side effects of myelosuppression and immunosuppression with lymphocyte dysfunction that persists beyond treatment, fludarabine has a limited role in the treatment of MF/SS outside of its role in conditioning regimens for stem cell transplant. Additional side effects include dose-dependent neurotoxicity, gastrointestinal (GI) symptoms, and pulmonary toxicity.[2] Secondary neoplasms have also been reported.

Cladribine

Similar to fludarabine, cladribine (2-chlorodeoxyadenosine, 2-CdA, or Leustatin) is an adenosine analog that inhibits DNA and RNA synthesis through its interaction with adenosine deaminase. Due to the high concentration of adenosine deaminase in T lymphocytes, cladribine acts preferentially in this cell population. It is FDA approved for hairy cell leukemia. In 1 of several early studies, 2 of 2 patients (stages not reported) treated with cladribine, 0.1 mg/kg/d for 7 days every 4 weeks, had a partial response (PR).[9] O'Brien reported on a complete response (CR) in 1/8 patients with stage I–IV MF treated with cladribine, 4 mg/m^2/d for 7 days every 28 days.[10] Kuzel and colleagues[11] performed a phase II study examining 0.1 mg/kg/d for 5 to 7 days and reported an ORR of 28%, including 3 with a CR (3/4 stage IB, 0/2 stage IIB, 2/5 stage III, 1/8 stage IVA, and 0/2 stage IVB). Low-dose cladribine, 0.06 mg/kg/d × 5 days every 4 weeks for up to 8 cycles, has been shown to provide some palliation (1/2 stage IIB and 1/6 stage IVA ORR).[12]

Similar to fludarabine, cladribine causes myelosuppression and protracted lymphopenia, with a decrease in CD4/CD8 ratio that can last 6 to 9 months after treatment.[2] Given the high degree of immunosuppression associated with advanced MF/SS,[13] this side effect limits the use of cladribine in MF/SS.

Pentostatin

Pentostatin (deoxycoformycin or Nipent) also inhibits adenosine deaminase, leading to a block in DNA synthesis. It is FDA approved for use in hairy cell leukemia. In one of the larger studies to examine pentostatin in advanced-stage (IIB or higher) disease, there was an ORR of 56% among 32 patients.[14] Dosing was 5 mg/m^2 for 3 days every 3 weeks. In an Eastern Cooperative Oncology Group (ECOG) study of 8 patients with CTCL (stages not reported), 4 of 8 had a response.[15] Dang-Vu and colleagues[16] reported on 1 patient with stage IIA MF treated with 5 mg/m^2/d for 3 days repeated at 35- to 71-day intervals who had a CR that lasted greater than 16 months off therapy. In a study by Greiner and colleagues[17] in 18 patients with stage I–IVB using 4 to 5 mg/m^2 every 1 to 4 weeks, there was an ORR of 39% (0/1 stage IA, 3/4 stage IIA, 1/3 stage IIB, 1/3 stage III, 2/6 stage IVA, and 0/1 stage IVB), including 2 CRs, with a median number of 5 cycles. In a study performed by the European Organisation for Research and Treatment of Cancer (EORTC), 22 patients with MF with lymphadenopathy or organomegaly and 21 patients with SS treated with pentostatin demonstrated 23% (5/22 patients) and 33% (7/21 patients) ORR, respectively.[18] Dosing in this trial was 4 mg/m^2 weekly for 3 weeks followed by every other week for 6 weeks. There was a monthly maintenance phase for 6 additional months at 4 mg/m^2. In a dose-adaptable study with a starting dose of 5 mg/m^2, Kurzrock and colleagues.[19] reported a response in 70% of 20 patients (10/14 SS and 4/6 tumor stage). Pentostatin (days 1 and 3 at 4 mg/m^2) has been combined with IFN (days 22 and 50 at 10 million units/m^2 and days 23 through 26 at 50 million units/m^2) in a phase II study of 41 patients (2 stage I–IIA, 5 stage IIB/III, 27 stage IVA, and 7 stage IVB) that showed an ORR of 41%.[20] Response in the blood, as defined by at least a 50% reduction in circulating atypical cells, was seen in 8 of 24 patients with blood involvement. None of the 7 patients with IVB (visceral involvement) had a response.

One retrospective study of 8 patients examined the use of pentostatin (4 mg/m^2 every 2 weeks) plus bexarotene (150 mg/m^2 × 14 days followed by 300 mg/m^2 × 14 days) plus cyclophosphamide (600 mg/m^2 every 2 weeks) for up to 8 cycles.[21] A median of 4 cycles was completed, with only 3 patients completing all 8 cycles. The response rate was 88% (1/1 stage IIA, 1/1 stage IIB, 2/2 stage III, 1/1 stage IVA, and 2/3 stage IVB); 5 patients demonstrated a CR, including the 2 patients with stage IVB. Unlike many prospective trials in MF/SS, however, most patients in this study had not been heavily pretreated (or were entirely treatment naïve).

Pentostatin can cause hematologic side effects, including a prolonged depression of CD4 count.[2] The bone marrow suppression with pentostatin typically occurs, however, in the initial cycles and is not as prolonged as observed with other adenosine deaminase inhibitors. GI distress, fevers, and transient liver function test abnormalities may also occur. Neurologic and pulmonary side effects have also been reported.[2]

Pyrimidine Analogs/Antagonists

Pyrimidine analogs are antimetabolites with a chemical structure that mimics pyrimidine bases (uracil and cytosine). Both DNA and RNA synthesis are inhibited, although similar to the purine analogs, it is uncertain which mechanism is most important in cytotoxicity and cell death.

5-Fluorouracil

5-Fluorouracil (5-FU or Adrucil) is an antimetabolite that mimics uracil and inhibits DNA synthesis through irreversible inhibition of thymidylate synthase.[22] There are few data on the use of IV 5-FU in the treatment of lymphoma. One study of 10 patients (1 stage IIA, 4 stage IIB, 1 stage III, 2 stage IVA, and 2 stage IVB) who were treated sequentially with methotrexate (MTX) (60–120 mg/m^2) followed by 5-FU (20 mg/kg per 24 hours for 36 hours) and leucovorin showed response in all patients treated.[23] The median survival for patients with tumors, regardless of stage, in this study was

5.25 years, compared with 3.3 years for patients not treated with this regimen.[24] There has been little follow-up, however, regarding these preliminary findings.

In a similar fashion, topical 5-FU has been reported to be of benefit in some patients with MF. Zackheim and Farber[25] considered the use of topical antimetabolites for the treatment of skin lymphoma more than 40 years ago. Only 1 trial with 6 patients (4 stage IA, 1 stage IB, and 1 stage IIB) has examined the use of topical 5-FU in MF/SS thus far. After daily topical treatment with 5-FU for 3 to 18 months, all 6 patients demonstrated a response.[26]

Cytosine arabinoside

Although there are data supporting the use of cytosine arabinoside (cytarabine or ara-C) in some NHLs, there are no data supporting its use in MF/SS. It is not recommended in the NCCN guidelines for treatment of CTCL.

Gemcitabine

Gemcitabine (2′,2′-dIfluorodeoxycytidine or Gemzar) is a pyrimidine nucleoside analog that mimics deoxycytidine. It is phosphorylated intracellularly and inhibits DNA synthesis. Gemcitabine is unique among the pyrimidine analogs in that it inhibits its own deamination (through interference of deoxycytidylate deaminase), thereby prolonging its activity.[27] It is FDA approved for use in breast, ovarian, lung, and pancreatic cancer. In a phase II study of 30 patients with stage T3 or T4,N0,M0 MF who had failed previous systemic therapy and were treated with 1200 mg/m^2 days 1, 8, and 15 monthly × 3 months, there was a 70% response rate.[28] In a follow-up from 1 of the centers in this study, Zinzani and colleagues reported on 19 patients with T3 or T4,N0,M0 MF who were followed for up to 10 years after treatment with gemcitabine (3–6 cycles at 1200 mg/m^2/d on days 1, 8, and 15 of a 28-day cycle). There was an ORR of 48% with a disease-free interval of 10, 18, and 120 months in 3 patients with a CR. In a multicenter phase II study of 26 patients with untreated MF/SS with advanced-stage disease (T3 or T4,N0,M0) treated with gemcitabine at 1200 mg/m^2 on days 1, 8, and 15 of a 28-day cycle for 6 cycles, an ORR of 73% was observed.[29] There was 1 patient in this trial with SS and that patient did not have a response.[29]

In another phase II study of gemcitabine in patients with MF, primarily stage IIB or greater, treated with 1000 mg/m^2 on days 1, 5, and 8 of a 28-day cycle, 20 of 31 (65%) had a response. Among those patients with stage IVA and IVB having B2 blood involvement (SS), 8 of 11 patients responded.[30] A retrospective study of 14 patients with MF with T3 or T4 disease (11 were transformed) and 6 patients with SS at 4 centers treated with 1000 mg/m^2 (with various schedules) showed 78% ORR in MF and 50% ORR in SS.[31] In a separate study, 3 patients with refractory tumor-stage MF demonstrated a response to gemcitabine, administered at 1000 mg/m^2 for multiple cycles, which was then decreased to 250 mg/m^2 weekly.[32] In all 3 patients, there was eventual progression of lymphoma within 4 months of stopping therapy (including 1 case with meningeal involvement), suggesting that low-dose gemcitabine is not useful as a maintenance therapy. These findings are in contrast to a separate case series reporting that 4 of 8 patients with refractory MF who had a response with lower-dose gemcitabine (150 mg/m^2).[30] The role of lower-dose gemcitabine in maintenance therapy requires further exploration. Finally, in a trial that combined gemcitabine, 1000 mg/m^2 IV on days 1 and 8 of a 21-day cycle for 4 cycles, with bexarotene, 300 mg/m^2 daily in 35 patients with MF/SS (5 stage IB, 2 stage IIA, 8 stage IIB, 8 stage III, and 12 stage IVA), the combination was not superior to gemcitabine alone.[33]

More common side effects of gemcitabine include elevations in liver function tests and bone marrow suppression with anemia, thrombocytopenia, and/or leukopenia. Other side effects include pulmonary toxicity, hemolytic uremic syndrome, exacerbation of radiation toxicity, capillary leak syndrome, hyperpigmentation, and posterior reversible encephalopathy,[2,34] all of which are rare.

Antifolates

Pralatrexate and MTX are discussed in the article by Wood and Wu elsewhere in this issue.

ALKYLATING AGENTS

Alkylating agents in chemotherapy were developed after it was noted that people exposed to the military agent, mustard gas, developed bone marrow suppression and lymphopenia. Nitrogen mustard was a less toxic agent that showed efficacy in various lymphomas.[35] There are 6 types of alkylating agents: (1) nitrogen mustards, (2) nitrosoureas, (3) alkyl sulfonates, (4) triazines, (5) ethylenimines, and (6) metal salts. The cellular enzyme O^6-methylguanine–DNA methyltransferase (MGMT) is able to repair the cyotoxic damage caused by alkylating agents, thereby introducing a mechanism for resistance to these compounds.

Nitrogen Mustards

Mechlorethamine

Mechlorethamine (Mustargen) is an alkylating agent that is currently infrequently used in a systemic form in the treatment of MF and SS. Karnofsky[36] and Van Scott and colleagues[37] reported 21 and 41 cases of MF/SS, respectively, treated with systemic nitrogen mustard. Karnofsky noted some benefit in the first cycle but later cycles were less effective.[36] Van Scott treated 46 patients with advanced cutaneous lymphomas, including 41 with MF or SS, with systemic Mustargen at various dosing regimens along with topical nitrogen mustard and reported a decrease in stage of disease in 34/41 MF/SS patients, including 12/41 (29%) with a CR.[37] These results with systemic nitrogen mustard ultimately led to the use of topical nitrogen mustard in the treatment of MF/SS.

Lymphopenia due to systemic mechlorethamine is common. Additional side effects include alopecia, tinnitus, nausea, vomiting, hypersensitivity, skin eruptions, and damage to reproductive organs/infertility. Thrombosis and thrombophlebitis may occur when the drug is infused IV.

Chlorambucil

Developed from nitrogen mustard, chlorambucil (Leukeran) is an alkylating agent that prevents DNA replication by cross-linking DNA, leading to DNA strand breaks. Chlorambucil was one of the first systemic treatments recognized to have activity specifically in SS[38,39] and since that time, there have been multiple case reports/series suggesting benefit in this setting.[40–42] Winkelmann developed the Winkelmann method, which consists of oral chlorambucil (2–6 mg/d) with prednisone (10–20 mg/d, weaned over time) for the treatment of SS.[39,43–45] It has also been adapted for the treatment of CLL, where it continues to be a common therapy.[45] Winkelmann reported that SS patients lived twice as long with chlorambucil therapy and 10 of 17 patients had a decreased peripheral blood Sézary cell count. Seven of 19 SS patients had a CR for at least 1 year on chlorambucil/corticosteroid.[44] Coors and colleagues[43] used chlorambucil with corticosteroids (chlorambucil 10–12 mg for 3 days and fluocortolone, first day 75 mg, second day 50 mg, and third day 25 mg) twice monthly and reported a 100% ORR in 13 patients with erythrodermic disease (8 stage III, 4 stage IVA, and 1 stage IVB). Moreover, a significant improvement in pruritus was also reported. McEvoy and colleagues[46] described 11 patients treated with combined chlorambucil-prednisone using the

Winkelmann method and adding leukapheresis with an ORR of 100%.

Lower doses of chlorambucil as utilized in the Winkelmann method are well tolerated. Leukopenia can occur and requires monthly blood counts.[2] Less common side effects include bone marrow suppression (thrombocytopenia, anemia, and leukopenia), drug fever, and hyperuricemia, which often occur soon after starting therapy. Additionally, because some patients remain on chlorambucil for longer periods of time, it is important to be aware of the delayed side effects, which include amenorrhea, azospermia, infertility, pulmonary interstitial fibrosis, cystitis, hepatotoxicity, and peripheral neuropathy. These toxicities are consistent among other alkylating agents. Although in a past, study doses above 1300 mg of chlorambucil were found leukomogenic,[47] more recently the risk of secondary malignancy in NHL after chlorambucil treatment was not found significant.[48]

Ifosfamide
Ifosfamide is an alkylating agent that has been combined with other chemotherapies in the treatment of NHL. It is part of ifosfamide, carboplatin, and etoposide (ICE) and ifosfamide and etoposide (IFE) multiagent chemotherapy. Although there are no data on its use in MF/SS, it has been reported (multiagent ICE regimen) in the treatment of non-MF CTCL.[49] It is also used as a second-line agent for aggressive T-cell lymphomas.[50]

Bendamustine
Bendamustine (Treanda) is a nitrogen mustard alkylating agent. Its chemical structure also makes it a purine analog.[51] This diversity in structure may explain why it is effective in a diverse range of cancers, including CLL[52]; multiple myeloma[53]; solid tumors, including breast and lung cancer[54,55]; and NHL.[56,57] It has a different antitumor effect than other alkylating agents (including cyclophosphamide, chlorambucil, or melphalan) and seems to function not only as an alkylating agent causing DNA breaks but also through effects on transcription and posttranslational events.[51] Bendamustine's structure and diversity of mechanism of action may make it less susceptible to drug resistance than other alkylating agents.[51] It is FDA approved for the treatment of indolent NHLs and CLL. Bendamustine, 120 mg/m^2/d over 30 to 60 minutes on days 1 and 2 every 3 weeks, for a total of 6 cycles, demonstrated benefit in T-cell lymphomas in an early phase II trial. This trial only included 2 MF patients (stage not defined) who were not analyzed as a subgroup. The ORR in the study (with most patients having peripheral T-cell lymphoma [PTCL]) was 50% (30 of 60 patients).[58] In a second trial that enrolled 3 patients with advanced-stage MF/SS, there were 2 with a PR at monotherapy doses of 60 to 100 mg/m^2.[59] The nonresponder, however, only received 1 cycle of bendamustine.

Myelosuppression requiring granulocyte colony-stimulating growth factors frequently occurs. Other hematologic abnormalities are also common, including lymphopenia, anemia, and thrombocytopenia. Infections, infusion reactions, and severe skin reactions, including toxic epidermal necrosis, have been reported. There are also reports of severe cytomegalovirus reactivation with treatment.[60] The most common nonhematologic side effects are nausea and vomiting.

Cyclophosphamide
Cyclophosphamide (Cytoxan) is an alkylating agent and derivative of mechlorethamine. Similar to other alkylating agents, it induces double-strand breaks in DNA. Although multiple studies have shown that single-agent cyclophosphamide has activity against MF/SS, the benefit is often low.[61–66] Abele and Dobson[61] reported 4 cases, mostly with early-stage disease, who showed a response. Van Scott and colleagues[66] subsequently reported 11 more cases, with 5 patients responding to single-agent cyclophosphamide at 50 to 300 mg/d for up to 117 days. Patients were treated until they developed leukopenia or anemia. There are multiple dose-limiting toxicities. Hemorrhagic cystitis, risk to reproductive capacity, and total alopecia are additional issues. Currently, single-agent cyclophosphamide is uncommonly used. As part of multiagent regimens (eg, CHOP), it remains a commonly used drug in MF/SS (see **Table 2**).

Melphalan
Melphalan (phenylalanine mustard, L-PAM, or Alkeran) is an alkylating agent and not used in the primary treatment of MF/SS but is used in combination in some conditioning regimens during stem cell transplantation.[67–69] This is discussed in the article by Virmani and colleagues elsewhere in this issue.

Lomustine
Lomustine (CeeNU) is an alkylating agent that is approved by the FDA for the treatment of brain tumors and Hodgkin lymphoma. It has not been studied in MF/SS but has been reported to have activity in 2 Tasmanian devils, 1 ground cuscus, and frequently in dogs with CTCL.[70–72] It is not recommended in the NCCN guidelines for treatment of NHL.

Nimustine

Similar to carmustine (BCNU), nimustine (ACNU or Nidran) has activity against MF, although the level of activity has been relatively undefined. It is not FDA approved for any use.[73]

Nitrosoureas

Carmustine

Carmustine is used IV for some lymphomas but not for MF/SS. It is compounded for topical application.

Alkyl Sulfonates

Busulfan

Busulfan (Busulfex or Myleran) is not used in the primary treatment of MF/SS but is used in combination in some conditioning regimens during stem cell transplantation.[67–69]

Triazines

Dacarbazine

Dacarbazine (DTIC or DTIC-Dome) is an alkylating agent that is not used as a single agent in MF/SS but is part of the doxorubicin, bleomycin, vincristine, and dacarbazine (ABVD) multiagent chemotherapy, a first-line therapy for Hodgkin lymphoma. Its benefit in MF/SS has not been established.

Temozolomide

Temozolomide (TMZ or Temodar) is an oral alkylating agent and a derivative of dacarbazine that is FDA approved for the treatment of certain brain cancers. In several small studies it has been shown to have activity in MF/SS. One patient with advanced MF was part of a study of 42 patients examining TMZ therapy for advanced cancer. The patient had a CR that lasted 7 months.[74] In a study of 9 patients with stage IIB or III MF, there was an ORR of 33% (3 of 9).[75] In the most recent trial, which examined TMZ at 200 mg/m^2 for 5 days every 28 days in stage IB–IVA MF/SS, there was an ORR in 7 of 26 (27%) in patients with treatment refractory disease.[76] Response was assessed at the 2nd cycle and responders were treated with TMZ through 1 year. The median disease-free survival, however, was only 4 months.

Myelopsuppression is common and requires dose reduction. The drop in neutrophils commonly occurs on day 22 after the initial dose. Nausea, vomiting, hepatotoxicity, and infections can also occur. Prophylaxis for pneumocystis pneumonia is required.

Procarbazine

Procarbazine (Matulane) has not been reported in the primary treatment of MF/SS but is used in certain multiagent regimens, such as MOPP (see **Table 2**).

Ethylenimines

Thiotepa

Thiotepa (Thioplex) is not used in the primary treatment of MF/SS but is used in combination in some conditioning regimens during stem cell transplantation.[67–69]

Metal Salts

Carboplatin

Carboplatin (Paraplatin) is not used in the primary treatment of MF/SS but is used in multiagent ICE therapy. ICE is generally reserved, however, for use only in transformed MF/SS as a second-line therapy.[50]

Cisplatin

Cisplatin (Platinol) is not used in the primary treatment of MF/SS but is used in multiagent (eg, etoposide, methyprednisilone, cytarabine, cisplatin [ESHAP]) therapy. ESHAP is generally reserved, however, for use only in second- or third-line salvage therapy in transformed MF/SS. Moreover, its risk/benefit has been questioned by a past study in patients with aggressive CTCL, which included 1 SS and 1 MF patient, due to high recurrence and low duration of response.[77] There was 1 PR in the MF patient, but that patient demonstrated disease progression within 2 months.

TOPOISOMERASE INHIBITORS
Anthracyclines

Anthracyclines were first developed from a compound found in the soil bacteria *Streptomyces*.[78] They are 1 of the most important class of drugs in the treatment of hematologic cancers[79] and work mainly by DNA intercalation and inhibition of topoisomerase II.[80] Although there is a strong antitumor effect, cardiotoxicity has been a common side effect that has historically limited use. Newer delivery systems that involve liposome encapsulation prolong the half-life of drug in circulation and alter the biodistribution such that there is increased deposition in tumor tissue with decreased deposition in normal tissues, with resultant decreased toxicity.[81–83] Pegylation additionally improves pharmacodynamics and pharmacokinetics of the drug. These formulations with decreased cardiotoxicity have allowed anthracyclines to be important agents in the treatment of MF/SS.

Doxorubicin and pegylated liposomal doxorubicin

Doxorubicin (AAN, hydroxydaunorubicin, or Adriamycin) is currently the most commonly used anthracycline for advanced CTCL. It is used for the treatment of NHL as part of the CHOP regimen. It is also FDA approved for the treatment of HIV-related Kaposi sarcoma. Doxorubicin monotherapy in MF was first reported by Levi and colleagues in 1977.[84] Thirteen patients with MF (described as "advanced disease," including 10 with tumors, 8 with lymph node involvement, and 4 with visceral involvement) were treated with a single IV dose of 60 mg/m^2, repeated in 21-day intervals, and continued for 3 doses beyond maximum clinical response for those who achieved remission. The investigators reported an ORR of 85%, including 23% CR. One patient with preexisting heart disease experienced cardiotoxicity with fatal congestive heart failure. In a dose-escalation study with pegylated liposomal doxorubicin (Doxil or Caelyx), Wollina and colleagues[85] reported 30 patients with stage I–IV MF and 1 patient with SS treated with 20 to 40 mg/m^2 1 to 2 times monthly; 26 of 30 patients with MF and the 1 patient with SS achieved a PR with an ORR of 87%, including 43% CR. Di Lorenzo and colleagues[86] reported on 10 patients with stage IVB MF treated with pegylated liposomal doxorubicin 20 mg/m^2 IV every 4 weeks. Unlike the patients in Wollina and colleagues' study, no subjects were noted to have a CR; 3 patients experienced a PR with an ORR of 30%. The investigators attribute the difference in response between the 2 studies to the fact that those in the latter study were characterized uniformly by advanced-stage disease. In a multicenter phase II trial with pegylated liposomal doxorubicin,[87] 19 patients, including 16 patients with MF/SS and 3 with PTCL, were treated with 20 mg/m^2 every 4 weeks for 2 to 8 treatments. The investigators reported an ORR of 81.2% (13/16) in the MF/SS patients, including a CR in 1 of 4 patients with stage I–IIA MF, 6 of 9 patients with stage IIB–IV MF, and 1 of 3 patients with SS. In another study with 25 patients with stage IIB–IVB MF and SS, subjects were administered pegylated liposomal doxorubicin at 40 mg/m^2 monthly for 8 cycles.[88] There was an ORR of 56%, with 5 patients achieving CR and 9 patients achieving PR. Of patients with SS, 1 had CR and 5 experienced PR. In those patients who responded, a median progression-free survival (PFS) of 5 months was observed. In an EORTC-initiated phase II trial for pegylated liposomal doxorubicin, Dummer and colleagues[89] studied a cohort of 49 patients with stage IIA–IVB MF from 9 centers in 6 countries. The patients were treated with 20 mg/m^2 IV on days 1 and 15 every 28 days (1 cycle) for up to 6 cycles. The ORR was 40.8%, including 3 patients with CR and 17 patients with PR. PFS was approximately 6 months in those who responded. In 2014, Straus and colleagues[90] published results of a phase II trial using doxorubicin hydroxychloride liposome injection in 37 patients with stage IB–IV disease, including 10 patients with SS. Subjects were treated with 20 mg/m^2 IV every 2 weeks for 16 weeks. All patients who did not progress also received bexarotene, 300 mg/m^2 daily, starting at week 16 for an additional 16 weeks; 41% responded with a CR observed in 2 patients (both stage IV) and a PR in 12 patients. The median overall survival duration was 18 months; there were 22 deaths after discontinuation of protocol treatment.

As discussed previously, cardiotoxicity may occur with doxorubicin, the risk of which may be reduced by limiting the cumulative dose to 450 to 550 mg/m^2.[91] Additional side effects include dose-dependent hematologic toxicity (including severe neutropenia), GI symptoms, palmoplantar erythrodysesthesia, and alopecia.

Daunorubicin and liposomal daunorubicin

Similar to doxorubicin, daunorubicin (daunomycin or Cerubidine) is a topoisomerase inhibitor anthracycline.[78] Although there has been more utilization of liposomal doxorubicin in MF/SS, liposomal daunorubicin (DaunoXome) also has shown activity in MF/SS. In a case series of 3 patients with tumor stage MF receiving liposomal daunorubicin, at 20 to 40 mg/m^2 once every 3 to 4 weeks, all 3 patients responded.[92]

Liposomal daunorubicin is FDA approved for the treatment of advanced HIV-associated Kaposi sarcoma. Myelosuppression, infections, alopecia, neuropathy, and cardiotoxicity occur, although grade 3 and 4 reactions are less common.

Epirubicin (Ellence)

The anthracycline, epirubicin (Ellence), is comparable to doxorubicin and has been described in a multiagent regimen similar to CHOP but without vincristine.[93] In the patient reported, however, who had stage IB disease, skin-directed therapies are standard and not multiagent chemotherapy. Several other cases with modified CHOP regimens have also been described replacing epirubicin for doxorubicin.[94,95] It is currently not known if epirubicin has any advantage over doxorubicin in multiagent regimens for MF/SS. Moreover, foregoing vincristine is not known to be significantly safer or superior to standard CHOP.

Idrarubicin

Idrarubicin (4-demethoxydaunorubicin or Idrarubicin) is an anthracycline approved by the FDA for the combination treatment of acute myeloid leukemia in adults. It is currently not known if idrarubicin has any advantage over doxorubicin in the treatment of MF/SS. It has been reported in combination with etoposide, idarubicin, cyclophosphamide, vincristine, prednisone, and bleomycin (VICOP-B) in advanced MF, but there were no responses observed in SS[96] (see **Table 2**).

Etoposide

Etoposide (VP-16, VP-16-213, or epipodophyllotoxin) is a semisynthetic derivative of podophyllotoxin, a plant toxin. It is FDA approved for small cell lung cancer, treatment of testicular tumors, and part of combination chemotherapy regimens for hematologic malignancies. It is available in both oral and IV formulations. Etoposide functions primarily via reversible binding to DNA topoisomerase II, which results in the inability of this enzyme to repair double-stranded DNA breaks and subsequent cell death. Additionally, it induces single-strand and double-stranded DNA breaks.[2]

Etoposide as monotherapy in MF/SS is not well studied and consists predominantly of single case reports. Jacobs and colleagues,[97] in 1975, reported a patient with tumor-stage MF who experienced CR to etoposide, 60 mg/m^2 IV for 5 days, given every 2 weeks. The total duration of treatment was not reported. The investigators also reported a second patient[98] with stage III MF who achieved CR with the same induction regimen for a total of 5 infusions, followed by monthly maintenance courses of 60 mg/m^2 IV and oral etoposide 100 mg/m^2 twice weekly for 3 weeks. Molin and colleagues[99] treated 9 patients with MF/SS (1/9 plaque stage and 8/9 tumor stage) with etoposide, 100 mg IV daily × 5 days every 2 to 3 weeks induction therapy, followed by 100 mg daily × 5 days during maintenance. Four of these patients also received concomitant cyclophosphamide. CR occurred in 2 patients and PR in 3; of these, 1 CR and 1 PR were treated with single-agent etoposide. In all responders, disease progression eventually occurred after 4 to 6 months. Nasuhara and colleagues[100] described a patient with MF with pulmonary involvement who experienced CR of over 2 years' duration with oral etoposide, 200 mg weekly, and prednisolone. He had previously been treated with combination chemotherapy with CHOP without any impact on skin lesions. Onozuka and colleagues[101] reported a patient with stage III MF treated with 150 mg IV, 3 times per week for 9 weeks, followed by oral etoposide, 25 mg daily for 21 days every 4 weeks; this therapy was continued for 60 months, 36 of which he experienced CR. Miyoshi and Noda[102] described a patient with SS (criteria not defined) who experienced CR for 4 years with oral etoposide; the dose used was not specified, however. Hirayama and colleagues[103] also reported a patient with SS who experienced CR with etoposide therapy; he was administered 25 mg orally with concomitant MTX of 10 mg weekly, with response maintained for 4 years.

Etoposide is generally well tolerated. Side effects predominantly involve myelosuppression and may be dose limiting. Other adverse effects include GI symptoms (nausea and vomiting), mucositis, and alopecia.[2] Chronic etoposide therapy has also been associated with acute myeloid leukemia. This complication has been reported 15 to 100 months after initiation of therapy, with increased risk associated with total cumulative dose as well as increased treatment frequency (ie, weekly or twice-weekly therapy compared with alternate week therapy).[102,104,105]

INTERLEUKINS
Interleukin-2

Interleukin (IL)-2 (aldesleukin or Proleukin) is a 15-kD polypeptide produced by activated CD4$^+$ lymphocytes. Overall, IL-2 stimulates activation, proliferation, and maintenance of T-helper lymphocytes in vivo and in vitro.[106] Although its antitumor effects are not well understood, they have been observed in various tumors. In MF/SS, IL-2 is thought to prevent and control disease progression through a favorable influence on cytokine milieu, including T-helper cytokine balance in immune responses.[107] IL-2 is FDA approved for the treatment of metastatic renal cell carcinoma and metastatic melanoma.

Nagatani and colleagues[108] first reported the successful treatment of a patient with tumor-stage MF treated first with intralesional IL-2 and then systemic IL-2 monthly. He maintained CR for 13 months. Rybojad and colleagues[109] reported a patient with stage IIB MF with a cytotoxic immunophenotype (CD8$^+$ and CD4$^-$) post–total skin electron beam radiation and autologous bone marrow transplant who underwent induction therapy with IL-2 IV infusion of 10 million units/m^2/d for 5, 4, and 3 consecutive days every 2 weeks followed by 5 monthly maintenance courses of 10 million units/m^2/d for 2 days. The patient achieved a CR and remained without evidence of disease 10 months after discontinuation of therapy. Marolleau and colleagues[110] evaluated 3 patients with MF and 3 with SS treated with IV

IL-2 20 million units/m² on days 1 to 5, 14 to 17, and 28 to 30 (induction) followed by 2 days per month for 5 months (consolidation). At the end of consolidation, 2 of 3 patients with MF (stages IIB–IVA) experienced a CR; a PR was seen in 1 of 3 SS patients. In a follow-up letter, it was observed that 2 of the patients with a CR continued to have response at 56 and 63 months post-treatment.[111]

Gisselbrecht and colleagues[112] performed a phase II study with 5 patients with MF (all stage IV) and 2 patients with SS treated with IV infusions of 20 million units/m²/d for 5, 4, and 3 days on weeks 1, 3, and 5 followed by an optional monthly maintenance therapy of 5 days. One patient had CR and 4 had a PR with an ORR of 71%. The patient with CR had a continued response for 29 months after initial response. In a phase II study using subcutaneous injections, Querfeld and colleagues[107] evaluated 22 patients with MF. Eleven MUs were injected for 4 consecutive days per week × 6 weeks followed by 2 weeks' observation and repeated for 8 weeks as tolerated. Only 4 patients responded (18%; 1/1 stage IA, 1/6 stage IB, 0/1 stage IIA, 1/3 stage IIB, 1/4 stage III, and 0/7 stage IVA/SS) and no CR was noted. The median event-free survival was 3 months.

Side effects include flulike illness (fever, chills, and fatigue), GI symptoms (nausea and vomiting), weight gain, elevated creatinine, hypotension, cytopenia, vascular leak syndrome, neurologic symptoms, and cardiac toxicity.[2,107,110]

Interleukin-12

IL-12 acts as a potent inducer of IFN-γ by T cells and natural killer cells and directly stimulates cytotoxic T-cell activity.[106,113] In advanced stages of CTCL, peripheral blood dendritic cells (which are producers of IL-12) are depleted in number and function with a concomitant decrease in IL-12 production.[106,114–116] Additionally, diminished IL-12 levels may occur due to increased IL-10 production by malignant T cells.[113] Recombinant human IL-12 has been evaluated in the treatment of MF/SS. Currently, there are no FDA-approved uses for IL-12.

In a phase I dose-escalation trial, 7 patients with MF (2 with T1, 3 with T2, 2 with T3, 2 with T4 skin stages, and 3 with SS) received 50, 100, or 300 ng/kg of IL-12 subcutaneously twice weekly for up to 24 weeks.[117] Each patient with T3 disease received the injections directly into tumor lesions. The ORR was 56% with 2 patients achieving CR (both T2) and 3 with PR (2 with T1 skin stage and 1 SS). In patients with tumors, there was flattening and/or resolution of the tumors treated intralesionally, but new lesions developed at other sites. In a

phase II trial, Rook and colleagues[118] evaluated 23 patients with stage IA–IIA MF treated with subcutaneous IL-12 100 ng/kg twice weekly × 2 weeks with subsequent increase to 300 ng/kg twice weekly for up to 24 weeks.[119] There was an ORR of 43% (10/23), all of which were PRs. Although no CRs were observed, many of those with a PR had extensive clearing of skin lesions.

Adverse effects of IL-12 are generally mild and short lived. These include fatigue, headache, myalgias, injection site reaction, neutropenia, diarrhea, depression, and anxiety.[113,117–119] One death from autoimmune hemolytic anemia has been observed,[119] but it was unclear if this was directly due to IL-12 administration or secondary to an infection.

PURINE NUCLEOSIDE PHOSPHORYLASE INHIBITORS: FORODESINE

Purine nucleoside phosphorylase (PNP) catalyzes phosphorolysis of deoxyguanosine to guanine and ribose 1-phosphate[120,121] Inhibition of PNP in T lymphocytes results in the accumulation of deoxyguanosine triphosphate, which in turn inhibits DNA synthesis with resultant suppression of cell proliferation.[121,122] Selective T-cell depletion occurs with PNP inhibition due to a relatively high level of kinase and low level of nucleotidase activity compared with those in other cells.[123–125] Forodesine (BCX-1777 or immucillin H) is a potent inhibitor of PNP that is available orally and in IV formulation. It has been shown to inhibit the proliferation of T lymphocytes in vivo and in vitro.[121,122,126] Forodesine has been examined in several studies for the treatment of MF/SS.

In a study of 13 patients (described as stage IIB–IV with all but 1 ≥ stage III), IV forodesine of 40 to 320 mg/m² was administered on day 1 followed by 8 doses every 12 hours (1 cycle) and repeated in 16-day intervals for a total of 3 cycles at 2-week intervals. Nine patients (69%) showed some degree of response.[127] Duvic and colleagues[128] reported a phase I/II trial of 37 patients with stage IB or greater CTCL. Patients were treated with oral forodesine, 40 to 320 mg/m² daily for 4 weeks. It was not reported how many of these patients represented MF/SS versus other cutaneous lymphomas. In patients with IIB or greater disease, the ORR was 53.6%, including 1 patient with a CR and 9 with a PR. The median duration of response was 127 days. Dummer and colleagues[129] recently published a phase II multicenter study of forodesine in 144 individuals, in whom 101 patients with stage IIB or greater disease were assessed for efficacy of the drug. Patients were administered 200 mg orally daily (approximately equivalent to 80 mg/m^2). An ORR of 11% was noted. The lower response rate compared with prior studies was thought possibly due to the lower dose of medication administered in this study.

Forodesine is generally well tolerated. Side effects include nausea, fatigue, reversible lymphopenia, and cutaneous infections.[127,129]

PROTEASOME INHIBITORS: BORTEZOMIB

Bortezomib (Velcade) is a cell-permeable dipeptide boronic acid that reversibly inhibits the β5 subunit of the proteasome. Multiple pro-oncogenic factors are under proteasome control, such as transcription factors, cyclins, cyclin-dependent kinase inhibitors, and apoptotic factors.[130–132] The antitumor acitivity of bortezomib likely varies among tumor types. It is FDA approved for IV treatment of multiple myeloma and mantle cell lymphoma. Only 1 study has evaluated the efficacy of bortezomib in MF. In a phase II trial, Zinzani and colleagues[133] evaluated 10 patients with MF (1 stage IIA, 3 stage IIB, and 6 stage IVA/B) treated with 1.3 mg/m^2 twice weekly for 2 weeks followed by 1-week rest period for up to 6 cycles. A response was noted in 7 patients (70%), including 1 CR and 6 PR. The duration of response was 7 to 14 months; the patient with a CR continued to be in remission 12 months after initial response.

Bortezomib is generally well tolerated; toxicities include neutropenia, thrombocytopenia, and sensory neuropathy. In trials for multiple myeloma, asthenia, GI symptoms, and headache were also documented.[2]

MULTIAGENT CHEMOTHERAPY

Although there are no large controlled studies of multiagent chemotherapy regimens in MF/SS, multiagent chemotherapy is the first-line treatment, along with clinical trials, for most aggressive/rapidly progressive CTCLs (including transformed MF).[134] Although the mainstay is the CHOP regimen,[135] first-line treatment also includes multiagent etoposide, vincristine, doxorubicin, bolus cyclophosphamide, and oral prednisone (EPOCH)[136] and hyper–cyclophosphamide, vincristine, doxorubicin, and dexamethasone (CVAD) alternating with high-dose MTX and cytarabine.[137] For individuals who are candidates for cell transplant, second-line multiagent therapy includes dexamethasone, cisplatin, and cytarabine (DHAP); etoposide, methylprednisolone, cytarabine, and cisplatin (ESHAP); gemcitabine, dexamethasone, and cisplatin (GDP); gemcitabine

and oxaliplatin (GemOx); ICE; and mesna, ifosfamide, mitoxantrone, and etoposide (MINE).[50,134,138–143] Overall, however, the efficacy of multiagent chemotherapy in the treatment of MF/SS is not well established. Studies that have evaluated various multiagent treatment regimens have often included other concomitant treatments, such as photopheresis or IFN administration, further hindering evaluation of their efficacy. Additionally, despite oft-reported high initial response rates, the duration of response is frequently short lived. Studies that have used multiagent chemotherapy in MF/SS are summarized in **Table 2**.

SUMMARY

Despite recent advances in the development of more targeted therapies in MF/SS, traditional chemotherapies remain an important modality for induction therapy, with some agents used as maintenance therapy. These agents generally target proliferating cells and, therefore, have significant toxicities. Nevertheless, as a category, traditional chemotherapies provide remissions as good as most other therapies and, therefore, must be relied on until more targeted therapies are developed. Other agents, including ILs, phosphorylase inhibitors, and proteasome inhibitors, may have a more significant role in treatment after further study.

REFERENCES

1. Hughes CF, Khot A, McCormack C, et al. Lack of durable disease control with chemotherapy for mycosis fungoides and Sezary syndrome: a comparative study of systemic therapy. Blood 2015;125(1):71–81.
2. Olsen EA, Rook AH, Zic J, et al. Sezary syndrome: immunopathogenesis, literature review of therapeutic options, and recommendations for therapy by the United States Cutaneous Lymphoma Consortium (USCLC). J Am Acad Dermatol 2011; 64(2):352–404.
3. Horwitz SM, Olsen EA, Duvic M, et al. Review of the treatment of mycosis fungoides and sezary syndrome: a stage-based approach. J Natl Compr Canc Netw 2008;6(4):436–42.
4. Redman JR, Cabanillas F, Velasquez WS, et al. Phase II trial of fludarabine phosphate in lymphoma: an effective new agent in low-grade lymphoma. J Clin Oncol 1992;10(5):790–4.
5. Von Hoff DD, Dahlberg S, Hartstock RJ, et al. Activity of fludarabine monophosphate in patients with advanced mycosis fungoides: a Southwest Oncology Group study. J Natl Cancer Inst 1990; 82(16):1353–5.

6. Quaglino P, Fierro MT, Rossotto GL, et al. Treatment of advanced mycosis fungoides/Sezary syndrome with fludarabine and potential adjunctive benefit to subsequent extracorporeal photochemotherapy. Br J Dermatol 2004;150(2):327–36.

7. Foss FM, Ihde DC, Linnoila IR, et al. Phase II trial of fludarabine phosphate and interferon alfa-2a in advanced mycosis fungoides/Sezary syndrome. J Clin Oncol 1994;12(10):2051–9.

8. Scarisbrick JJ, Child FJ, Clift A, et al. A trial of fludarabine and cyclophosphamide combination chemotherapy in the treatment of advanced refractory primary cutaneous T-cell lymphoma. Br J Dermatol 2001;144(5):1010–5.

9. Betticher DC, Fey MF, von Rohr A, et al. High incidence of infections after 2-chlorodeoxyadenosine (2-CDA) therapy in patients with malignant lymphomas and chronic and acute leukaemias. Ann Oncol 1994;5(1):57–64.

10. O'Brien S, Kurzrock R, Duvic M, et al. 2-Chlorodeoxyadenosine therapy in patients with T-cell lymphoproliferative disorders. Blood 1994;84(3):733–8.

11. Kuzel TM, Hurria A, Samuelson E, et al. Phase II trial of 2-chlorodeoxyadenosine for the treatment of cutaneous T-cell lymphoma. Blood 1996;87(3):906–11.

12. Trautinger F, Schwarzmeier J, Honigsmann H, et al. Low-dose 2-chlorodeoxyadenosine for the treatment of mycosis fungoides. Arch Dermatol 1999;135(10):1279–80.

13. Jawed SI, Myskowski PL, Horwitz S, et al. Primary cutaneous T-cell lymphoma (mycosis fungoides and Sezary syndrome): part II. Prognosis, management, and future directions. J Am Acad Dermatol 2014;70(2):223.e1–17 [quiz: 240–2].

14. Tsimberidou AM, Giles F, Duvic M, et al. Phase II study of pentostatin in advanced T-cell lymphoid malignancies: update of an M.D. Anderson Cancer Center series. Cancer 2004;100(2):342–9.

15. Cummings FJ, Kim K, Neiman RS, et al. Phase II trial of pentostatin in refractory lymphomas and cutaneous T-cell disease. J Clin Oncol 1991;9(4):565–71.

16. Dang-Vu AP, Olsen EA, Vollmer RT, et al. Treatment of cutaneous T cell lymphoma with 2'-deoxycoformycin (pentostatin). J Am Acad Dermatol 1988;19(4):692–8.

17. Greiner D, Olsen EA, Petroni G. Pentostatin (2'-deoxycoformycin) in the treatment of cutaneous T-cell lymphoma. J Am Acad Dermatol 1997;36(6 Pt 1):950–5.

18. Ho AD, Suciu S, Stryckmans P, et al. Pentostatin in T-cell malignancies–a phase II trial of the EORTC. Leukemia Cooperative Group. Ann Oncol 1999;10(12):1493–8.

19. Kurzrock R, Pilat S, Duvic M. Pentostatin therapy of T-cell lymphomas with cutaneous manifestations. J Clin Oncol 1999;17(10):3117–21.

20. Foss FM, Ihde DC, Breneman DL, et al. Phase II study of pentostatin and intermittent high-dose recombinant interferon alfa-2a in advanced mycosis fungoides/Sezary syndrome. J Clin Oncol 1992;10(12):1907–13.

21. Calderon Cabrera C, de la Cruz Vicente F, Marin-Niebla A, et al. Pentostatin plus cyclophosphamide and bexarotene is an effective and safe combination in patients with mycosis fungoides/Sezary syndrome. Br J Haematol 2013;162(1):130–2.

22. Longley DB, Harkin DP, Johnston PG. 5-Fluorouracil: mechanisms of action and clinical strategies. Nat Rev Cancer 2003;3(5):330–8.

23. Schappell DL, Alper JC, McDonald CJ. Treatment of advanced mycosis fungoides and Sezary syndrome with continuous infusions of methotrexate followed by fluorouracil and leucovorin rescue. Arch Dermatol 1995;131(3):307–13.

24. Kim YH, Liu HL, Mraz-Gernhard S, et al. Long-term outcome of 525 patients with mycosis fungoides and Sezary syndrome: clinical prognostic factors and risk for disease progression. Arch Dermatol 2003;139(7):857–66.

25. Zackheim HS, Farber EM. Topical antimetabolites. Annu Rev Med 1970;21:59–66.

26. Kannangara AP, Levitan D, Fleischer AB Jr. Six patients with early-stage cutaneous T-cell lymphoma successfully treated with topical 5-fluorouracil. J Drugs Dermatol 2010;9(8):1017–8.

27. Mini E, Nobili S, Caciagli B, et al. Cellular pharmacology of gemcitabine. Ann Oncol 2006;17(Suppl 5):v7–12.

28. Zinzani PL, Baliva G, Magagnoli M, et al. Gemcitabine treatment in pretreated cutaneous T-cell lymphoma: experience in 44 patients. J Clin Oncol 2000;18(13):2603–6.

29. Marchi E, Alinari L, Tani M, et al. Gemcitabine as frontline treatment for cutaneous T-cell lymphoma: phase II study of 32 patients. Cancer 2005;104(11):2437–41.

30. Duvic M, Talpur R, Wen S, et al. Phase II evaluation of gemcitabine monotherapy for cutaneous T-cell lymphoma. Clin Lymphoma Myeloma 2006;7(1):51–8.

31. Jidar K, Ingen-Housz-Oro S, Beylot-Barry M, et al. Gemcitabine treatment in cutaneous T-cell lymphoma: a multicentre study of 23 cases. Br J Dermatol 2009;161(3):660–3.

32. Buhl T, Bertsch HP, Kaune KM, et al. Low-dose gemcitabine efficacious in three patients with tumor-stage mycosis fungoides. Clin Lymphoma Myeloma 2009;9(5):E21–4.

33. Illidge T, Chan C, Counsell N, et al. Phase II study of gemcitabine and bexarotene (GEMBEX) in the treatment of cutaneous T-cell lymphoma. Br J Cancer 2013;109(10):2566–73.

34. Marrone LC, Marrone BF, de la Puerta Raya J, et al. Gemcitabine monotherapy associated with

posterior reversible encephalopathy syndrome. Case Rep Oncol 2011;4(1):82–7.

35. Rhoads CP. Nitrogen mustards in the treatment of neoplastic disease; official statement. J Am Med Assoc 1946;131:656–8.

36. Karnofsky DA. Nitrogen mustards in the treatment of neoplastic disease. Adv Intern Med 1950;4:1–75.

37. Van Scott EJ, Grekin DA, Kalmanson JD, et al. Frequent low doses of intravenous mechlorethamine for late-stage mycosis fungoides lymphoma. Cancer 1975;36(5):1613–8.

38. Libánský J, Trapl J. Chlorambucil in erythrodermia. Lancet 1960;275(7127):732–3.

39. Winkelmann RK, Linman JW. Erythroderma with atypical lymphocytes (Sézary syndrome). Am J Med 1973;55(2):192–8.

40. Holmes RC, McGibbon DH, Black MM. Mycosis fungoides: progression towards Sezary syndrome reversed with chlorambucil. Clin Exp Dermatol 1983;8(4):429–35.

41. Mante C, Brodkin RH, Cohen F. Chlorambucil in mycosis fungoides. Report of a case of successful treatment. Acta Derm Venereol 1968;48(1):60–3.

42. Hamminga L, Hartgrink-Groeneveld CA, van Vloten WA. Sezary's syndrome: a clinical evaluation of eight patients. Br J Dermatol 1979;100(3):291–6.

43. Coors EA, von den Driesch P. Treatment of erythrodermic cutaneous T-cell lymphoma with intermittent chlorambucil and fluocortolone therapy. Br J Dermatol 2000;143(1):127–31.

44. Winkelmann RK, Diaz-Perez JL, Buechner SA. The treatment of Sezary syndrome. J Am Acad Dermatol 1984;10(6):1000–4.

45. Winkelmann RK, Perry HO, Muller SA, et al. Treatment of Sezary syndrome. Mayo Clin Proc 1974; 49(8):590–2.

46. McEvoy MT, Zelickson BD, Pineda AA, et al. Intermittent leukapheresis: an adjunct to low-dose chemotherapy for Sezary syndrome. Acta Derm Venereol 1989;69(1):73–6.

47. Travis LB, Curtis RE, Stovall M, et al. Risk of Leukemia Following Treatment for Non-Hodgkin's Lymphoma. Natl Cancer Inst 1994;86(19):1450–7.

48. Mudie NY, Swerdlow AJ, Higgins CD, et al. Risk of second malignancy after non-hodgkin's lymphoma: a British cohort study. J Clin Oncol 2006;24(10): 1568–74.

49. Hosler GA, Liégeois N, Anhalt GJ, et al. Transformation of cutaneous gamma/delta T-cell lymphoma following 15 years of indolent behavior. J Cutan Pathol 2008;35(11):1063–7.

50. Zelenetz AD, Hamlin P, Kewalramani T, et al. Ifosfamide, carboplatin, etoposide (ICE)-based second-line chemotherapy for the management of relapsed and refractory aggressive non-Hodgkin's lymphoma. Ann Oncol 2003;14(Suppl 1):i5–10.

51. Leoni LM, Bailey B, Reifert J, et al. Bendamustine (Treanda) displays a distinct pattern of cytotoxicity and unique mechanistic features compared with other alkylating agents. Clin Cancer Res 2008; 14(1):309–17.

52. Bergmann MA, Goebeler ME, Herold M, et al. Efficacy of bendamustine in patients with relapsed or refractory chronic lymphocytic leukemia: results of a phase I/II study of the German CLL Study Group. Haematologica 2005;90(10):1357–64.

53. Knop S, Straka C, Haen M, et al. The efficacy and toxicity of bendamustine in recurrent multiple myeloma after high-dose chemotherapy. Haematologica 2005;90(9):1287–8.

54. Ponisch W, Mitrou PS, Merkle K, et al. Treatment of bendamustine and prednisone in patients with newly diagnosed multiple myeloma results in superior complete response rate, prolonged time to treatment failure and improved quality of life compared to treatment with melphalan and prednisone–a randomized phase III study of the East German Study Group of Hematology and Oncology (OSHO). J Cancer Res Clin Oncol 2006;132(4):205–12.

55. von Minckwitz G, Chernozemsky I, Sirakova L, et al. Bendamustine prolongs progression-free survival in metastatic breast cancer (MBC): a phase III prospective, randomized, multicenter trial of bendamustine hydrochloride, methotrexate and 5-fluorouracil (BMF) versus cyclophosphamide, methotrexate and 5-fluorouracil (CMF) as first-line treatment of MBC. Anticancer Drugs 2005;16(8):871–7.

56. Friedberg JW, Cohen P, Chen L, et al. Bendamustine in patients with rituximab-refractory indolent and transformed non-Hodgkin's lymphoma: results from a phase II multicenter, single-agent study. J Clin Oncol 2008;26(2):204–10.

57. Rummel MJ, Al-Batran SE, Kim SZ, et al. Bendamustine plus rituximab is effective and has a favorable toxicity profile in the treatment of mantle cell and low-grade non-Hodgkin's lymphoma. J Clin Oncol 2005;23(15):3383–9.

58. Damaj G, Gressin R, Bouabdallah K, et al. Results from a prospective, open-label, phase II trial of bendamustine in refractory or relapsed T-cell lymphomas: the BENTLY trial. J Clin Oncol 2013; 31(1):104–10.

59. Zaja F, Baldini L, Ferreri AJ, et al. Bendamustine salvage therapy for T cell neoplasms. Ann Hematol 2013;92(9):1249–54.

60. Hosoda T, Yokoyama A, Yoneda M, et al. Bendamustine can severely impair T-cell immunity against cytomegalovirus. Leuk Lymphoma 2013;54(6): 1327–8.

61. Abele DC, Dobson RL. The treatment of mycosis fungoides with a new agent, cyclophosphamide (Cytoxan). Arch Dermatol 1960;82:725–31.

62. Auerbach R. Mycosis fungoides successfully treated with cyclophosphamide (Cytoxan). Arch Dermatol 1970;101(5):611.

63. Maguire A. Treatment of mycosis fungoides with cyclophosphamide and chlorpromazine. Br J Dermatol 1968;80(1):54–7.

64. Mendelson D, Block JB, Serpick AA. Effect of large intermittent intravenous doses of cyclophosphamide in lymphoma. Cancer 1970;25(3):715–20.

65. Suter DE. Follow-up case mycosis fungoides treated with cyclophosphamide (cytoxan). Arch Dermatol 1964;89:616.

66. Van Scott EJ, Auerbach R, Clendenning WE. Treatment of mycosis fungoides with cyclophosphamide. Arch Dermatol 1962;85:499–501.

67. Molina A, Zain J, Arber DA, et al. Durable clinical, cytogenetic, and molecular remissions after allogeneic hematopoietic cell transplantation for refractory Sezary syndrome and mycosis fungoides. J Clin Oncol 2005;23(25):6163–71.

68. Duarte RF, Canals C, Onida F, et al. Allogeneic hematopoietic cell transplantation for patients with mycosis fungoides and sézary syndrome: a retrospective analysis of the lymphoma working party of the european group for blood and marrow transplantation. J Clin Oncol 2010;28(29):4492–9.

69. Polansky M, Talpur R, Daulat S, et al. Long-Term complete responses to combination therapies and allogeneic stem cell transplants in patients with Sezary Syndrome. Clin Lymphoma Myeloma Leuk 2015;15(5):e83–93.

70. Fontaine J, Heimann M, Day MJ. Canine cutaneous epitheliotropic T-cell lymphoma: a review of 30 cases. Vet Dermatol 2010;21(3):267–75.

71. Goodnight AL, Couto CG, Green E, et al. Chemotherapy and radiotherapy for treatment of cutaneous lymphoma in a ground cuscus (Phalanger gymnotis). J Zoo Wildl Med 2008;39(3):472–5.

72. Scheelings TF, Dobson EC, Hooper C. Cutaneous T-cell lymphoma in two captive Tasmanian devils (Sarcophilus harrisii). J Zoo Wildl Med 2014;45(2):367–71.

73. Jimbow K, Horikoshi T, Kamimura M. [Topical application of ACNU for the treatment of mycosis fungoides]. Gan To Kagaku Ryoho 1982;9(7):1231–6 [in Japanese].

74. Newlands ES, Blackledge GR, Slack JA, et al. Phase I trial of temozolomide (CCRG 81045: M&B 39831: NSC 362856). Br J Cancer 1992;65(2):287–91.

75. Tani M, Fina M, Alinari L, et al. Phase II trial of temozolomide in patients with pretreated cutaneous T-cell lymphoma. Haematologica 2005;90(9):1283–4.

76. Querfeld C, Rosen ST, Guitart J, et al. Multicenter phase II trial of temozolomide in mycosis fungoides/sezary syndrome: correlation with O(6)-methylguanine-DNA methyltransferase and mismatch repair proteins. Clin Cancer Res 2011;17(17):5748–54.

77. Mebazaa A, Dupuy A, Rybojad M, et al. ESHAP for primary cutaneous T-cell lymphomas: efficacy and tolerance in 11 patients. Hematol J 2005;5(7):553–8.

78. Minotti G, Menna P, Salvatorelli E, et al. Anthracyclines: molecular advances and pharmacologic developments in antitumor activity and cardiotoxicity. Pharmacol Rev 2004;56(2):185–229.

79. Hoffman R. Hematology: basic principles and practice. 6th edition. Philadelphia: Saunders/Elsevier; 2013.

80. Binaschi M, Bigioni M, Cipollone A, et al. Anthracyclines: selected new developments. Curr Med Chem Anticancer Agents 2001;1(2):113–30.

81. Crawford J. Clinical uses of pegylated pharmaceuticals in oncology. Cancer Treat Rev 2002;28(Suppl A):7–11.

82. Waterhouse DN, Tardi PG, Mayer LD, et al. A comparison of liposomal formulations of doxorubicin with drug administered in free form: changing toxicity profiles. Drug Saf 2001;24(12):903–20.

83. Working PK, Dayan AD. Pharmacological-toxicological expert report. CAELYX. (Stealth liposomal doxorubicin HCl). Hum Exp Toxicol 1996;15(9):751–85.

84. Levi JA, Diggs CH, Wiernik PH. Adriamycin therapy in advanced mycosis fungoides. Cancer 1977;39(5):1967–70.

85. Wollina U, Dummer R, Brockmeyer NH, et al. Multicenter study of pegylated liposomal doxorubicin in patients with cutaneous T-cell lymphoma. Cancer 2003;98(5):993–1001.

86. Di Lorenzo G, Di Trolio R, Delfino M, et al. Pegylated liposomal doxorubicin in stage IVB mycosis fungoides. Br J Dermatol 2005;153(1):183–5.

87. Pulini S, Rupoli S, Goteri G, et al. Pegylated liposomal doxorubicin in the treatment of primary cutaneous T-cell lymphomas. Haematologica 2007;92(5):686–9.

88. Quereux G, Marques S, Nguyen JM, et al. Prospective multicenter study of pegylated liposomal doxorubicin treatment in patients with advanced or refractory mycosis fungoides or Sezary syndrome. Arch Dermatol 2008;144(6):727–33.

89. Dummer R, Quaglino P, Becker JC, et al. Prospective international multicenter phase II trial of intravenous pegylated liposomal doxorubicin monochemotherapy in patients with stage IIB, IVA, or IVB advanced mycosis fungoides: final results from EORTC 21012. J Clin Oncol 2012;30(33):4091–7.

90. Straus DJ, Duvic M, Horwitz SM, et al. Final results of phase II trial of doxorubicin HCl liposome injection followed by bexarotene in advanced cutaneous T-cell lymphoma. Ann Oncol 2014;25(1):206–10.

91. Hortobagyi GN. Anthracyclines in the treatment of cancer. An overview. Drugs 1997;54(Suppl 4):1–7.

92. Wollina U, Hohaus K, Schonlebe J, et al. Liposomal daunorubicin in tumor stage cutaneous T-cell lymphoma: report of three cases. J Cancer Res Clin Oncol 2003;129(1):65–9.

93. Akinbami AA, Osikomaiya BI, John-Olabode SO, et al. Mycosis fungoides: case report and literature review. clinical medicine insights. Case Rep 2014;7:95–8.

94. Ishida M, Mochizuki Y, Saito Y, et al. CD8(+) mycosis fungoides with esophageal involvement: a case report. Oncol Lett 2013;5(1):73–5.

95. Liu YQ, Zhu WY, Shu YQ, et al. A case of advanced mycosis fungoides with comprehensive skin and visceral organs metastasis: sensitive to chemical and biological therapy. Asian Pac J Trop Med 2012;5(8):669–72.

96. Fierro MT, Doveil GC, Quaglino P, et al. Combination of etoposide, idarubicin, cyclophosphamide, vincristine, prednisone and bleomycin (VICOP-B) in the treatment of advanced cutaneous T-cell lymphoma. Dermatology 1997;194(3):268–72.

97. Jacobs P, King HS, Gordon W. Letter: Epipodophyllotoxin in mycosis fungoides. Lancet 1975;1(7898):111–2.

98. Jacobs P, King HS, Gordon W. Letter: Chemotherapy of mycosis fungoides. S Afr Med J 1975;49(32):1286.

99. Molin L, Thomsen K, Volden G, et al. Epipodophyllotoxin (VP-16-213) in mycosis fungoides: a report from the Scandinavian mycosis fungoides study group. Acta Derm Venereol 1979;59(1):84–7.

100. Nasuhara Y, Kobayashi S, Munakata M, et al. A case of mycosis fungoides with pulmonary involvement: effect of etoposide and prednisolone. Nihon Kyobu Shikkan Gakkai Zasshi 1995;33(9):1013–8 [in Japanese].

101. Onozuka T, Yokota K, Kawashima T, et al. An elderly patient with mycosis fungoides successfully treated with chronic low-dose oral etoposide therapy. Clin Exp Dermatol 2004;29(1):91–2.

102. Miyoshi N, Noda M. Complication of topoisomerase II inhibitor-related acute promyelocytic leukemia with t(1;10) (q21;q26) in a patient with Sezary syndrome. Rinsho Ketsueki 2006;47(5):399–401 [in Japanese].

103. Hirayama Y, Nagai T, Ohta H, et al. Sezary syndrome showing a stable clinical course for more than four years after oral administration of etoposide and methotrexate. Rinsho Ketsueki 2000;41(9):750–4 [in Japanese].

104. Pui CH. Epipodophyllotoxin-related acute myeloid leukaemia. Lancet 1991;338(8780):1468.

105. Pui CH, Ribeiro RC, Hancock ML, et al. Acute myeloid leukemia in children treated with epipodophyllotoxins for acute lymphoblastic leukemia. N Engl J Med 1991;325(24):1682–7.

106. Rook AH, Kuzel TM, Olsen EA. Cytokine therapy of cutaneous T-cell lymphoma: interferons, interleukin-12, and interleukin-2. Hematol Oncol Clin North Am 2003;17(6):1435–48, ix.

107. Querfeld C, Rosen ST, Guitart J, et al. Phase II trial of subcutaneous injections of human recombinant interleukin-2 for the treatment of mycosis fungoides and Sezary syndrome. J Am Acad Dermatol 2007;56(4):580–3.

108. Nagatani T, Kin ST, Baba N, et al. A case of cutaneous T cell lymphoma treated with recombinant interleukin 2 (rIL-2). Acta Derm Venereol 1988;68(6):504–8.

109. Rybojad M, Marolleau JP, Flageul B, et al. Successful interleukin-2 therapy of advanced cutaneous T-cell lymphoma. Br J Dermatol 1992;127(1):63–4.

110. Marolleau JP, Baccard M, Flageul B, et al. High-dose recombinant interleukin-2 in advanced cutaneous T-cell lymphoma. Arch Dermatol 1995;131(5):574–9.

111. Baccard M, Marolleau JP, Rybojad M. Middle-term evolution of patients with advanced cutaneous T-cell lymphoma treated with high-dose recombinant interleukin-2. Arch Dermatol 1997;133(5):656.

112. Gisselbrecht C, Maraninchi D, Pico JL, et al. Interleukin-2 treatment in lymphoma: a phase II multicenter study. Blood 1994;83(8):2081–5.

113. Rook AH, Kubin M, Cassin M, et al. IL-12 reverses cytokine and immune abnormalities in Sezary syndrome. J Immunol 1995;154(3):1491–8.

114. Wysocka M, Zaki MH, French LE, et al. Sezary syndrome patients demonstrate a defect in dendritic cell populations: effects of CD40 ligand and treatment with GM-CSF on dendritic cell numbers and the production of cytokines. Blood 2002;100(9):3287–94.

115. Vowels BR, Cassin M, Vonderheid EC, et al. Aberrant cytokine production by Sezary syndrome patients: cytokine secretion pattern resembles murine Th2 cells. J Invest Dermatol 1992;99(1):90–4.

116. Asadullah K, Docke WD, Haeussler A, et al. Progression of mycosis fungoides is associated with increasing cutaneous expression of interleukin-10 mRNA. J Invest Dermatol 1996;107(6):833–7.

117. Rook AH, Wood GS, Yoo EK, et al. Interleukin-12 therapy of cutaneous T-cell lymphoma induces lesion regression and cytotoxic T-cell responses. Blood 1999;94(3):902–8.

118. Rook AH, Zaki MH, Wysocka M, et al. The role for interleukin-12 therapy of cutaneous T cell lymphoma. Ann N Y Acad Sci 2001;941:177–84.

119. Duvic M, Sherman ML, Wood GS, et al. A phase II open-label study of recombinant human interleukin-12 in patients with stage IA, IB, or IIA mycosis fungoides. J Am Acad Dermatol 2006;55(5):807–13.

120. Krenitsky TA. Purine nucleoside phosphorylase: kinetics, mechanism, and specificity. Mol Pharmacol 1967;3(6):526–36.

121. Gandhi V, Balakrishnan K. Pharmacology and mechanism of action of forodesine, a T-cell targeted agent. Semin Oncol 2007;34(6 Suppl 5): S8–12.

122. Kicska GA, Long L, Horig H, et al. Immucillin H, a powerful transition-state analog inhibitor of purine nucleoside phosphorylase, selectively inhibits human T lymphocytes. Proc Natl Acad Sci U S A 2001;98(8):4593–8.

123. Duvic M, Foss FM. Mycosis fungoides: pathophysiology and emerging therapies. Semin Oncol 2007; 34(6 Suppl 5):S21–8.

124. Bantia S, Kilpatrick JM. Purine nucleoside phosphorylase inhibitors in T-cell malignancies. Curr Opin Drug Discov Devel 2004;7(2):243–7.

125. Bantia S, Miller PJ, Parker CD, et al. Purine nucleoside phosphorylase inhibitor BCX-1777 (Immucillin-H)–a novel potent and orally active immunosuppressive agent. Int Immunopharmacol 2001;1(6):1199–210.

126. Gandhi V, Kilpatrick JM, Plunkett W, et al. A proof-of-principle pharmacokinetic, pharmacodynamic, and clinical study with purine nucleoside phosphorylase inhibitor immucillin-H (BCX-1777, forodesine). Blood 2005;106(13):4253–60.

127. Lansigan F, Foss FM. Current and emerging treatment strategies for cutaneous T-cell lymphoma. Drugs 2010;70(3):273–86.

128. Duvic M, Forero-Torres A, Foss F, et al. Oral Forodesine (Bcx-1777) Is Clinically Active in Refractory Cutaneous T-Cell Lymphoma: Results of a Phase I/II Study. ASH Annual Meeting Abstracts. 2006;108(11):2467. November 1, 2006.

129. Dummer R, Duvic M, Scarisbrick J, et al. Final results of a multicenter phase II study of the purine nucleoside phosphorylase (PNP) inhibitor forodesine in patients with advanced cutaneous T-cell lymphomas (CTCL) (Mycosis fungoides and Sezary syndrome). Ann Oncol 2014;25(9):1807–12.

130. Fernandez Y, Miller TP, Denoyelle C, et al. Chemical blockage of the proteasome inhibitory function of bortezomib: impact on tumor cell death. J Biol Chem 2006;281(2):1107–18.

131. Adams J, Palombella VJ, Sausville EA, et al. Proteasome inhibitors: a novel class of potent and effective antitumor agents. Cancer Res 1999; 59(11):2615–22.

132. Elliott PJ, Zollner TM, Boehncke WH. Proteasome inhibition: a new anti-inflammatory strategy. J Mol Med (Berl) 2003;81(4):235–45.

133. Zinzani PL, Musuraca G, Tani M, et al. Phase II trial of proteasome inhibitor bortezomib in patients with relapsed or refractory cutaneous T-cell lymphoma. J Clin Oncol 2007;25(27):4293–7.

134. National Comprehensive Cancer Network (U.S.). The complete library of NCCN oncology practice guidelines. Rockledge (PA): NCCN; 2000.

135. Savage KJ, Chhanabhai M, Gascoyne RD, et al. Characterization of peripheral T-cell lymphomas in a single North American institution by the WHO classification. Ann Oncol 2004;15(10):1467–75.

136. Wilson WH, Bryant G, Bates S, et al. EPOCH chemotherapy: toxicity and efficacy in relapsed and refractory non-Hodgkin's lymphoma. J Clin Oncol 1993;11(8):1573–82.

137. Escalon MP, Liu NS, Yang Y, et al. Prognostic factors and treatment of patients with T-cell non-Hodgkin lymphoma: the M. D. Anderson Cancer Center experience. Cancer 2005;103(10):2091–8.

138. Mey UJ, Orlopp KS, Flieger D, et al. Dexamethasone, high-dose cytarabine, and cisplatin in combination with rituximab as salvage treatment for patients with relapsed or refractory aggressive non-Hodgkin's lymphoma. Cancer Invest 2006; 24(6):593–600.

139. Velasquez WS, Cabanillas F, Salvador P, et al. Effective salvage therapy for lymphoma with cisplatin in combination with high-dose Ara-C and dexamethasone (DHAP). Blood 1988; 71(1):117–22.

140. Velasquez WS, McLaughlin P, Tucker S, et al. ESHAP–an effective chemotherapy regimen in refractory and relapsing lymphoma: a 4-year follow-up study. J Clin Oncol 1994;12(6):1169–76.

141. Crump M, Baetz T, Couban S, et al. Gemcitabine, dexamethasone, and cisplatin in patients with recurrent or refractory aggressive histology B-cell non-Hodgkin lymphoma: a Phase II study by the National Cancer Institute of Canada Clinical Trials Group (NCIC-CTG). Cancer 2004; 101(8):1835–42.

142. Dong M, He XH, Liu P, et al. Gemcitabine-based combination regimen in patients with peripheral T-cell lymphoma. Med Oncol 2013;30(1):351.

143. Lopez A, Gutierrez A, Palacios A, et al. GEMOX-R regimen is a highly effective salvage regimen in patients with refractory/relapsing diffuse large-cell lymphoma: a phase II study. Eur J Haematol 2008;80(2):127–32.

144. Zinzani PL, Venturini F, Stefoni V, et al. Gemcitabine as single agent in pretreated T-cell lymphoma patients: evaluation of the long-term outcome. Ann Oncol 2010;21(4):860–3.

145. Hallahan DE, Griem ML, Griem SF, et al. Combined modality therapy for tumor stage mycosis fungoides: results of a 10-year follow-up. J Clin Oncol 1988;6(7):1177–83.

146. Bunn PA Jr, Hoffman SJ, Norris D, et al. Systemic therapy of cutaneous T-cell lymphomas (mycosis fungoides and the Sezary syndrome). Ann Intern Med 1994;121(8):592–602.

147. Groth O, Molin L, Thomsen K. Tumour stage of mycosis fungoides treated with bleomycin and methotrexate: report from the Scandinavian mycosis fungoides study group. Acta Derm Venereol 1979;59(1):59–63.

148. Grozea PN, Jones SE, McKelvey EM, et al. Combination chemotherapy for mycosis fungoides: a Southwest Oncology Group study. Cancer Treat Rep 1979;63(4):647–53.

149. Lamberg SI, Green SB, Byar DP, et al. Status report of 376 mycosis fungoides patients at 4 years: Mycosis Fungoides Cooperative Group. Cancer Treat Rep 1979;63(4):701–7.

150. Fierro MT, Quaglino P, Savoia P, et al. Systemic polychemotherapy in the treatment of primary cutaneous lymphomas: a clinical follow-up study of 81 patients treated with COP or CHOP. Leuk Lymphoma 1998;31(5–6):583–8.

151. Molin L, Thomsen K, Volden G, et al. Combination chemotherapy in the tumour stage of mycosis fungoides with cyclophosphamide, vincristine, vp-16, adriamycin and prednisolone (cop, chop, cavop): a report from the Scandinavian mycosis fungoides study group. Acta Derm Venereol 1980;60(6):542–4.

152. Raafat J, Oster MW. Combination chemotherapy for advanced squamous cell carcinoma of the head and neck. Cancer Treat Rep 1980;64(1):187–9.

153. Lutzner M, Edelson R, Schein P, et al. Cutaneous T-cell lymphomas: the Sezary syndrome, mycosis fungoides, and related disorders. Ann Intern Med 1975;83(4):534–52.

154. Tirelli U, Carbone A, Zagonel V, et al. Staging and treatment with cyclophosphamide, vincristine and prednisone (CVP) in advanced cutaneous T-cell lymphomas. Hematol Oncol 1986;4(1):83–90.

155. Hamminga L, Hermans J, Noordijk EM, et al. Cutaneous T-cell lymphoma: clinicopathological relationships, therapy and survival in ninety-two patients. Br J Dermatol 1982;107(2):145–55.

156. Molin L, Thomsen K, Volden G, et al. Retinoids and systemic chemotherapy in cases of advanced mycosis fungoides. A report from the Scandinavian Mycosis Fungoides Group. Acta Derm Venereol 1987;67(2):179–82.

157. Zachariae H, Thestrup-Pedersen K. Combination chemotherapy with bleomycin, cyclophosphamide, prednisone and etretinate (BCPE) in advanced mycosis fungoides: a six-year experience. Acta Derm Venereol 1987;67(5):433–7.

158. Zachariae H, Grunnet E, Thestrup-Pedersen K, et al. Oral retinoid in combination with bleomycin, cyclophosphamide, prednisone and transfer factor in mycosis fungoides. Acta Derm Venereol 1982;62(2):162–4.

159. Akpek G, Koh HK, Bogen S, et al. Chemotherapy with etoposide, vincristine, doxorubicin, bolus cyclophosphamide, and oral prednisone in patients with refractory cutaneous T-cell lymphoma. Cancer 1999;86(7):1368–76.

160. Doberauer C, Ohl S. Advanced mycosis fungoides: chemotherapy with etoposide, methotrexate, bleomycin, and prednimustine. Acta Derm Venereol 1989;69(6):538–40.

161. Kaye FJ, Bunn PA Jr, Steinberg SM, et al. A randomized trial comparing combination electron-beam radiation and chemotherapy with topical therapy in the initial treatment of mycosis fungoides. N Engl J Med 1989;321(26):1784–90.

162. Braverman IM, Yager NB, Chen M, et al. Combined total body electron beam irradiation and chemotherapy for mycosis fungoides. J Am Acad Dermatol 1987;16(1 Pt 1):45–60.

163. Zakem MH, Davis BR, Adelstein DJ, et al. Treatment of advanced stage mycosis fungoides with bleomycin, doxorubicin, and methotrexate with topical nitrogen mustard (BAM-M). Cancer 1986;58(12):2611–6.

Hematopoietic Stem Cell Transplant for Mycosis Fungoides and Sézary Syndrome

Pooja Virmani, MBBS, MD[a,1], Jasmine Zain, MD[b,1], Steven T. Rosen, MD[b], Patricia L. Myskowski, MD[a], Christiane Querfeld, MD, PhD[b,c,d],*

KEYWORDS

- Cutaneous T-cell lymphoma • Mycosis fungoides • Sézary syndrome
- Autologous hematopoietic stem cell transplant • Allogeneic hematopoietic stem cell transplant
- Myeloablative • Reduced-intensity conditioning

KEY POINTS

- Autologous transplant has low treatment-related complications in mycosis fungoides (MF)/Sézary syndrome (SS), but high relapse rates.
- Allogeneic transplant has curative potential in MF/SS with lower relapse rates and improved survival.
- Allogeneic transplant induces an immune-mediated graft-versus-lymphoma (GvL) effect in MF/SS.
- Myeloablative conditioning (MAC) in MF/SS is associated with higher risk of treatment-related toxicities and acute graft-versus-host disease (GVHD) and is limited to younger and medically fit patients.
- Reduced-intensity conditioning (RIC) in MF/SS shows lower treatment-related complications and is increasingly used in older patients with comorbidities.
- There is no difference in chronic GVHD between MAC and RIC.
- Relapses following allogeneic transplant respond to GvL effect induced by decreased immunosuppression and donor lymphocyte infusion (DLI).

INTRODUCTION

Primary cutaneous T-cell lymphomas (CTCL) represent a heterogeneous group of non–Hodgkin lymphomas (NHLs) that manifest in the skin with no evidence of extracutaneous disease at the time of diagnosis. The exception is MF, the most common type of CTCL, which accounts for more than 50% of primary cutaneous lymphomas.[1] MF is generally associated with an indolent course with most of the patients presenting in early stage of the disease. However, about one-third of

Funding sources: none.
Conflict of interest: authors have no conflict of interest.
[a] Dermatology Service, Department of Medicine, Memorial Sloan Kettering Cancer Center, 16 East 60th Street, New York, NY 10022, USA; [b] Department of Hematology/Hematopoietic Cell Transplantation, City of Hope Comprehensive Cancer Center, 1500 East Duarte Road, Duarte, CA 91010, USA; [c] Department of Pathology, City of Hope Comprehensive Cancer Center, 1500 East Duarte Road, Duarte, CA 91010, USA; [d] Memorial Sloan Kettering Cancer Center, 16 East 60th Street, New York, NY 10022, USA
[1] First coauthors.
* Corresponding author. Department of Pathology, City of Hope Comprehensive Cancer Center, 1500 East Duarte Road, Duarte, CA 91010.
E-mail address: cquerfeld@coh.org

Dermatol Clin 33 (2015) 807–818
http://dx.doi.org/10.1016/j.det.2015.05.014

patients present with advanced stage (generally considered to be stage IIB and higher) and another 25% progress into higher stage in the course of their disease.[1–3] SS is the leukemic and most commonly encountered type of aggressive CTCL.[1]

Most patients with early-stage MF respond well to skin-directed therapies with reported long-term remissions. Treatment for patients with advanced disease includes various combinations of skin-directed therapies, biologic response modifiers, histone deacetylase (HDAC) inhibitors, investigational agents, as well as single-agent and/or multi-agent chemotherapy regimens.[4,5] None of these treatment options have been shown to prolong disease-specific survival or overall survival (OS) and often lead to short-term disease control with a median survival ranging from 1.4 to 4.7 years in patients with advanced stages (IIB–IVB) of MF and SS.[6] Borrowing from the paradigm of aggressive lymphomas, hematopoietic stem cell transplant (HSCT) has been explored as a treatment option in patients with advanced-stage MF/SS and other subtypes. The data for using high-dose therapy and autologous HSCT (ASCT) remain disappointing, but the results of allogeneic stem cell transplant are encouraging for the treatment of CTCL. The data series are small, and there is little consensus on conditioning regimens and other aspects of the transplants that are largely driven by institutional preferences. This article discusses the role of allogeneic stem cell transplant in the care of patients with CTCL and presents relevant data to support its use.

OVERVIEW OF HEMATOPOIETIC STEM CELL TRANSPLANT

HSCT, formerly known as bone marrow transplant (BMT), is a medical procedure in which multipotent stem cells derived from the bone marrow, peripheral blood, or umbilical cord are infused into a patient for treatment of hematological disorders and malignancies. This procedure requires that the patient's own hematopoietic and immune function be suppressed enough to accept the infused cells and allow homing of these cells to the marrow spaces and establishment of a donor-derived hematopoietic system in the host. This procedure can be accomplished either by chemotherapy alone or by combination of chemotherapy with radiation therapy called conditioning or preparative regimen given before stem cell infusion. The establishment of a donor-derived hematopoietic system requires some time during which the patient remains pancytopenic and entirely depends on supportive measures to prevent and treat the complication of pancytopenia as well as the conditioning regimen.

The stem cells can be derived from the patient's own hematopoietic system (autologous) or from an HLA-matched donor (allogeneic) who can be a sibling (related) or a matched unrelated donor. Other sources now extend to haploidentical family members and cord blood stem cells and are discussed below. Major indications for stem cell transplant include hematologic malignancies such as leukemia, lymphoma, multiple myeloma, and other myeloproliferative disorders. According to the Center for International Blood and Marrow Transplant Research (CIBMTR) data, approximately 12,000 autologous and 8000 allogeneic transplants were performed in the year 2013 and the numbers are increasing.[7]

STEM CELL SOURCES

Hematopoietic stem cells express properties of multipotency and self-renewal and reside in bone marrow niches supported by cytokines and other microenvironmental factors. Human hematopoietic stem cells express CD34, CD38, CD90, CD133, CD105, CD45, and also c-kit (CD117), the receptor for stem cell factor, and these cells test negative for the markers that are used for the detection of lineage commitment. Historically, stem cell collection was performed in the operating room under general anesthesia using a large trocar to collect bone marrow from the pelvic bones in adults and long bones in children. This procedure has now given way to peripheral blood as a source of stem cells through a process called apheresis.[8] The peripheral blood stem cells can be mobilized into the circulation either by chemotherapy (in case of autologous collections) or by injections of hematopoietic growth factors, that is, granulocyte colony-stimulating factor supplemented by CXR4 inhibitors such as plexiafor,[9] and collected. Most autologous stem cells are cryopreserved in dimethyl sulfoxide before infusion in contrast to allogeneic stem cells that are usually infused fresh on the day of collection. Umbilical cord blood (UCB), which is rich in hematopoietic stem cells, can be cryopreserved and used in an appropriate patient. However, because a cord can yield only small amounts of blood (approximately 50 mL), a single cord can only provide adequate stem cells for a child or small adult. Generally, 2 UCB units need to be combined for adult transplants, and there is now a significant body of data to support the safety and efficacy of this approach.

DONOR SELECTION

HLA typing is required to match a donor and recipient for allogeneic stem cell transplants. The major

HLA genes fall into 2 categories (Type I and Type II), and serologic and molecular matching is performed on the basis of variability at 6 loci of the HLA gene. A perfect match at these loci is desirable to ensure engraftment and prevent complications of GVHD. Mismatches of the Type I genes (ie, HLA-A, HLA-B, or HLA-C) increase the risk of graft rejection. A mismatch of an HLA Type II gene (ie, HLA-DR, or HLA-DQB1) increases the risk of GVHD. Molecular methods are increasingly being used to increase the accuracy of tissue typing to ensure optimal matching. Sibling donors have a 25% chance of being a match with the recipient. Rarely, patients have a syngeneic donor, that is, a monozygotic twin who is perfectly matched at all HLA loci. Most other patients need to rely on an unrelated HLA-matched donor who may be found through the National Marrow Donor Program and other such worldwide registries.[10] Unfortunately, these registries have marked underrepresentation of specific ethnic and minority racial groups. This underrepresentation has driven the need to look for alternative donors. A haploidentical donor is a partially matched first-degree relative of the patient (child, parent, or sibling).[11] The advantage of haploidentical transplant is immediate and permanent availability of the donor for current and future therapies. Initially, the 3 antigen mismatches in these transplants led to unacceptably high transplant-related toxicity, but with the use of T-cell depletion techniques, improved immunosuppression, and supportive care, haploidentical transplants are increasingly being offered to patients who lack an HLA-matched donor.[12] Umbilical cords provide immunologically naive stem cells and a reduced risk of GVHD and are a relatively accessible source of stem cell transplants. The main disadvantage is the small number of stem cells that may by themselves be inadequate in number for successful engraftment in an adult. Ex vivo expansion, double cord transplants, and combined haploidentical and cord transplants have resulted in improved outcomes for these patients.[13,14] According to the European Bone Marrow Transplant Registry survey of 2013, as many as 43% of all HSCTs done that year were allogeneic and there was a notable increase in the use of alternate donors.[15]

CONDITIONING REGIMENS

The preparative regimen given before stem cell infusion is called a conditioning regimen and has a 2-fold purpose depending on the type of transplant. In the case of an autologous stem cell transplant, the conditioning regimen consists of chemotherapy with or without radiation and is designed to give a high dose of antitumor therapy for cytotoxic purposes. The hematopoietic system damaged by chemotherapy is then reconstituted with transplanted autologous stem cells. The state of immunosuppression created by the conditioning regimen improves with time, and the patient does not have any GVHD. In allogeneic transplant, conditioning treatment is required for engraftment and prevention of GVHD by suppressing host immunity in addition to antitumor effects. Regimens can be fully MAC for maximal antitumor effects and generally include high-dose cytoxan, busulfan, high-dose etoposide, and/or total body irradiation (TBI). These regimens can have significant immediate toxicity that can contribute to significant regimen-related morbidity and mortality in the immediate posttransplant period.[16,17] Nonrelapse mortality (NRM) of 22% was reported in a cohort of 60 patients with advanced CTCL (clinical stage IIB–IVB) treated with allogeneic stem cell transplant. In multivariate analysis, MAC was associated with a higher NRM (hazard ratio, 4.5; $P = .1$)[18] RIC or nonmyeloablative transplants are less cytotoxic and mostly immunosuppressive, resulting in decreased immediate transplant-related toxicity and allowing older and more frail patients to undergo transplant.[19] These regimens consist of purine analogs such as fludarabine and cladribine as well as low-dose TBI and rely on the GVHD effect for their antitumor effects. These regimens are associated with decreased immediate transplant-related toxicity and less-acute GVHD, but there has been no change in the incidence of chronic GVHD with RIC.[20] Use of RIC has extended the use of allogeneic stem cell transplants to patients into their 70s and 80s if they are otherwise in good health. CIBMTR data confirm the increasing use of RIC for allogeneic stem cell transplants and the increasing age of transplant recipients in the United States.[15]

COMPLICATIONS

Several complications are associated with HSCT depending on the type of conditioning, type of transplant, and engraftment phase.[21] The most common cause of transplant-related morbidity and mortality is GVHD, followed by infections. GVHD remains a challenge in the care of patients undergoing allogeneic stem cell transplant. Classically, acute GVHD occurs within the first 100 days of transplant and manifests itself primarily in the skin, gastrointestinal tract, and liver. However, the development of various conditioning regimens and the use of DLI after transplant have changed the time course and presentation for acute and chronic GVHD.

The pathogenesis of acute GVHD is initiated by recipient tissue damage occurring from conditioning regimen leading to release of inflammatory cytokines that lead to the expansion of donor lymphocytes following contact with host and donor antigen-presenting cells that express disparate antigens resulting in alloreactive T cells that induce tissue damage. The incidence of acute GVHD varies from 20% to 70% and is directly related to the degree of mismatch between HLA proteins. The incidence ranges from 35% to 45% in recipients of full-matched sibling donor grafts to 60% to 80% in recipients of one-antigen HLA-mismatched unrelated donor grafts. The same degree of mismatch causes less GVHD using UCB grafts, and the incidence of acute GVHD is lower following the transplant of partially matched UCB units and ranges from 35% to 65%.[22] Chronic GVHD is the major cause of late nonrelapse death following transplant. Older recipient age and a history of acute GVHD are the greatest risk factors for chronic GVHD. Incidence ranges from 60% to 80%, and manifestations of chronic GVHD are protean and often resemble an autoimmune disorder.[22] The National Institutes of Health proposed standard criteria in 2005 for diagnosis, organ scoring, and global assessment of chronic GVHD severity to establish a common platform for subclassifying chronic GVHD.[23]

Prevention strategies using immunosuppressive agents including calcineurin inhibitors, methotrexate, mammalian target of rapamycin inhibitors, or novel agents begin before stem cell infusion and are maintained for some time after allogeneic transplant. Treatment of GVHD is initiated when any sign of GVHD appears and consists of high-dose steroids and other strategies for immunosuppression. Prolonged immunosuppression delays immune reconstitution of the host and increases the risk of serious infections leading to high morbidity and mortality rates. Other complications after stem cell transplant can be related to conditioning regimens causing end-organ toxicity, secondary malignancies, and psychosocial issues related to chronic medical problems. Even with improved supportive care measures, there is a significant morbidity and mortality associated with stem cell transplant, which in the case of allogeneic stem cell transplants can range from 20% to 40% depending on the patient's comorbidities, donor type, degree of HLA mismatch, underlying disease, and conditioning regimen.[24] Autologous stem cell transplants are associated with a much lower risk of death at less than 5% in most centers, but there is a higher incidence of disease relapse. When determining the eligibility for HSCT, these risks have to be weighed against the risk of death and morbidity posed by the disease.

GRAFT-VERSUS-LYMPHOMA EFFECT

The existence of an immunologic GvL reaction associated with allogeneic stem cell transplant is well established.[25,26] Allogeneic transplant is successful partly because of the GvL effect of the donor graft, independent of the conditioning regimen. Evidence for GvL effects is based on the following criteria: RIC resulting in long-term disease control, increased risk of relapse associated with T-cell depletion, withdrawal of immunosuppression, use of DLIs to eradicate documented disease relapse after allogeneic transplant, and association of disease control with GVHD. A GvL effect against CTCL has been established and is discussed in later sections.

AUTOLOGOUS STEM CELL TRANSPLANT FOR MYCOSIS FUNGOIDES AND SÉZARY SYNDROME

High-dose therapy and ASCT have curative potential in aggressive chemotherapy-sensitive relapsed lymphomas. Using similar approaches, ASCT has been performed in cases of advanced CTCL in order to establish long-term remissions. Conditioning regimens have incorporated high-dose chemotherapy either with or without TBI. Some investigators have reported the use of total skin electron beam (TSEB) therapy to provide improved control of skin disease in patients with CTCL before initiating ASCT and avoid the generalized organ toxicity of TBI. Bigler and colleagues[27] first reported on 6 patients with MF who underwent TBI or TSEB-based regimens followed by ASCT: 5 patients achieved complete remission (CR) but 3 showed relapse in less than 100 days, whereas 2 remained in persistent CR after 1 year. Results demonstrated that the procedure was feasible, and increased transplant-related mortality (TRM) or transplant-related morbidity was not reported for these patients. A few other case reports showed early relapses within the first 100 days.[28–31] The largest series by Ingen-Housz-Oro et al[32] reported on 10 patients with CTCL that included 1 patient with MF; 8 patients with peripheral T-cell lymphoma (PTCL), unspecified (PTCL, not otherwise specified [NOS]); and 1 patient with subcutaneous panniculitis-like T-cell lymphoma including patients with systemic disease in addition to skin manifestations. Conditioning was TBI based and 7 of 10 patients achieved a CR. However, in 6 patients, the condition relapsed in less than 4 months and in 1, it relapsed at 7 years (PTCL, NOS). Remaining patients experienced fatal progression. Of note, some of the relapses responded to local and biologic therapies.

Another case series was reported by Olavarria and colleagues[33] on 9 patients with MF consisting of 5 patients with stage IIB and 4 patients with stage IVA disease; 8 patients demonstrated a T-cell clone in the peripheral blood. This study was a pilot study of T-cell depletion and ASCT in these patients using double CD34-positive and CD4/CD8-negative selection by immunomagnetic methods. TBI was given to only 2 patients, and the others were conditioned with chemotherapy only. Of the 9 patients, the condition relapsed in 7 patients at a median of 7 months, mostly with limited disease that responded to conventional therapy; 4 patients were analyzed for T-cell receptor rearrangement after transplant and had detectable clone before or at the time of relapse. There is one report of a patient with SS receiving autologous HSCT.[28] This patient was conditioned with the combination of chemotherapy and TBI. He showed relapse after 3 months and died after 15 months of infectious complications. Moreau and colleagues[34] reported successful transplant in 1994 on 4 cases of CTCL other than MF/SS (including 2 patients with a CD30 + lymphoproliferative disorder [CD30 + LPD]) using a TBI-based regimen with CR at 22, 41, 46, 44, and 51 months. This report predates the 2008 World Health Organization classification, and it is unclear from the publication whether patients were diagnosed with primary cutaneous anaplastic large cell lymphoma (PCALCL) or lymphomatoid papulosis or both. No specific data are available for the use of ASCT in large cell transformation (LCT)-MF, although these cases tend to be treated as systemic T-cell lymphomas and are likely included in the series of transplants for systemic diseases.

These limited data show that ASCT is feasible, but in most cases, the responses are not sustained except possibly for CD30 + LPD; however, these entities have already a favorable long-term outcome without the need of aggressive therapies.[1] The duration of remission does not seem to be related to the stage of the disease or the absence of a detectable T-cell clone in the harvest. Although the numbers are very small, the use of TBI did not seem to predict improved outcomes. These early relapses point to the inability of high-dose therapy to control disease pointing to the need for improved targeted therapies. However, some of the relapses seemed to be less aggressive and could be managed with local and biologic therapies for a while. The use of high-dose therapy and ASCT has essentially been abandoned with a belief that this is not a curative approach and that the inherent chemoresistance of these tumors contributes to the low success rate of this approach.

ALLOGENEIC STEM CELL TRANSPLANT FOR MYCOSIS FUNGOIDES AND SÉZARY SYNDROME

Allogeneic stem cell transplant has been shown to achieve durable CRs and provide long-term remissions and a potentially curative treatment option in CTCL through a proposed GvL. One of the earliest allogeneic transplants was reported by Koeppel and colleagues[35] in 1994 and supported the feasibility of the procedure in spite of the general state of immunosuppression and compromised skin barrier in these patients. Several case reports and series have been published since then as indicated in **Table 1**.[18,36–46] However, the experience of allogeneic transplant for treatment of MF/SS is limited to small retrospective studies with small number of patients usually lumped together with transplant data for subtypes of T cell and other NHL. The following discussion attempts to tease out data specific to CTCL and its subtypes.

There are no prospective studies for allogeneic stem cell transplants in CTCL. In 2005, the City of Hope Comprehensive Cancer Center published the first larger single-center retrospective series of allogeneic stem cell transplant in 8 patients with advanced MF/SS (IIB = 1, IVA = 7) including 1 patient with transformed MF and 4 patients with SS.[36] Patients were heavily pretreated with a median of 7 treatments before transplant including skin-directed therapies. A total of 4 patients received full-intensity conditioning, whereas the remaining 4 received fludarabine- and melphalan-based RIC regimens. All patients achieved complete clinical and molecular remission after transplant within 2 months; 6 of 8 had durable remission and were alive at a median follow-up of 7 years, and 1 patient with SS died of chronic GVHD and another with tumor MF died of respiratory syncytial virus pneumonia with a TRM of 25%. At a median follow-up of 56 months, 6 of 8 were alive with no evidence of disease. Even though the numbers were small, there seemed to be no difference in outcome based on intensity of conditioning and TBI seemed to be associated with increased skin toxicity in the posttransplant period.

A large multicenter center study from the European Bone Marrow transplant registry reported on a 10-year allotransplant experience of 60 patients with advanced MF (n = 36, 20 stage IV and 16 with IIB/III) and SS (n = 24) by Duarte and colleagues.[18] In this study, 73% (44/60) received RIC, 27% had MAC, and 42% (25/60) had T-cell depletion before transplant. Patients were followed up for a median of 7 years with the longest follow-up being of 12 years. There was no significant difference in outcome for patients with MF and SS. An

Table 1
List of larger case series and retrospective studies on allogeneic transplant in patients with MF/SS

Reference	No of Patients	Patient Characteristics	Conditioning Regimen	Follow up	OS (2 y/5 y)	PFS	Relapse Rate	Morbidity	Mortality
Molina et al,[36] 2005	8	4 MF (IIB = 1; IVA = 3) 4 SS (IVA = 4)	4 MAC 4 RIC 4 HLA-matched sibs 4 unrelated donors	56 mo	—	—	—	—	25% (2/8) died 1/2: chronic GVHD 1/2: RSV pneumonia
Wu et al,[37] 2009	20	14 MF (IB = 1, IIB = 3, IVA = 10) 6 SS (IIIA = 1, IVA = 5)	9 MAC 11 RIC	38 mo	1-y OS: 85% 5-y OS: 80%	1 y: 65% 5 y: 60%	25% (5/20): relapsed (2 in MAC and 3 in RIC)	75% (15/20): GVHD	20% (4/20) died 2/4: infection 2/4: GVHD (similar in MAC and RIC)
Duvic et al,[38] 2010	19	8 MF (IIB = 3, IVA = 4, IVB = 1, LCT = 2) 11 SS (IVA = 2, IVB = 9, LCT = 6)	19/19 RIC 15/19 TSEB	1.7 y	2-y OS: 79%	2 y: 53%	39%: relapse Median time 50 d (28–718 d)	67% acute GVHD 67% chronic GVHD	31.5% (6/19) died 4/6 in CR 2/6 died of progressive disease
Paralkar et al,[39] 2012	12	5 MF (IIB = 2, IIIB = 1, IVA2 = 1, IVB = 1, LCT = 1) 4 SS (IVA1 = 1, IVA2 = 3, LCT = 1) 3 GDTL	10/12 RIC 2/12 MAC	15 mo (all patients) 22 mo (alive patients)	2-y OS 58% Median OS 37 m Median PFS 5.3 m	—	40% (4/10) showed relapse 2/4 reachieved CR with DLI/ decreased immunosuppression	75 acute GVHD	17% died of sepsis and active disease
Shiratori et al,[40] 2014	9	7 MF (IIB = 2, IVA2 = 4, IVB = 1) 2 SS (IIB, IVA2) LCT = 8	RIC	—	3 y OS: 86%	3 y: 44%	56% (5/9) (80% only in skin)	11%: acute GVHD 67%: chronic GVHD	—

Study	No.	Patients	Conditioning	Follow-up					GVHD	
Duarte et al,[18] 2014	60	36 MF, 24 SS; IIB = 3, III = 13, IVA = 31, IVB = 13	73% RIC, 27% MAC	7–12 y	1 y: 66%, 5 y: 46%, 7 y: 44%	—	5 y: 32%, 7 y: 30%, 8/27: alive at 8 y	45% (27/60) had relapse at 4 m	69%: acute GVHD, 44%: chronic GVHD; 46% (11/24), 77% (8/11) died shortly due to complications	22% NRM
Polansky et al,[41] 2015	13 (217)	13 SS (IVA = 3, IVB = 10)	TSEB: 13/16	—	—				—	
de Masson et al,[42] 2014	37	5 MF, 1 FMF, 5 SS (IIB = 11, IIIA = 2, IVA1 = 2, IVA2 = 11, IVB = 5), 19 LCT-MF (IIB = 7, IIIA = 1, IVA2 = 9, IVB = 2), 1 LCT-SS (IVA1), 5 PCALCL, 1 PTCL, NOS	12 MAC, 25 RIC	29 mo	57%	51%			59% acute cutaneous GVHD; • In first year • Mostly in skin • 50% as less-severe form	18%
Lechowicz et al,[43] 2014	129	Registry data	83/129 RIC, 46/129 MAC	32–39 mo	1 y: 54%, 5 y: 32%, No difference between MAC & RIC	1 y: 31%, 5 y: 17%	1 y: 50%, 5 y: 61%		41% acute GVHD, 43% chronic GVHD at 3 y	1 y: 19%, 5 y: 22%, No difference between AC & RIC

Abbreviations: FMF, folliculotropic MF; GDTCL, gamma delta T-cell lymphoma; PFS, progression-free survival; RSV, respiratory syncytial virus.

OS of 44% was reported at 7 years with a progression-free survival (PFS) of 30%. About 45% patients showed relapse at a median of 3.8 months with only 2 relapses occurring later than 2 years after transplant. All but one patient with relapse achieved CR with DLI and/or salvage therapies. The NRM at 7 years was 22% with all deaths occurring within 14 months of transplant. The investigators concluded that advanced-phase disease and T-cell depletion were associated with increased risk of relapse and progression. Patients with low performance scores before transplant and those receiving MAC had higher NRM. Transplant from unrelated donors had a marginal effect on NRM, but the PFS and OS were significantly reduced when compared with related donors. Finally, RIC had better OS (63% vs 29% at 3 years) and lower NRM (14% vs 49%) when compared with MAC with no significant difference in the relapse rates. The series identified disease status, type of conditioning, and donor type as the main factors affecting the outcome of allogeneic transplant in MF/SS.

Duvic and colleagues[38] have reported the largest single-center study using reduced-intensity allogeneic transplant in 19 patients (median age 50 years) with advanced MF/SS. There were 3 patients with stage IIB MF, 2 with IVA/B MF, and 14 patients with SS as determined by the worst stage before transplant; 8 patients had LCT including 3 with CD30 + LCT. Of note, in this study, TSEB was used in 15 patients to improve control of skin disease along with the conditioning regimen that was based mostly on fludarabine and melphalan. The CR rate of 58% was similar to the 60.5% rate reported by Duarte and colleagues.[18] At the end of the median follow-up period of 1.7 years, 13 patients (68%) were alive with 11 were in complete clinical and molecular remission. Patients in whom the condition relapsed were treated with DLI and/or tapering immunosuppression to induce secondary remission. Of the 6 patients who died, 4 were in CR; 2 patients with SS died due to progressive disease and acute GVHD, precluding treatment with DLI. Sex, stem cell source, and SS were not predictive of relapse or OS (79% at 2 years). The study concluded that TSEBT combined with reduced-intensity allogeneic HSCT is an effective treatment option in advanced MF/SS. Subsequently, there have been several studies further exploring the role of RIC with allogeneic transplant in MF/SS. In 2014, Shiratori and colleagues[40] reiterated the role of allogeneic transplant in downstaging the lymphoma in subsequent relapses with significantly low NRM rates associated with RIC. Shorter duration of remission was, however, noted by Herbert and colleagues[44] in 3 patients with advanced-stage refractory disease treated with reduced-intensity allografts. The relapses responded to DLI and reduction in immunosuppression, but the response was not sustained. One of them showed relapse with high-grade disease and another died of chronic GVHD. The investigators concluded that GvL effect is insufficient for high-grade disease and that reduced-intensity allografting should be considered early in the disease course with prior tumor debulking preferably with prior ASCT.

Other notable studies include the report from the French Study Group on Cutaneous Lymphomas by de Masson and colleagues.[42] Their multicenter retrospective analysis included 37 patients with advanced MF. Patient characteristics were as follows: 31 patients had MF or SS including 20 (54%) with LCT with 10 cases of CD30-positive LCT; 5 patients had PCALCL including 3 cases that were ALK (anaplastic lymphoma kinase)-1 negative, 1 alk-positive case, and 1 alk-unknown case. All patients with epidermotropic T-cell lymphoma had failed skin-directed therapies; 22(59%) had received combination chemotherapy.

Both MAC (32%) and RIC (68%) were used for these patients. Relapse rate was high in this group of patients with advanced disease. The 2-year estimated PFS was 31% and OS was 57%. In this study, the use of antithymocyte globulin significantly reduced PFS ($P = .01$) in univariate and multivariate analysis. Lechowicz and colleagues[43] have published the outcomes of allogeneic transplant in 129 patients with CTCL, diagnosed with MF/SS and reported to CIBMTR between 2000 and 2009. Most (64%) patients received nonablative conditioning or RIC. PFS at 1 year and 5 years was 31% and 17%, respectively, and was lower than that reported by Duarte and colleagues[18]; the NRM of both the studies were similar (22% at 5 years). The study, however, concluded that the conditioning intensity did not have any impact on NRM or OS, unlike the previous study. The relapse rate was quite high with most relapses occurring within the first year of transplant (50% at 1 year and 61% at 5 years). The study did not differentiate between outcomes for patients with MF and SS.

Overall, the results of allogeneic transplant are encouraging when compared with autologous transplant and conventional treatment options in terms of sustained remission and high rates of PFS and OS after the procedure. A comparison done by Wu and colleagues[37] in 2009 revealed a 5-year OS of 80% in allogeneic versus 23% in autologous transplant group with similar clinical characteristics in both groups. While 60% remained disease free at 5 years postallogeneic transplant, all patients in the autologous group showed relapse at a median of 2.5 months (range 1–14 months). In this meta-analysis, most patients (70%) had persistent GVHD after receiving alloge-neic transplant for the treatment of MF/SS.[37] All 4 patients with myeloablative allogeneic transplant treated by the group at City of Hope developed relatively severe acute GVHD progressing into chronic disease, whereas none of the patients in the reduced-intensity group developed acute GVHD greater than grade 2. One of the patients in the myeloablative group eventually died because of complications of treatment of GVHD.[36] Duvic and colleagues[38] reported GVHD in 62% patients treated with reduced-intensity allogeneic transplant. The disease was, however, noted to be less severe as a result of prior tumor debulking with TSEBT, leading to only 1 GVHD-related death. Similar rates of GVHD were re-ported by de Masson and colleagues[42]; however, no difference was noted between the different conditioning regimens.

The high rates of NRM because of GVHD and in-fections associated with myeloablative regimens have improved with the use of reduced-intensity and nonmyeloablative regimens, which have been proved to be equally efficacious if used early in the disease at a low tumor bulk. Advanced-phase disease has been suggested as an independent adverse factor for relapse in various studies.[18,44] The outcomes of these studies highlight the fact that reduced-intensity transplants are promising and merit further investigation. Strategies such as pretransplant tumor bulk reduction with TSEBT or prior autologous transplants can be used to pro-vide additional benefit and to avoid the toxicity associated with full-dose myeloablation in patients with high-grade disease.

The selection of the appropriate patient for transplant still remains challenging with no unifying criteria except physician judgments.

SUMMARY AND FUTURE DIRECTIONS

Cutaneous lymphomas remain clinically chal-lenging, and many patients show a slowly pro-tracted indolent course that would never require a stem cell transplant for disease control. For advanced-stage MF with relapse/refractory dis-ease or aggressive subtypes such as SS, stem cell therapy needs to be considered. ASCT has been largely abandoned because of high numbers of early relapses, whereas allogeneic HSCT has shown to result in complete clearance of skin le-sions, blood involvement, and other evidence of disease with some patients achieving long-term remissions. GvL effect has been demonstrated by the successful use of RIC regimens, use of

DLI, and withdrawal of immunosuppression in cases of disease relapse after transplant. Although most studies are small, with marked heterogenic-ity in treated disease stage, histology, prior thera-pies, and transplant-related procedures, the outcome data do not suggest any difference be-tween MF or SS and the numbers for other sub-types are too small to draw any conclusions. There is no consensus about the degree of remis-sion needed before transplant for a successful outcome. Both related and unrelated matched do-nors have been used, and there are now support-ing data using cord blood as a source of stem cells. There is still no consensus on conditioning regimens, but remissions have been achieved us-ing RIC even in patients with advanced and refrac-tory disease states indicating that the intensity of the conditioning regimen may not be required for response. TSEB before transplant may be associ-ated with improved skin control. Relapses still occur after allogeneic transplants but have been treated successfully with adjustment of immuno-suppression, DLI infusion, or skin-directed treat-ments. The use of allogeneic stem cell transplant is associated with higher incidence of complica-tions including GVHD, infections, and death.

At present, there are no clear guidelines to select appropriate patients for stem cell trans-plant. Historical data have suggested that trans-plant has been performed for patients who have required multiple lines of systemic therapy after failing skin-directed therapies, especially combi-nation chemotherapy, usually with tumor stage/ nodal or systemic disease. However, the approval of new targeted therapies for CTCL including HDAC inhibitors and other targeted therapies now allows for more patients to be treated and maintained on noncytotoxic therapies. Talpur and colleagues[47] have published improved out-comes in patients with MF and SS at all stages including improved PFS and OS. The use of ge-netic profiling and gene sequencing is likely to allow better prognostic characterization of these tumors beyond clinical features of LCT and histo-logic subtype and may allow better selection of patients who require transplant for disease control.[48]

As with other hematologic malignancies, dedi-cated transplant protocols should be developed in multicenter trials to address the needs of pa-tients with CTCL with improved conditioning re-gimes and supportive care measures. In addition, transplant physicians need to be aware of the unique disease features of patients with the various types of CTCL and need to develop strate-gies for improved disease control to prevent re-lapses and reduce posttransplant complications.

The increasing numbers of targeted agents for the treatment of CTCL, notably HDAC inhibitors, including vorinostat,[49,50] and romidepsin,[51,52] brentuximab vedotin,[53] and various immune checkpoint inhibitors should be incorporated into transplant protocols either in conditioning regimens or as maintenance strategies. Selection of the appropriate patient for allogeneic stem cell transplant remains challenging, and guidelines are needed for the treating physicians for appropriate referrals to specialized transplant centers. Autologous transplant in the setting of therapeutic advances, particularly immune modulation, should be revisited as a potential therapeutic approach because of its low risk for complications.

REFERENCES

1. Willemze R, Jaffe ES, Burg G, et al. WHO-EORTC classification for cutaneous lymphomas. Blood 2005;105(10):3768–85.
2. Kim YH, Liu HL, Mraz-Gernhard S, et al. Long-term outcome of 525 patients with mycosis fungoides and Sezary syndrome: clinical prognostic factors and risk for disease progression. Arch Dermatol 2003;139(7):857–66.
3. Kim YH, Willemze R, Pimpinelli N, et al, ISCL and the EORTC. TNM classification system for primary cutaneous lymphomas other than mycosis fungoides and Sezary syndrome: a proposal of the international society for cutaneous lymphomas (ISCL) and the cutaneous lymphoma task force of the European Organization of Research and Treatment of Cancer (EORTC). Blood 2007;1102(2):479–84.
4. Olsen EA, Rook AH, Zic J, et al. Sézary syndrome: immunopathogenesis, literature review of therapeutic options, and recommendations for therapy by the United States Cutaneous Lymphoma Consortium (USCLC). J Am Acad Dermatol 2011; 64(2):352–404.
5. Wilcox RA. Cutaneous T-cell lymphoma: 2014 update on diagnosis, risk-stratification, and management. Am J Hematol 2014;89(8):837–51.
6. Agar NS, Wedgeworth E, Crichton S, et al. Survival outcomes and prognostic factors in mycosis fungoides/Sézary syndrome: validation of the revised international society for cutaneous lymphomas/European Organisation for Research and Treatment of Cancer staging proposal. J Clin Oncol 2010; 28(31):4730–9.
7. Pasquini MC, Zhu X. Current use and outcome of hematopoietic stem cell transplantation: CIBMTR Summary Slides. 2014. Available at: http://www.cibmtr. org. Accessed March 25, 2015.
8. Schmitz N, Dreger P, Suttorp M, et al. Primary transplantation of allogeneic peripheral blood progenitor cells mobilized by filgrastim (granulocyte colony-stimulating factor). Blood 1995;85:1666–72.
9. Keating GM. Plerixafor: a review of its use in stem cell mobilization in patients with Lymphoma or Multiple Myeloma. Drugs 2011;71(12):1623–47.
10. Gratwohl A, Baldomero H, Aljurf M, et al. Worldwide network of blood and marrow transplantation. Hematopoietic stem cell transplantation: a global perspective. JAMA 2010;303(16):1617–24.
11. Koh LP, Chao N. Haploidentical hematopoietic cell transplantation. Bone Marrow Transpl 2008; 42(Suppl 1):S60–3.
12. Kekre N, Antin JH. Hematopoietic stem cell transplantation donor sources in the 21st century: choosing the ideal donor when a perfect match does not exist. Blood 2014;124(3):334–43.
13. Alpdogan O, Grosso D, Flomenberg N. Recent advances in haploidentical stem cell transplantation. Discov Med 2013;16(88):159–65.
14. Eapen M, O'Donnell P, Brunstein CG, et al. Mismatched related and unrelated donors for allogeneic hematopoietic cell transplantation for adults with hematologic malignancies. Biol Blood Marrow Transplant 2014;20(10):1485–92.
15. Passweg JR, Baldomero H, Bader P, et al. Hematopoietic SCT in Europe 2013: recent trends in the use of alternative donors showing more haploidentical donors but fewer cord blood transplants. Bone Marrow Transplant 2015;50(4):476–82.
16. Baronciani D, Depau C, Targhetta C, et al. Treosulfan-fludarabine-thiotepa conditioning before allogeneic haemopoietic stem cell transplantation for patients with advanced lympho-proliferative disease. A single centre study. Hematol Oncol 2015, in press.
17. Bensinger WI. High-dose preparatory regimens. In: Appelbaum FR, Forman SJ, editors. Thomas' hematopoietic cell transplantation: stem cell transplantation. 4th edition. Oxford (United Kingdom): Wiley-Blackwell; 2009. ch 22;p. 316–32.
18. Duarte RF, Boumendil A, Onida F, et al. Long-term outcome of allogeneic hematopoietic cell transplantation for patients with mycosis fungoides and Sézary syndrome: a European society for blood and marrow transplantation lymphoma working party extended analysis. J Clin Oncol 2014;32(29):3347–8.
19. Baron F, Labopin M, Peniket A, et al. Reduced-intensity conditioning with fludarabine and busulfan versus fludarabine and melphalan for patients with acute myeloid leukemia: a report from the acute leukemia working party of the European Group for Blood and Marrow Transplantation. Cancer 2015; 121(7):1048–55.
20. Bearman SI. Reduced-intensity allogeneic stem cell transplantation. Curr Hematol Rep 2003;2(4): 277–86.
21. Hamadani M, Craig M, Awan FT, et al. How we approach patient evaluation for hematopoietic

stem cell transplantation. Bone Marrow Transpl 2010;45(8):1259–68.

22. Ferrara JL, Levine JE, Reddy P, et al. Graft-versus-host disease. Lancet 2009;373(9674):1550–61.

23. Filipovich AH, Weisdorf D, Pavletic S, et al. National Institutes of Health consensus development project on criteria for clinical trials in chronic graft-versus-host disease: I. Diagnosis and staging working group report. Biol Blood Marrow Transplant 2005; 11(12):945–56.

24. Defor TE, Majhail NS, Weisdorf DJ, et al. A modified comorbidity index for hematopoietic cell transplantation. Bone Marrow Transplant 2010;45:933–8.

25. Barnes DW, Corp MJ, Loutit JF, et al. Treatment of murine leukemia with X rays and homologous bone marrow; preliminary communication. Br Med J 1956;2(4993):626–7.

26. Jones RJ, Ambinder RF, Piantadosi S, et al. Evidence of a graft-versus-lymphoma effect associated with allogeneic bone marrow transplantation. Blood 1991;77(3):649–53.

27. Bigler RD, Crilley P, Micaily B, et al. Autologous bone marrow transplantation for advanced stage mycosis fungoides. Bone Marrow Transplant 1991;7:133–7.

28. Sterling JC, Marcus R, Burrows NP, et al. Erythrodermic mycosis fungoides treated with total body irradiation and autologous bone marrow transplantation. Clin Exper Dermatol 1995;20:73–5.

29. FerraFerrà C, Servitje O, Pétriz L, et al. Autologous haematopoietic progenitor transplantation in advanced mycosis fungoides. Br J Dermatol 1999; 140(6):1188–9.

30. Russell-Jones R, Child F, Olavarria E, et al. Autologous peripheral blood stem cell transplantation in tumor-stage mycosis fungoides: predictors of disease-free survival. Ann NY Acad Sci 2001;941:147–54.

31. Chen YC, Wang CH, Huang SC, et al. Autologous bone marrow transplantation after supralethal dose of total body irradiation in a case of mycosis fungoides. Taiwan Yi Xue Hui Za Zhi 1986;85(3):304–14.

32. Ingen-Housz-Oro S, Bachéeles H, Verola O, et al. High-dose therapy and autologous stem cell transplantation in relapsing cutaneous lymphoma. Bone Marrow Transpl 2004;33:629–34.

33. Olavarria E, Child F, Woolford A, et al. T-cell depletion and autologous stem cell transplantation in the management of tumour stage mycosis fungoides with peripheral blood involvement. Br J Haematol 2001;114(3):624–31.

34. Moreau P, LeTortorec S, Mahé MA, et al. Autologous bone marrow transplantation using TBI and CBV for disseminated high/intermediate grade cutaneous non-epidermotropic non-Hodgkin's lymphoma. Bone Marrow Transplant 1994;14:775–8.

35. Koeppel MC, Stoppa AM, Resbeut M, et al. Mycosis fungoides and allogenic bone marrow transplantation. Acta Derm Venereol 1994;74(4):331–2.

36. Molina A, Zain J, Arber DA, et al. Durable clinical, cytogenetic, and molecular remissions after allogeneic hematopoietic cell transplantation for refractory Sezary syndrome and mycosis fungoides. J Clin Oncol 2005;23(25):6163–71.

37. Wu PA, Kim YH, Lavori PW, et al. A meta-analysis of patients receiving allogeneic or autologous hematopoietic stem cell transplant in mycosis fungoides and Sézary syndrome. Biol Blood Marrow Transplant 2009;15(8):982–90.

38. Duvic M, Donato M, Dabaja B, et al. Total skin electron beam and non-myeloablative allogeneic hematopoietic stem-cell transplantation in advanced mycosis fungoides and Sezary syndrome. J Clin Oncol 2010;28(14):2365–72.

39. Paralkar VR, Nasta SD, Morrissey K, et al. Allogeneic hematopoietic SCT for primary cutaneous T cell lymphomas. Bone Marrow Transplant 2012;47(7):940–5.

40. Shiratori S, Fujimoto K, Nishimura M, et al. Allogeneic hematopoietic stem cell transplantation following reduced-intensity conditioning for mycosis fungoides and Sezary syndrome. Hematol Oncol 2014, in press.

41. Polansky M, Talpur R, Daulat S, et al. Long-term complete responses to combination therapies and allogeneic stem cell transplants in patients with Sézary syndrome. Clin Lymphoma Myeloma Leuk 2015; 15(5):e83–93.

42. de Masson A, Beylot-Barry M, Bouaziz JD, et al, French Study Group on Cutaneous Lymphomas and Société Française de Greffe de Moëlle et Thérapie Cellulaire. Allogeneic stem cell transplantation for advanced cutaneous T-cell lymphomas: a study from the French Society of Bone Marrow Transplantation and French Study Group on Cutaneous Lymphomas. Haematologica 2014;99(3):527–34.

43. Lechowicz MJ, Lazarus HM, Carreras J, et al. Allogeneic hematopoietic cell transplantation for mycosis fungoides and Sezary syndrome. Bone Marrow Transplant 2014;49(11):1360–5.

44. Herbert KE, Spencer A, Grigg A, et al. Graft-versus-lymphoma effect in refractory cutaneous T-cell lymphoma after reduced-intensity HLA-matched sibling allogeneic stem cell transplantation. Bone Marrow Transplant 2004;34:521.

45. Gabriel IH, Olavarria E, Jones RR, et al. Graft versus lymphoma effect after early relapse following reduced-intensity sibling allogeneic stem cell transplantation for relapsed cytotoxic variant of mycosis fungoides. Bone Marrow Transplant 2007;40(4): 401–3.

46. Duarte RF, Schmitz N, Servitje O, et al. Haematopoietic stem cell transplantation for patients with primary cutaneous T-cell lymphoma. Bone Marrow Transpl 2008;41(7):597–604.

47. Talpur R, Singh L, Daulat S, et al. Long-term outcomes of 1,263 patients with mycosis fungoides

and Sezary syndrome from 1982 to 2009. Clin Cancer Res 2012;18(18):5051–60.

48. Sekulic A, Liang WS, Tembe W, et al. Personalized treatment of Sezary syndrome by targeting a novel CTLA4:Cd28 fusion. Mol Genet Genomic Med 2015;3(2):130–6.

49. Kakizaki A, Fujimura T, Mizuashi M, et al. Successful treatment of syringotropic CD8+ mycosis fungoides accompanied by hypohidrosis with vorinostat and retinoids. Australas J Dermatol 2013;54:e82–4.

50. Duvic M, Olsen EA, Breneman D, et al. Evaluation of the long-term tolerability and clinical benefit of vorinostat in patients with advanced cutaneous T-cell lymphoma. Clin Lymphoma Myeloma 2009;9(6): 412–6.

51. Prince HM, Dickinson M, Khot A. Romidepsin for cutaneous T-cell lymphoma. Future Oncol 2013; 9(12):1819–27.

52. Li JY, Horwitz S, Moskowitz A, et al. Management of cutaneous T cell lymphoma: new and emerging targets and treatment options. Cancer Manag Res 2012;4:75–89.

53. Mehra T, Ikenberg K, Moos RM, et al. Brentuximab as a treatment for CD30+ mycosis fungoides and Sézary syndrome. JAMA Dermatol 2015;151(1): 73–7.

Practical Management of CD30⁺ Lymphoproliferative Disorders

Lauren C. Hughey, MD

KEYWORDS

- Lymphomatoid papulosis • Primary cutaneous anaplastic large cell cutaneous lymphoma
- Mycosis fungoides with large cell transformation • CD30⁺ cutaneous lymphoproliferative disorders

KEY POINTS

- The CD30⁺ cutaneous lymphoproliferative disorders can look similar both clinically and histologically. Evaluation by a clinician and dermatopathologist with expertise in cutaneous lymphomas is invaluable in the correct classification of these disorders.
- Correct classification sets the stage for choosing an appropriate treatment regimen for each of these disorders. Lymphomatoid papulosis (LyP) rarely requires systemic therapy, whereas refractory or multifocal cutaneous anaplastic large cell lymphoma (cALCL) and mycosis fungoides (MF) with large cell transformation (LCT) may require systemic therapy in combination with skin-directed therapy.
- Given the chronic nature and typical good prognosis of most CD30⁺ lymphoproliferative disorders (LPDs), the clinician should take into account possible deleterious long-term side effects of treatment options.

INTRODUCTION

Primary cutaneous CD30⁺ LPDs account for approximately 25% of cutaneous lymphomas.[1] The peak incidence is in the fifth and sixth decades. Although these CD30⁺ LPDs are clinically heterogeneous, they can be indistinguishable histologically. The 2 CD30⁺ primary cutaneous LPDs listed in the World Health Organization European Organization for Research and Treatment of Cancer (EORTC) classification scheme are LyP and primary cALCL[2]; however, it is important to include LCT of MF in this discussion as these 3 CD30⁺ LPDs can mimic, be mistaken for, and occur concomitantly with each other. Recognizing and differentiating these CD30⁺ entities can be challenging, but correct classification is imperative for developing an effective treatment protocol. There is no definitive test to differentiate these 3

CD30⁺ LPDs; therefore, assimilating clinical and pathologic data remains the best method to date. By observing the primary lesion morphology, distribution on the body, the natural course of the lesions, the histology, and the immunohistochemical data, more often than not, one can correctly categorize the disorder.

Many different treatment strategies have been used for the CD30⁺ LPDs; however, given the rarity of these diseases, there are little accumulated data for evidence-based guidelines. Most studies are case reports, small series, or retrospective reviews. There are very few prospective studies. However, the EORTC, International Society for Cutaneous Lymphomas (ISCL), and the US Cutaneous Lymphoma Consortium (USCLC) recently convened an expert multidisciplinary panel and offered recommendations for treatment of LyP and cALCL based on literature analysis and

Author disclosures: Investigator for Kyowa and Eisai.
University of Alabama at Birmingham, 1530 3rd Avenue South, EFH 414, Birmingham, AL 35294, USA
E-mail address: lchughey@uab.edu

Dermatol Clin 33 (2015) 819–833
http://dx.doi.org/10.1016/j.det.2015.05.013
0733-8635/15/$ – see front matter © 2015 Elsevier Inc. All rights reserved.

derm.theclinics.com

discussion by clinicians.[3] The National Comprehensive Cancer Network (NCCN) guidelines are also a great Web-based reference to aid in the workup and treatment of CD30[+] LPDs (www. nccn.org).

The following discussion offers practical pearls to differentiate entities, addresses most of the treatment options, and addresses the treatment of MF with LCT, which was not discussed in the prior review.

LYMPHOMATOID PAPULOSIS

Whether to classify LyP as benign or malignant remains a controversy. However, most experts in the field think of LyP as an indolent cutaneous lymphoma on the same spectrum as cALCL. LyP incidence peaks in the fifth decade and has an excellent prognosis with a 10-year survival approaching 100% (LyP).[1] Up to70% of LyP cases are associated with +TCR gene rearrangements.[4] The classic clinical description of LyP is crops of erythematous papules (often at different stages of development) most often on the trunk or proximal extremities that progress to central necrosis and heal spontaneously over weeks to possibly months (**Fig. 1**). The histology can be variable with predominant CD4[+] or CD8[+] T cells and is categorized into 5 different subtypes (A–E) (**Table 1**), although a single patient may exhibit several of these histologic patterns. These subtypes are not predictive of clinical course or of severity of disease. However, it is important to be knowledgeable about these histologic subtypes as they mimic the histology of other more concerning LPDs and may lead to misdiagnosis and possibly more aggressive treatment than is needed.

The most common type A LyP histology resembles wedge-shaped clusters of CD30[+] large atypical lymphocytes interspersed between a mixed

inflammatory infiltrate of neutrophils, histiocytes, eosinophils, and smaller lymphoctyes, and epidermotropism is typically absent. The rarer type B LyP exhibits histologic features reminiscent of MF, with a bandlike infiltrate and epidermotropism of small to medium atypical lymphocytes that may be CD30[-]. Type C LyP is described as cALCL-like with larger clusters or sheets of large anaplastic CD30[+] atypical lymphocytes without the mixed inflammatory infiltrate seen in type A. Type D LyP has a more worrisome histologic appearance and can mimic CD8[+] aggressive epidermotropic cutaneous T-cell lymphoma (CTCL) with large CD8[+], CD30[+] lymphocytes that stain for cytotoxic markers, including T-cell intracellular antigen-1 (TIA-1), granzyme, and perforin.[5] These cases do not usually have necrosis and ulceration but may lose expression of T-cell antigens including CD2, CD3, CD5, and CD7. Recently reported type E LyP is described as angioinvasive with small, medium, and large angiocentric CD30[+] atypical lymphocytes that invade the walls of small to medium vessels in the dermis and less so in the subcutis, often with associated necrosis.[6] Clinically, the initial papules in type E LyP quickly progress to larger hemorrhagic and necrotic ulcers, but even these cases follow the typical course of LyP and spontaneously resolve.[7,8] In addition, one case series describes LyP type F, which exhibits perifollicular infiltrates of CD30[+] atypical cells with folliculotrophism with or without follicular mucinosis.[9]

LyP may occur in conjunction with other lymphomas in about 20% of cases.[10] There have been reported cases of LyP in association with cALCL, MF, Hodgkin disease, systemic ALCL, and other systemic lymphomas. In some of these cases, the same clone is responsible for both diseases, suggesting a possible common origin in the precursor lymphoid stem cell.[11–13] The coexistence of these disorders can lead to confusing clinical presentations making accurate diagnosis challenging. In these situations, it is important to remember that performing multiple biopsies of each different primary lesion morphology and observing the course of individual lesions can be helpful in deciphering these cases. In addition, if LyP nodules begin to exceed 1 cm, one should be suspicious for progression to another subtype of cutaneous lymphoma.[13]

Treatment of Lymphomatoid Papulosis

Despite the excellent prognosis of LyP, the recurrent nature of the lesions is typically bothersome for patients, and most desire treatment (**Box 1**). Although topical corticosteroid therapy does not

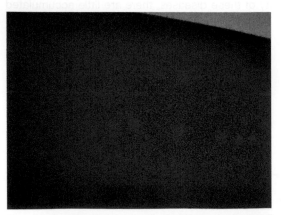

Fig. 1. Lymphomatoid papulosis: crops of clustered papules often with central eschar.

Table 1
Lymphomatoid papulosis subtypes

LyP Subtypes	Histologic Description
Type A	Wedge-shaped clusters CD30⁺ large atypical lymphocytes interspersed with a mixed inflammatory infiltrate of neutrophils, histiocytes, and eosinophils
Type B	MF-like with bandlike infiltrate and epidermotropism of smaller atypical lymphocytes that may be CD30⁻
Type C	cALCL-like with larger clusters or sheets of large anaplastic CD30⁺ cells without the interspersed mixed infiltrate of Type A
Type D	CD8⁺ epidermotropic CTCL-like with large CD8⁺, CD30⁺ lymphocytes that often stain with cytotoxic markers (TIA-1, granzyme, perforin)
Type E	Angioinvasive with small to large angiocentric CD30⁺ atypical lymphocytes that invade walls of small to medium vessels in dermis or SQ
Type F	Perifollicular infiltrates of CD30⁺ atypical cells with folliculotrophism with or without follicular mucinosis

Abbreviations: CTCL, cutaneous T-cell lymphoma; SQ, subcutaneous; TIA-1, T-cell intracellular antigen-1.

prevent lesions or change the natural history of the disease, spot treatment with a high-potency topical steroid can be helpful to reduce the size and to hasten involution of papules. For those patients with frequent outbreaks of many LyP lesions, treatment options that may prevent occurrence of new lesions are often desirable and may include single-agent systemic immunomodulators, chemotherapy, and/or phototherapy. However, given the excellent prognosis of LyP, the long-term sequela of these therapies should be considered. There is no role for multiagent chemotherapy for LyP, as the risks likely outweigh the benefits.

According to the EORTC, ISCL, and USCLC recent review,[3] topical corticosteroids, methotrexate (MTX), and psoralen + ultraviolet A (PUVA) are all first-line therapies successful at obtaining a partial response (PR) or complete response (CR)

Box 1
Lymphomatoid papulosis treatment options

Skin-directed treatment options
- Observation
- Topical corticosteroids
- Phototherapy
- Topical imiquimod
- Topical nitrogen mustard
- Interferon intralesional (IL)

Systemic treatment options
- Methotrexate
- Oral retinoids
- Interferon

in LyP. Thus, the decision on which of these treatments to choose depends on the extent of the patient's disease (Is it too widespread for topical treatment?), where the patient lives (Are they within driving distance of a phototherapy unit?), their insurance situation (Are they insured and does their insurance cover the pharmacy cost of psoralen?), and their comorbidities (Is any preexisting liver disease or poor kidney function making them a poor candidate for MTX?). Other second- and third-line treatment options are also discussed.

Topical corticosteroids
Although monotherapy with topical corticosteroids does not prevent new lesions, they do typically help the lesions remain smaller and resolve faster and therefore are a good option for patients with limited and infrequent disease outbreaks. Topical corticosteroids are also used often as adjunctive treatment along with MTX or PUVA. Of the 25 patients with LyP reviewed by Kempf and colleagues,[3] only 3 had a CR with topical corticosteroids reflecting that, although helpful, monotherapy with topical corticosteroids rarely achieve CRs in LyP. Given the chronic nature of LyP, the risks outweigh the benefits for oral systemic corticosteroids, and they have not been shown to be effective in LyP.[14]

Phototherapy
There is a lack of published data on the use of phototherapy (PUVA) for LyP, but there is ample anecdotal evidence and small case series to strongly support its use as a first-line treatment modality for LyP.[15] Kempf and colleagues[3] reported in their review of 19 patients with LyP published in the literature that 68% had a PR and 27% had a CR

with PUVA therapy. Relapses occurred in all patients shortly after discontinuing light therapy. An example of a typical PUVA regimen for patients with LyP or MF begins with treatments 3 times weekly according to institution protocols and skin type of the patient. Once the patient has substantial improvement, PUVA frequency can be decreased to twice per week, then to once per week, then to once every other week, then once every third week, and so on until reaching the minimum maintenance dose appropriate to keep that patient's disease not 100% clear but rather well controlled. Discussing realistic expectations with patients is important. It may take a year or more to reach the desired maintenance frequency with PUVA. The minimum frequency of PUVA maintenance therapy is typically once every 8 weeks.

There are also reports of effectiveness with ultraviolet B (UVB) phototherapy in 6 of 7 children with LyP.[16] Although UVB therapy does not penetrate to the depth that PUVA reaches to treat thicker lesions, it still may be effective for thinner LyP lesions. Broadband UVB (BBUVB) and narrowband UVB (NBUVB) also typically start with a 3-times-per-week treatment regimen until the patient substantially improves. Then one can further decrease the frequency to twice per week, then to once per week, and then every other week. Further decreases in BBUVB and NBUVB may lead to loss of efficacy and increased potential for phototoxicity. This every-other-week maintenance UVB regimen may be safely continued for extended periods in an effort to control disease. Although PUVA is associated with increased risk of both melanoma and nonmelanoma skin cancers, NBUVB does not have this same association.[17–19]

One case report heralded the success in treating refractory LyP lesions with methyl aminolevulinate photodynamic therapy (MAL PDT) with a 630-nm light source after 3 hours of incubation under occlusion. MAL PDT was repeated 1 week later, and refractory lesions resolved 7 days after the second treatment without recurrence of lesions in the treated area during an 11-month follow-up period.[20] PDT treatment may prove useful as field treatment in patients with recurrent or refractory lesions of LyP within a localized area.

The 308-nm excimer laser has been used for the treatment of localized LyP lesions. A total of 13 treatments given 3 times weekly with a maximum fluence of 500 mJ/cm^2 induced clearance in 75% of treated lesions in one report; however, duration of response was not addressed.[21]

In one LyP case, extracorporeal photopheresis with 8-methoxypsoralen was used on 2 consecutive days once monthly to achieve a PR, albeit temporary, in this refractory case of diffuse LyP.[22]

Methotrexate

MTX is a folate antagonist that inhibits purine and pyrimidine synthesis. Despite few published reports,[23–26] MTX is an accepted first-line treatment of CD30$^+$ LPDs, and there are ample anecdotal successes in controlling CD30$^+$ LPDs with low-dose MTX. Effective doses range from 10 to 25 mg oral once weekly typically with concomitant folic acid, 1 mg, each day. The largest study using MTX included cALCL as well as LyP. Of 45 patients, 39 (87%) had satisfactory long-term control of their disease.[27] Doses in some patients reached 60 mg per week; however, the investigators found that patients responded equally well with lower doses in the range of 15 to 20 mg per week. The patients typically responded within 4 weeks of beginning therapy. Once improvement was seen, MTX frequency was reduced in an effort to retain control of disease while reducing risk of drug toxicity. In some patients MTX could be reduced to once every 10 to 28 days with good control of CD30$^+$ lesions but with less control of the MF patches (in the patients with coexisting MF). Median total duration of MTX therapy exceeded 39 months (range, 2–205 months). After MTX was discontinued, 10 patients remained free of disease from 24 to 227 months. The most common side effects reported were fatigue (47%), elevated liver transaminase levels (27%), and nausea (22%). Of 10 patients treated with MTX for more than 3 years, 5 had evidence of hepatic fibrosis.[27]

Subcutaneous (SQ) administration of MTX can be considered in patients not responding to oral dosing.[13] There is one report of topical MTX use in a patient with LyP who moistened his MTX tablet with tap water and applied it to some of his LyP lesions. He essentially used his other LyP lesions as a control and found that the lesions treated with topical MTX resolved faster and stayed smaller than the controls. MTX is known to have poor percutaneous systemic absorption; therefore, the effect of the MTX is thought to be local in this case.[28] Given the issues with cutaneous absorption, no commercially available topical MTX exists, making this treatment modality difficult to replicate; however, a previous phase 1/2 trial of a topical MTX-laurocapram topical hydrophilic gel did show some efficacy in CTCL, and similar compounds may hold promise for the future.[29]

Bexarotene

Bexarotene is an oral retinoid with a high affinity for the retinoid X receptor (RXR). It was approved by the US Food and Drug Administration (FDA) for the treatment of CTCL in 1999. In a prospective study of 10 patients with LyP treated with either topical or oral bexarotene, 300 mg/m^2/d, all patients had a response in regards to decreased number or duration of lesions, with an objective response seen in 8 of 10 patients (1 CR in a patient using oral bexarotene, with all lesions clearing and no new lesions during continued therapy; 1 CR and 5 PRs in treated lesions in patients using bexarotene gel; and 1 PR in a patient using both oral and topical bexarotene).[30] The use of bexarotene gel was associated with more rapid disappearance (average of 3 days to resolve compared with 2–4 months for lesion resolution), less necrosis, and overall fewer lesions than before the patient started using bexarotene gel. One patient with recurrent LyP lesions in a localized area experienced a reduction of new lesions after field treating the area with bexarotene gel, suggesting that bexarotene gel may be useful in treating active lesions as well as preventing new lesions. Bexarotene gel can cause an intense retinoid dermatitis in some patients; therefore, counseling patients on what to expect, allowing a reduction from the recommended 4 times a day dosing for MF, and prescribing a topical corticosteroid to calm retinoid dermatitis can encourage patient compliance and continued therapy.[30]

A more extensive review of bexarotene is offered by Dr. Huen AO; however, it is important to mention here the central hypothyroidism and hypertriglyceridemia seen with oral bexarotene. Thyroid-stimulating hormone remains low throughout oral bexarotene therapy because of central hypothyroidism; therefore, it is the free T4 that must be followed to titrate the thyroid supplementation dose. Communicating with the patient's primary doctor is of utmost importance in patients administered oral bexarotene so that there is joint understanding of the thyroid tests used to monitor these patients. For lipid control, a fenofibrate or statin should be administered at the same time as oral bexarotene with subsequent monitoring of the fasting lipid panel to adjust these medications as needed.

Interferon

There are little published data about the use of interferons (IFNs) for CD30+ LPDs.[31] In an open trial of patients with LyP, 5 patients were treated with IFN-α SQ injection 3 times per week for 6 weeks (1 with 15 million units (MU) 3 times per week, 4 with 3 MU 3 times per week). There were 4 CRs and 1 PR. The 2 of 5 patients who had recurrent disease shortly after IFN discontinuation were only treated with 5 to 7 months of IFN suggesting that it is difficult to alter the chronic recurring nature of LyP with only short-term IFN use. One of these patients was then able to regain CR with subsequent additional 17 months of IFN therapy and has

maintained remission for 3 years. The other patient with recurrent disease was treated with an additional 12 months of IFN and still has stable disease 31 years later. The other 3 patients were treated for longer 12- to 13-month intervals with IFN and were able to maintain their remission throughout the follow-up period after drug discontinuation (from 1 to 11 years) and did not require any retreatment, suggesting that treating with IFN for at least 1 year may yield better long-term results.[32]

Intralesional IFN has been used successfully for larger, more refractory lesions. One report described 1 MU intralesional injection of IFN-α2b into 3 LyP lesions (3 MU total) 3 times weekly. Lesions smaller than 0.5 cm resolved after 3 injections. The larger lesions took up to 3 to 10 intralesional injections. After resolution of lesions, maintenance therapy was continued with 3 MU SQ injection into the abdomen 3 times weekly. The patient reported some skin recurrences; however, overall number and size of skin lesions were reduced while on IFN therapy.[33]

Imiquimod

Imiquimod is a Toll-like receptor 7 and 8 agonist. This topical immune response modifier enhances the T_H1 response leading to increased production of IFN-α, interleukin 12, IFN-γ, and other cytokines thereby having an antitumor effect and balancing the T_H2 profile of CTCL.[34,35] One report of topical imiquimod application 3 times a week in a patient with LyP, who was already administered low-dose MTX, noted a faster regression of lesions from his typical 2 months down to 2 weeks.[36] Imiquimod seemed to have only a local effect as new lesions appeared elsewhere in the patient, but this topical immunomodulator provides a good option for adjunctive treatment of refractory LyP lesions.

Topical nitrogen mustard

Despite a lack of published data, topical nitrogen mustard is used often in clinical practice for refractory LyP lesions. A review of CD30+ LPD treatments found that only 1 of 17 patients with LyP had a sustained response with topical nitrogen mustard.[3] However, sustained responses are often not plausible in this chronic, relapsing, and remitting disease, and nitrogen mustard should be considered in the armamentarium of LyP treatments. More studies need to be done to assess whether its use leads to faster resolution of lesions.

PRIMARY CUTANEOUS ANAPLASTIC LARGE CELL LYMPHOMA

Primary cALCL typically presents as a solitary or few tumor nodules without evidence of extracutaneous disease at the time of diagnosis (**Fig. 2**).

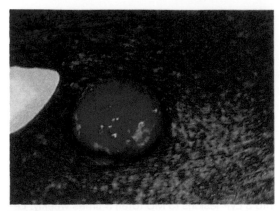

Fig. 2. Primacy cutaneous anaplastic large cell lymphoma tumor.

These nodules may progress to ulceration, and, although up to 25% to 44% may show partial regression over time, they less commonly completely resolve on their own.[1,10] Despite various treatment strategies, up to 60% of patients with cALCL have recurrences of skin nodules.[3,37] Regional lymph node involvement may infrequently occur and is typically not associated with a worse prognosis. Widespread systemic involvement is rare,[1] and when it occurs, the patient would be considered to have systemic ALCL. cALCL has an excellent prognosis of more than 90% 10-year survival; however, patients with multifocal cALCL (lesions in more than 1 anatomic area) are more at risk for extracutaneous spread.[38] In addition, extensive extremity involvement can prove refractory to therapy and may be associated with a worse prognosis.[39] Histologically, these tumors comprise large sheets of anaplastic, pleomorphic, or immunoblastic T cells with irregularly shaped nuclei and pale cytoplasm, which extend into the deep dermis or SQ tissue and are CD30[+] and anaplastic lymphoma kinase (ALK-1) negative. Surrounding eosinophils and small reactive lymphocytes may be seen at the periphery of the infiltrate. By definition, CD30 is expressed by greater than 75% of the large tumor cells.[2]

Treatment of Cutaneous Anaplastic Large Cell Lymphoma

Approximately one-fourth of cALCL lesions may spontaneously improve or even resolve (**Box 2**).[1,13,40,41] Surgical excision and/or local radiation therapy are reasonable options for the treatment of solitary or localized cALCL. There is no literature to suggest that radiation following excision has a better outcome than either treatment modality alone. However, despite these 2 treatment options, cALCL recurs in about 40% of patients either in the same or in a new location. Multifocal lesions or frequent recurrences leading to multiple surgical excisions and radiation exposures become less appealing. In these situations, moving from a skin-directed to a systemic single-agent immunomodulator or chemotherapeutic treatment regimen offers a good alternative. Low-dose MTX, oral retinoids (isotretinoin, acitretin, or bexarotene), brentuximab vedotin, gemcitabine, IFN, or etoposide have data to support their efficacy in this condition and are discussed in detail.

Multiagent chemotherapies do not offer better long-term response rates nor do they offer fewer relapses compared with excision and/or radiotherapy. Weighing risks versus benefits of the long-term sequela of aggressive multiagent chemotherapy regimens in this disease with excellent prognosis is important. In a review article summarizing several studies, multiagent C: cytoxan (cyclophosphamide), H: adriamycin (hydroxy doxorubicin), O: vincristine (Oncovin), P: prednisone (CHOP) chemotherapy offered CRs in approximately 85% of patients receiving that therapy; however, relapse rates in the various reviewed studies approached 71%, and the median duration of response for some of these patients was as short as 6 weeks.[1,3] Multiagent CHOP chemotherapy has not been shown to be superior, and in fact may lead to more frequent subsequent relapses than other treatment regimens.[1,38] Although its use is not addressed further in this article, it may be used for the rare case of refractory or widespread extracutaneous disease.

Excision

Surgical excision is a well-accepted and first-line treatment strategy for solitary cALCL of reasonable size.[3,38] There is no consensus on margins for tumor removal. Removal of clinically abnormal-appearing skin with small margins are accepted; however, Mohs surgery does not likely offer any benefit, as it is difficult to decipher margin of tumor compared with surrounding inflammatory lymphocytes on frozen section, which may lead to larger-than-necessary margins. Whether there is any significance of leaving positive margins is not known.

Radiotherapy

Local radiation therapy is a first-line monotherapy for single or few localized lesions of cALCL. A recent review found that successful local electron beam radiation doses typically ranged from 30 to 46 Gy. About 2- to 4-cm margins of uninvolved skin were included in the radiation field. Radiation dermatitis and other side effects such as skin atrophy, sweat gland dysfunction, alopecia, and edema were mild and tolerable. Although 95% of patients in the review had a CR, 41% recurred within the follow-up period of 22 months. Of 11 patients treated with surgical excision followed by radiation, 67% experienced a sustained CR, but 64% had recurrence within 54 months.[42]

Brentuximab vedotin

SGN-30, the monoclonal antibody without any chemotherapy attachment, is no longer available; therefore, this discussion concentrates on SGN-35 (brentuximab vedotin [BV]). BV is a CD30 monoclonal antibody conjugated to the chemotherapy monomethyl auristatin E, which inhibits microtubule polymerization, leading to cell death. This antibody-drug conjugate has been successful in treating CD30+ LPDs. BV is only FDA-approved drug for CD30+ systemic ALCL and relapsed/refractory Hodgkin lymphoma; however, data support its use in other CD30+ LPDs.[43–49] A phase 2 single-center trial of 56 patients with CD30+ CTCL (MF with LCT, n = 28; LyP, n = 9; cALCL, n = 2; and patients with mixed lesions unable to be classified clearly, n = 9) treated with BV revealed objective response rates (PR plus CR) of 73% across all disease types. Dosing in this phase 2 trial was 1.8 mg/kg intravenously (IV) over 30 minutes every 21 days with dose reduction to 1.2 mg/kg if needed for adverse effect management. Of 56 patients, 12 (21%) required dose adjustments secondary to peripheral neuropathy (9 patients), liver dysfunction (2 patients), and arthralgias (2 patients). Both patients with cALCL had CRs, and 5 of 9 (55%) patients with LyP had CR, with the remaining having greater than 50%

reduction in lesion count. Of 9 patients with mixed lesions, 8 (88%) had CRs, and the remaining patient had a PR. Median time to response was 3 weeks (range, 3–9 weeks), and median duration of response was 26 weeks (range, 6–44) for cALCL, LyP, and mixed lesions. Disease recurred in most cases when BV was discontinued. Nausea and neutropenia were the only grade 3 adverse events, but overall, most adverse events were mild. Although 65% of patients experienced peripheral neuropathy, it resolved in 45% of patients after a median of 41.5 weeks.[50]

These trial data have led to using BV in the clinical setting. For cALCL, as long as the patient does not have peripheral neuropathy or other adverse effects, the 1.8-mg/kg dosing every 21 days can be continued until lesions are clear and then followed with 2 additional doses, after which a wait and see approach is taken. If new lesions occur or old lesions recur, 1 to 2 additional doses of BV can be given. Using BV on an as-needed basis can extend the use of this drug while reducing likelihood of side effects. This same plan can be used with the lower 1.2-mg/kg dosing regimen if neuropathies are an issue. Finding an end point for BV in the treatment of LyP is more difficult given the recurrent crops of lesions that tend to recur once BV is discontinued. In addition, although rare, there have been at least 8 reported cases of progressive multifocal leukoencephalopathy associated with BV (2 of whom had CTCL).[51] Therefore, BV may be best used to gain control over severe LyP cases to bridge them to other maintenance therapy, but its use in indolent low-level disease is likely not warranted.

Methotrexate

Oral MTX experience with cALCL has already been discussed earlier in the LyP section; however, to summarize, doses of 15 to 20 mg once weekly is typically effective for controlling cALCL. Dose frequency may be decreased as disease responds. Intralesional MTX has also been used with varying dosing regimens.[24] One report noted a CR to a cALCL leg lesion with 12.5 mg MTX intralesional injection followed by another 10-mg injection 1 week later. No recurrence of the tumor nodule was noted in the 9-month follow-up period. Pain at the injection site can be ameliorated with topical or injected anesthetic agents before MTX injections.[52] Low-dose MTX may also be used as maintenance therapy after excision or radiation of cALCL lesions to prevent recurrence.[27]

Oral retinoids

There are only case reports or small series of retinoid use in cALCL, but anecdotally, they have been successful.[53–56] Bexarotene doses are typically low dose, ranging from 225 to 450 mg/d. Isotretinoin doses range from 0.5 to 1.0 mg/kg, and acitretin doses from 20 to 50 mg/d.[38,56] The mechanism of action and pharmacokinetics of retinoids are addressed elsewhere in this issue.

Gemcitabine

Gemcitabine, a pyrimidine analogue that halts DNA replication and leads to cell apoptosis, is successfully used for the treatment of refractory or advanced CTCLs.[57] Typical gemcitabine dosing for refractory CTCL is 1000 to 1200 mg/m² IV over 30 minutes on days 1, 8, and 15 of a 28-day cycle.[58] This dosing regimen is appropriate and useful in CD30+ LPDs; however, results can sometimes be achieved with lower-dose regimens (750 mg/m²) or lower frequency of dosing (every 14–21 days). Gemcitabine is typically well tolerated in this patient population, but reported side effects include hematologic, cardiac, hepatic, and gastrointestinal effects.

Etoposide

Etoposide is a cytotoxic topoisomerase inhibitor successfully used in refractory cALCL. In a recent review, there were 3 PRs and 4 CRs in the 7 cALCL cases treated with oral etoposide, 50 mg/d.[59] Etoposide remains a well-tolerated therapeutic option for refractory, multifocal cALCL.

Interferon

There is a paucity of literature,[31,60,61] but some reports do support the use of the immunomodulating agent IFN to promote return of T_H1 cytokine profile and improve skin lesions in CD30+ LPDs including cALCL.[31,60] IFN may be used by intralesional, SQ, or IV routes. Doses range from 9 to 18 MU each week given in divided doses. A common regimen is 3 MU 3 times weekly intralesional injection for refractory cALCL lesions, although fewer units and less frequent dosing can also be used.

Imiquimod

Success with the topical immunomodulator imiquimod has been reported in several cases of cALCL.[62] Two patients with solitary cALCL lesions (10-mm nodule and 2 × 4-cm tumor), which had been present for 6 and 10 months without resolution, were treated with topical imiquimod 5% cream to the lesions 3 times weekly for 6 weeks. Both patients had a CR, with no recurrence during the 8-month follow-up.[63] In another report, imiquimod was used 3 times weekly on a patient with cALCL, and CR was achieved.[64]

Phototherapy

The 308-nm excimer UVB laser has been successfully used in the past for refractory patches or plaques of MF, especially those that are in sanctuary areas or those that have not responded to topical medications. Similar scenarios could be considered for the use of excimer laser in localized or refractory CD30+ LPDs. One report described the use of the excimer laser to treat a solitary CD30+ LPD nodule (likely cALCL) twice weekly during 12 sessions starting at 150 mJ and increasing to 500 mJ by the end of the course. There was no recurrence of the lesion in a 15-month follow-up period.[65]

Background data suggest that the photosensitizing agent used in photodynamic therapy is preferentially absorbed by the activated T lymphocytes in cutaneous lymphomas and that PDT can cause inhibition of and apoptosis in these T cells.[66–68] PDT is not widely used nor is there a prescribed regimen for its use in CD30+ LPDs; however, this treatment modality may be an option to consider for tumor debulking in patients with cALCL. One report described a dramatic reduction in size of a cALCL tumor. Histology showed massive degeneration of lymphoma cells after PDT treatments with 20% 5-aminolevulinic acid occluded for 6 hours and then treated with visible light in the spectrum of 630 to 700 nm for 20 minutes once daily on 9 consecutive days.[69]

Combination therapies

A combination of bexarotene and IFN-α has been reported and is commonly used with success. In one case report, low doses of each were used (150 mg/d bexarotene and 3 MU SQ IFN-α 3 times weekly) to achieve a rapid and complete remission sustained during a 12-month follow-up period in a patient with multifocal cALCL.[60]

Although there are reports of benefit of denileukin diftitox for CD30+ LPDs, the discussion of this has been omitted from this article as this drug is currently not available.

MYCOSIS FUNGOIDES WITH LARGE CELL TRANSFORMATION

The classic clinical presentation of LCT in MF occurs as a new solitary pink to violaceous nodule within a long-standing MF patch or plaque, abrupt onset of multiple pink scattered nodules, or a new or enlarging tumor nodule of MF (**Fig. 3**).[70] However, LCT occurring in patches or plaques of MF does not necessarily signify a change in disease stage. LCT occurs in 8% to 55% of MF cases and is more common in advanced disease. In an article retrospectively studying long-term

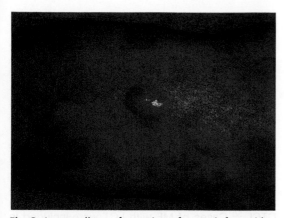

Fig. 3. Large cell transformation of mycosis fungoides.

outcomes of patients with LCT, the investigators found that 1.4% of stage I-IIA, 26% stage IIb, 2.8% stage III, 55% stage IVA, and 66% stage IVB developed transformation.[71] In addition to advanced stage, histologic transformation within the first 2 years of diagnosis also portends a worse prognosis.[72] Although the transformed clone often matches the original MF clone in these patients, the risk factors for LCT are largely unknown.[73,74] The classification of LCT of MF is made histologically when greater than 25% of lymphocytes are large (>4 times the size of a normal lymphocyte). These cells may be immunoblastic, pleomorphic, or Reed-Sternberg cell–like in appearance and are more often than not CD30+. MF with LCT can be more refractory to treatment, and most agree that transformed MF portends a worse prognosis compared with those MF patients without transformed disease especially if transformation is found in the lymph nodes in addition to the skin. For these reasons, more aggressive therapy is typically warranted in these patients. Median survival times from transformation to death ranges from 19 to 36 months in most reports; however, one study found median survival of 8.3 years.[75] The reason for this discrepancy is difficult to decipher; however, it is known that differentiating MF with LCT from concomitant cALCL can be challenging, or perhaps these patients with MF had earlier recognition and more aggressive treatment leading to improved overall survival. Most patients with MF and LCT benefit from a combination of skin-directed and systemic therapies. Bexarotene, IFN, and MTX are options from NCCN guidelines category A drugs for those patients with more indolent LCT. NCCN guidelines suggest choosing a category C systemic drug for MF with LCT that has more aggressive behavior (liposomal doxorubicin, gemcitabine, romidepsin, or pralatrexate).

Treatment of Mycosis Fungoides with Large Cell Transformation

Pralatrexate

Pralatrexate is a folate analogue therapy with a higher affinity for tumor cells than MTX (**Box 3**). Pralatrexate gained FDA approval for the indication of peripheral T-cell lymphoma (PTCL) and transformed MF in September 2009. A subgroup analysis of the original pralatrexate in patients with relapsed or refractory peripheral T-cell lymphoma (PROPEL) study reviewed effectiveness of pralatrexate in 12 patients with MF with LCT.[76] About 25% of patients had an objective response by independent central review; however, 58% of patients had a response by investigator assessment. In this study, pralatrexate was well tolerated. A median of 10 pralatrexate injections were given at a dose of 30 mg/m^2 once weekly for 6 weeks of a 7-week cycle. Median duration of response was 4.4 months, and median progression-free survival was 5.3 months by investigator assessment. Median survival in this study was 13 months. Mucositis occurred in 58% of patients; however, the only grade 4 adverse events were fatigue (1 patient) and thrombocytopenia (1 patient). There were no toxicity-related discontinuations in this study; however, mucositis was a dose-limiting toxicity.

In a separate study, dose-limiting mucositis was an issue in the patient population with CTCL, and therefore, a lower-dose regimen, 15 mg/m^2, given

---

Box 3
Mycosis fungoides with large cell transformation treatment options

Skin-directed treatment options (may be used adjunctively with some systemic therapies)

- Topical nitrogen mustard
- Topical retinoids
- Phototherapy

Systemic treatment options

- Methotrexate
- Interferon
- Oral retinoids
- Pralatrexate
- Gemcitabine
- Pegylated liposomal doxorubicin
- Brentuximab vedotin
- Romidepsin
- Allogenic stem cell transplant

by IV push for 3 weeks of a 4-week cycle seemed to be better tolerated and had an overall response rate of 45% (MF with LCT was not specifically discussed in this study).[76] In addition, starting supplementation with 1 mg B_{12} intramuscular injection every 8 to 10 weeks (several weeks before starting pralatrexate) and daily folic acid, 1 mg, oral supplementation (started at least 10 days before pralatrexate) also helps to reduce mucositis issues. Warm salt water rinses 4 times daily and a bland diet are also helpful in reducing mucositis. In addition, prescription mouthwashes containing antacids, antihistamines, antifungals, and anesthetic agents may be used.

Preemptive leucovorin use has been reported to minimize pralatrexate toxicity without sacrificing efficacy in a study of 3 patients with MF with LCT.[77] Leucovorin, 50 mg, IV single dose was given 24 hours after each dose of pralatrexate, 30 mg/m². There was no mucositis noted in these 3 patients.

Gemcitabine

Gemcitabine, a purine analogue, has been reported to be successful with intermittent low doses in the treatment of transformed MF.[78] In this study of 3 patients, doses ranged from 750 to 1000 mg/m² given by typical regimen on days 1, 8, and 15 of a 28-day cycle and also by dosing from every other week to even more intermittent dosing when needed based on tumor growth. Grade 3 thrombocytopenia was noted in 1 patient, and all 3 patients experienced grade 4 neutropenia requiring treatment with granulocyte-macrophage colony-stimulating factor. Gemcitabine can be continued long term in a patient with well-controlled disease and can be combined easily with skin-directed therapy.

Pegylated liposomal doxorubicin

Pegylated liposomal doxorubicin contains doxorubicin encapsulated within liposomes allowing for accumulation in the area of the neoplasm, and the pegylation reduces clearance. This formulation of doxorubicin has fewer cardiac and renal side effects than nonpegylated formulations. A prospective multicenter study evaluated patients with advanced or refractory CTCL treated with pegylated liposomal doxorubicin once monthly at a dose of 40 mg/m² IV.[79] Of the 25 patients, 10 had transformed CTCL in this study. In this subset of transformed disease, overall response rate was 50% (5 of 10) after 8 treatment cycles (1 was a CR). The other 5 had progressive disease after 2 to 8 cycles of doxorubicin. The median progression-free survival time in these patients with transformed CTCL was 2 months. About 80% of the side effects were grade 1 or 2. The most common side effects were anemia (36%), asthenia (20%), and nausea/vomiting (20%). Only 2 patients experienced grade 4 side effects, one with hyperthermia and the other with hemophagocytosis. The use of doxorubicin is limited by the maximum life-time dose, given the associated cardiac side effects with long-term use of this chemotherapy.

Brentuximab vedotin

The mechanism of action and dosing of this CD30 monoclonal antibody tagged with a chemotherapeutic agent was discussed earlier as were the details of the phase 2 study using BV for patients with CTCL.[50] Cases of MF with LCT were included in this study. Overall response rate (ORR) was 73%, median time to response was 12 weeks (range, 3–39 weeks), and median duration of response was 32 weeks (range, 3–93 weeks) for patients with MF. Of 28 patients with MF, 15 (54%) achieved a 50% reduction in the modified severity weighted assessment tool score with 2 CRs. Patients with MF responded despite differences in CD30 staining. There was no correlation found between the extent of CD30 expression and response. For MF with LCT, BV tends to work well for the LCT nodules and tumors but less so for the MF patches and plaques. Therefore, BV may be combined with skin-directed modalities for MF to achieve better overall response.

Romidepsin

Romidepsin is a histone deacetylase (HDAC) inhibitor. There are no specific reports of romidepsin use for MF with LCT; however, it is listed in the category C systemic therapies suggested for MF with LCT in the NCCN guidelines, as this treatment modality may be effective for tumor lesions and patients with refractory CTCL.[80–82] The typical dose is 14 mg/m² IV on days 1, 8, and 15 of a 28-day cycle. The HDAC inhibitors can be used in combination with total skin electron beam (TSEB) and phototherapy, making them a useful option when a systemic therapy and skin-directed therapy are needed at the same time.[83]

Bexarotene

Oral bexarotene has been used successfully in the treatment of MF with LCT and can be used safely in the long term without immunosuppression and with few side effects, making this an attractive treatment option. The maximum daily recommended dose is 300 mg/m²; however, lower doses are often effective.[84]

Alemtuzumab

Alemtuzumab is a humanized anti-CD52 monoclonal antibody proposed to be effective in the treatment of refractory CTCL, although it is approved by the FDA only for the treatment of chronic lymphocytic leukemia. A multicenter retrospective analysis of alemtuzumab in advanced CTCL included 11 patients with transformed disease among the 39 patients in the study.[85] Alemtuzumab, 30 mg, was given 2 to 3 times per week for a median duration of 12 weeks, and the dose was then transitioned to once weekly for the maintenance phase thereafter (21% IV, 79% SQ injection). All patients received sulfamethoxazole/trimethoprim and valacyclovir prophylaxis. The overall response rate was 51% (70% in sezary syndrome [SS] and 25% in MF); however, in the 11 patients with transformed disease before alemtuzumab administration, only 1 had clinical response to skin tumors. There were 5 additional patients with SS who experienced transformation of their CTCL in the skin during the alemtuzumab treatment. Most patients experienced severe lymphopenia, and 69% of patients had at least 1 grade 3 side effect, including 62% with infections. The conclusion of this study proposed alemtuzumab as an effective treatment option in SS but ineffective in MF and transformed CTCL. In a previous study of 8 patients treated with alemtuzumab, 1 of 8 had LCT MF; however, cytomegalovirus infection occurred after the sixth week of treatment, necessitating discontinuation of therapy.[86] Given these findings, alemtuzumab is not a first-line treatment of MF with LCT.

Allogeneic stem cell transplant

Autologous stem cell transplant has been disappointing in the primary cutaneous CD30⁺ LPDs secondary to high relapse rates; however, allogeneic transplants have been more successful. A multicenter retrospective analysis of 37 cases of advanced-stage primary CTCLs treated with allogeneic stem cell transplantation included 20 (54%) transformed MF cases.[87] Of these latter cases, there was a 22% transplant-related mortality, 56% relapse or progression, 26% progression-free survival, and 60% overall survival at 2 years. Previously, success with TSEB and nonmyeloablative (reduced intensity) allogeneic hematopoietic stem-cell transplantation had been reported in a series of 19 patients, 8 of whom had MF with LCT.[88] Of these 8 with LCT, 1 died of progressive disease, 3 were deceased with CR, and 4 were alive with 3 CR and 1 PR at the median follow-up period of 1.7 years (range, 0.8–7.9 years). In both these series, graft-versus-lymphoma effect was thought to play a role in the success of this treatment regimen. Allogenic stem cell transplant remains an option for severe, refractory MF with LCT.

Combination therapies

Although it is not specifically reported in the literature, skin-directed therapy used for MF combined with systemic agents likely provides additional value in these patients with LCT.

The combination of pralatrexate and bexarotene was compared with pralatrexate monotherapy in 26 patients, with a reported overall response rate of 50% versus 33%, respectively. Two patients with MF with LCT were included in this study, both of whom had a PR. Pralatrexate, 15 mg/m², combined with bexarotene, 150 mg/m², seemed to be the best dosing regimen with most acceptable adverse event profile. Mucositis was the most common adverse effect. Leucovorin was used in 3 patients, but this did not seem to affect the mucositis in the opinion of the investigators.[89]

Bexarotene in combination with MTX was used to achieve a CR in a patient with refractory MF with LCT. Doses started with bexarotene 450 mg/d and MTX 50 mg each week; however, these doses were reduced secondary to side effects to bexarotene 300 mg/d and MTX 30 mg each week. CR was obtained in 9 months with this regimen.[90]

SUMMARY/PEARLS

Accurate diagnosis and classification of patients cannot be overemphasized when dealing with CD30⁺ LPDs. It is important to look for different types of primary lesions, including in sun-protected areas. Papules, papules with necrotic eschars, scaly erythematous patches, plaques, nodules, and tumors may all coexist, and each may be a clue to the patient's diagnosis. The distribution of lesions on the body is also important, with potential patterns including crops of clustered papules (suggestive of LyP), solitary or few tumor nodules (suggestive of cALCL or tumor stage MF), and tumors in association with patches (suggestive of MF with or without LCT). Understanding that the CD30⁺ LPDs may coexist, multiple biopsies are often helpful in these patients to fully evaluate the clinical picture. Close communication with a dermatopathologist experienced with cutaneous lymphoma is imperative in these challenging cases.[91] It is hoped that the patient's diagnosis will be clear after clinical evaluation and biopsy; however, many times, a classification cannot be made right away. Patience and observing the natural course of the disease eventually leads to an accurate diagnosis in most patients. For example, it is unlikely for MF to have any spontaneous improvement, whereas this is not uncommon with cALCL. However, there are always those who do not fit the box and who may have features of 2 of these CD30$^+$ entities. In those cases, it is best to choose a treatment that is acceptable for both diagnoses.

One should remember the key concept of treating CTCL: aggressive chemotherapy yields no better results than conservative sequential therapy.[92] Skin-directed regimens should be used whenever possible, but one should also recognize that widespread, multifocal disease likely requires systemic therapy. When treating a treatment-refractory case, NCCN guidelines may be used to help guide the use of a combination regimen if monotherapy is not successful. Finally, a specialized CTCL multidisciplinary clinic can be invaluable for diagnosis and development of a treatment plan for these patients.

REFERENCES

1. Bekkenk MW, Geelen FA, van Voorst Vader PC, et al. Primary and secondary cutaneous CD30(+) lymphoproliferative disorders: a report from the Dutch Cutaneous Lymphoma Group on the long-term follow-up data of 219 patients and guidelines for diagnosis and treatment. Blood 2000;95(12):3653–61.

2. Willemze R, Jaffe ES, Burg G, et al. WHO-EORTC classification for cutaneous lymphomas. Blood 2005;105(10):3768–85.

3. Kempf W, Pfaltz K, Vermeer MH, et al. EORTC, ISCL, and USCLC consensus recommendations for the treatment of primary cutaneous CD30-positive lymphoproliferative disorders: lymphomatoid papulosis and primary cutaneous anaplastic large-cell lymphoma. Blood 2011;118(15):4024–35.

4. Greisser J, Palmedo G, Sander C, et al. Detection of clonal rearrangement of T-cell receptor genes in the diagnosis of primary cutaneous CD30 lymphoproliferative disorders. J Cutan Pathol 2006;33(11):711–5.

5. Bertolotti A, Pham-Ledard AL, Vergier B, et al. Lymphomatoid papulosis type D: an aggressive histology for an indolent disease. Br J Dermatol 2013; 169(5):1157–9.

6. Saggini A, Gulia A, Argenyi Z, et al. A variant of lymphomatoid papulosis simulating primary cutaneous aggressive epidermotropic CD8+ cytotoxic T-cell lymphoma. Description of 9 cases. Am J Surg Pathol 2010;34(8):1168–75.

7. Kempf W, Kazakov DV, Scharer L, et al. Angioinvasive lymphomatoid papulosis: a new variant simulating aggressive lymphomas. Am J Surg Pathol 2013;37(1):1–13.

8. Sharaf MA, Romanelli P, Kirsner R, et al. Angioinvasive lymphomatoid papulosis: another case of a newly described variant. Am J Dermatopathol 2014;36(3):e75–7.

9. Kempf W, Kazakov DV, Baumgartner HP, et al. Follicular lymphomatoid papulosis revisited: a study of 11 cases, with new histopathological findings. J Am Acad Dermatol 2013;68(5):809–16.

10. Beljaards RC, Willemze R. The prognosis of patients with lymphomatoid papulosis associated with malignant lymphomas. Br J Dermatol 1992;126(6):596–602.

11. Wood GS, Crooks CF, Uluer AZ. Lymphomatoid papulosis and associated cutaneous lymphoproliferative disorders exhibit a common clonal origin. J Invest Dermatol 1995;105(1):51–5.

12. Davis TH, Morton CC, Miller-Cassman R, et al. Hodgkin's disease, lymphomatoid papulosis, and cutaneous T-cell lymphoma derived from a common T-cell clone. N Engl J Med 1992;326(17):1115–22.

13. Drews R, Samel A, Kadin ME. Lymphomatoid papulosis and anaplastic large cell lymphomas of the skin. Semin Cutan Med Surg 2000;19(2):109–17.

14. Sanchez NP, Pittelkow MR, Muller SA, et al. The clinicopathologic spectrum of lymphomatoid papulosis: study of 31 cases. J Am Acad Dermatol 1983;8(1):81–94.

15. Wantzin GL, Thomsen K. PUVA-treatment in lymphomatoid papulosis. Br J Dermatol 1982;107(6):687–90.

16. de Souza A, Camilleri MJ, Wada DA, et al. Clinical, histopathologic, and immunophenotypic features of lymphomatoid papulosis with CD8 predominance in 14 pediatric patients. J Am Acad Dermatol 2009;61(6):993–1000.

17. Archier E, Devaux S, Castela E, et al. Carcinogenic risks of psoralen UV-A therapy and narrowband UV-B therapy in chronic plaque psoriasis: a systematic literature review. J Eur Acad Dermatol Venereol 2012;26(Suppl 3):22–31.

18. Stern RS, Laird N. The carcinogenic risk of treatments for severe psoriasis. Photochemotherapy follow-up study. Cancer 1994;73(11):2759–64.

19. Lee E, Koo J, Berger T. UVB phototherapy and skin cancer risk: a review of the literature. Int J Dermatol 2005;44(5):355–60.

20. Rodrigues M, McCormack C, Yap LM, et al. Successful treatment of lymphomatoid papulosis with photodynamic therapy. Australas J Dermatol 2009; 50(2):129–32.

21. Kontos AP, Kerr HA, Malick F, et al. 308-nm Excimer laser for the treatment of lymphomatoid papulosis and stage IA mycosis fungoides. Photodermatol Photoimmunol Photomed 2006;22(3):168–71.

22. Wollina U. Lymphomatoid papulosis treated with extracorporeal photochemotherapy. Oncol Rep 1998;5(1):57–9.

23. Fujita H, Nagatani T, Miyazawa M, et al. Primary cutaneous anaplastic large cell lymphoma successfully treated with low-dose oral methotrexate. Eur J Dermatol 2008;18(3):360–1.

24. Yokoi I, Ishikawa E, Koura A, et al. Successful treatment of primary cutaneous anaplastic large cell lymphoma with intralesional methotrexate therapy. Acta Derm Venereol 2014;94(3):319–20.

25. Oliveira LS, Nobrega MP, Monteiro MG, et al. Primary cutaneous anaplastic large-cell lymphoma – case report. An Bras Dermatol 2013;88(6 Suppl 1):132–5.

26. Nandini A, Mysore V, Sacchidanand S, et al. Primary cutaneous anaplastic large cell lymphoma arising from lymphomatoid papulosis, responding to low dose methotrexate. J Cutan Aesthet Surg 2009;2(2):97–100.

27. Vonderheid EC, Sajjadian A, Kadin ME. Methotrexate is effective therapy for lymphomatoid papulosis and other primary cutaneous CD30-positive lymphoproliferative disorders. J Am Acad Dermatol 1996;34(3):470–81.

28. Bergstrom JS, Jaworsky C. Topical methotrexate for lymphomatoid papulosis. J Am Acad Dermatol 2003;49(5):937–9.

29. Demierre MF, Vachon L, Ho V, et al. Phase 1/2 pilot study of methotrexate-laurocapram topical gel for the treatment of patients with early-stage mycosis fungoides. Arch Dermatol 2003;139(5):624–8.

30. Krathen RA, Ward S, Duvic M. Bexarotene is a new treatment option for lymphomatoid papulosis. Dermatology 2003;206(2):142–7.

31. Yagi H, Tokura Y, Furukawa F, et al. Th2 cytokine mRNA expression in primary cutaneous CD30-positive lymphoproliferative disorders: successful treatment with recombinant interferon-gamma. J Invest Dermatol 1996;107(6):827–32.

32. Schmuth M, Topar G, Illersperger B, et al. Therapeutic use of interferon-alpha for lymphomatoid papulosis. Cancer 2000;89(7):1603–10.

33. Proctor SJ, Jackson GH, Lennard AL, et al. Lymphomatoid papulosis: response to treatment with recombinant interferon alfa-2b. J Clin Oncol 1992;10(1):170.

34. Suchin KR, Junkins-Hopkins JM, Rook AH. Treatment of stage IA cutaneous T-cell lymphoma with topical application of the immune response modifier imiquimod. Arch Dermatol 2002;138(9):1137–9.

35. Huen AO, Rook AH. Toll receptor agonist therapy of skin cancer and cutaneous T-cell lymphoma. Curr Opin Oncol 2014;26(2):237–44.

36. Hughes PS. Treatment of lymphomatoid papulosis with imiquimod 5% cream. J Am Acad Dermatol 2006;54(3):546–7.

37. Liu HL, Hoppe RT, Kohler S, et al. CD30+ cutaneous lymphoproliferative disorders: the Stanford experience in lymphomatoid papulosis and primary cutaneous anaplastic large cell lymphoma. J Am Acad Dermatol 2003;49(6):1049–58.

38. Shehan JM, Kalaaji AN, Markovic SN, et al. Management of multifocal primary cutaneous CD30 anaplastic large cell lymphoma. J Am Acad Dermatol 2004;51(1):103–10.

39. Woo DK, Jones CR, Vanoli-Storz MN, et al. Prognostic factors in primary cutaneous anaplastic large cell lymphoma: characterization of clinical subset with worse outcome. Arch Dermatol 2009;145(6):667–74.

40. Diamantidis MD, Myrou AD. Perils and pitfalls regarding differential diagnosis and treatment of primary cutaneous anaplastic large-cell lymphoma. ScientificWorldJournal 2011;11:1048–55.

41. Willemze R, Beljaards RC. Spectrum of primary cutaneous CD30 (Ki-1)-positive lymphoproliferative disorders. A proposal for classification and guidelines for management and treatment. J Am Acad Dermatol 1993;28(6):973–80.

42. Yu JB, McNiff JM, Lund MW, et al. Treatment of primary cutaneous CD30+ anaplastic large-cell lymphoma with radiation therapy. Int J Radiat Oncol Biol Phys 2008;70(5):1542–5.

43. Desai A, Telang GH, Olszewski AJ. Remission of primary cutaneous anaplastic large cell lymphoma after a brief course of brentuximab vedotin. Ann Hematol 2013;92(4):567–8.

44. Broccoli A, Derenzini E, Pellegrini C, et al. Complete response of relapsed systemic and cutaneous anaplastic large cell lymphoma using brentuximab vedotin: 2 case reports. Clin Lymphoma Myeloma Leuk 2013;13(4):493–5.

45. Mody K, Wallace JS, Stearns DM, et al. CD30-positive cutaneous T-cell lymphoma and response to brentuximab vedotin: 2 illustrative cases. Clin Lymphoma Myeloma Leuk 2013;13(3):319–23.

46. Kaffenberger BH, Kartono Winardi F, Frederickson J, et al. Periocular cutaneous anaplastic large cell lymphoma clearance with brentuximab vedotin. J Clin Aesthet Dermatol 2013;6(8):29–31.

47. Patsinakidis N, Kreuter A, Moritz RK, et al. Complete remission of refractory, ulcerated, primary cutaneous CD30+ anaplastic large cell lymphoma following brentuximab vedotin therapy. Acta Derm Venereol 2015;95(2):233–4.

48. Saintes C, Saint-Jean M, Renaut JJ, et al. Dramatic efficacy of brentuximab vedotin in 2 patients with epidermotropic cutaneous T-cell lymphomas after treatment failure despite variable CD30 expression. Br J Dermatol 2015;172(3):819–21.

49. Mehra T, Ikenberg K, Moos RM, et al. Brentuximab as a treatment for CD30+ mycosis fungoides and Sezary syndrome. JAMA Dermatol 2015;151(1):73–7.

50. Duvic M, Tetzlaff M, Clos AL, et al. Phase II trial of brentuximab vedotin for CD30+ cutaneous T-cell lymphomas and lymphoproliferative disorders. Blood 2013;122(21 suppl) [ASH abstract: 367].

51. Carson KR, Newsome SD, Kim EJ, et al. Progressive multifocal leukoencephalopathy associated with brentuximab vedotin therapy: a report of 5 cases from the Southern Network on Adverse Reactions (SONAR) project. Cancer 2014;120(16):2464–71.

52. Blume JE, Stoll HL, Cheney RT. Treatment of primary cutaneous CD30+ anaplastic large cell lymphoma

with intralesional methotrexate. J Am Acad Dermatol 2006;54(5 Suppl):S229–30.

53. Oliveira A, Fernandes I, Alves R, et al. Primary cutaneous CD30 positive anaplastic large cell lymphoma – report of a case treated with bexarotene. Leuk Res 2011;35(11):e190–2.

54. Aldaoud A. Long-term bexarotene monotherapy in large cell CD30+ pleomorphic T-cell lymphoma. Dermatol Clin 2008;26(Suppl 1):15–7.

55. Keun YK, Woodruff R, Sangueza O. Response of CD30+ large cell lymphoma of skin to bexarotene. Leuk Lymphoma 2002;43(5):1153–4.

56. Chou WC, Su IJ, Tien HF, et al. Clinicopathologic, cytogenetic, and molecular studies of 13 Chinese patients with Ki-1 anaplastic large cell lymphoma. Special emphasis on the tumor response to 13-cis retinoic acid. Cancer 1996;78(8):1805–12.

57. Pellegrini C, Stefoni V, Casadei B, et al. Long-term outcome of patients with advanced-stage cutaneous T cell lymphoma treated with gemcitabine. Ann Hematol 2014;93(11):1853–7.

58. Duvic M, Talpur R, Wen S, et al. Phase II evaluation of gemcitabine monotherapy for cutaneous T-cell lymphoma. Clin Lymphoma Myeloma 2006;7(1):51–8.

59. Yamane N, Kato N, Nishimura M, et al. Primary cutaneous CD30+ anaplastic large-cell lymphoma with generalized skin involvement and involvement of one peripheral lymph node, successfully treated with low-dose oral etoposide. Clin Exp Dermatol 2009;34(5):e56–9.

60. French LE, Shapiro M, Junkins-Hopkins JM, et al. Regression of multifocal, skin-restricted, CD30-positive large T-cell lymphoma with interferon alfa and bexarotene therapy. J Am Acad Dermatol 2001; 45(6):914–8.

61. Hazneci E, Aydin NE, Dogan G, et al. Primary cutaneous anaplastic large cell lymphoma in a young girl. J Eur Acad Dermatol Venereol 2001;15(4): 366–7.

62. Ehst BD, Dreno B, Vonderheid EC. Primary cutaneous CD30+ anaplastic large cell lymphoma responds to imiquimod cream. Eur J Dermatol 2008; 18(4):467–8.

63. Didona B, Benucci R, Amerio P, et al. Primary cutaneous CD30+ T-cell lymphoma responsive to topical imiquimod (Aldara). Br J Dermatol 2004;150(6): 1198–201.

64. Coors EA, Schuler G, Von Den Driesch P. Topical imiquimod as treatment for different kinds of cutaneous lymphoma. Eur J Dermatol 2006;16(4):391–3.

65. Meisenheimer JL. Novel use of 308-nm excimer laser to treat a primary cutaneous CD30+ lymphoproliferative nodule. J Drugs Dermatol 2007;6(4):440–2.

66. Boehncke WH, Konig K, Ruck A, et al. In vitro and in vivo effects of photodynamic therapy in cutaneous T cell lymphoma. Acta Derm Venereol 1994;74(3): 201–5.

67. Boehncke WH, Ruck A, Naumann J, et al. Comparison of sensitivity towards photodynamic therapy of cutaneous resident and infiltrating cell types in vitro. Lasers Surg Med 1996;19(4):451–7.

68. Rittenhouse-Diakun K, Van Leengoed H, Morgan J, et al. The role of transferrin receptor (CD71) in photodynamic therapy of activated and malignant lymphocytes using the heme precursor delta-aminolevulinic acid (ALA). Photochem Photobiol 1995;61(5):523–8.

69. Umegaki N, Moritsugu R, Katoh S, et al. Photodynamic therapy may be useful in debulking cutaneous lymphoma prior to radiotherapy. Clin Exp Dermatol 2004;29(1):42–5.

70. Herrmann JL, Hughey LC. Recognizing large-cell transformation of mycosis fungoides. J Am Acad Dermatol 2012;67(4):665–72.

71. Arulogun SO, Prince HM, Ng J, et al. Long-term outcomes of patients with advanced-stage cutaneous T-cell lymphoma and large cell transformation. Blood 2008;112(8):3082–7.

72. Diamandidou E, Colome-Grimmer M, Fayad L, et al. Transformation of mycosis fungoides/Sezary syndrome: clinical characteristics and prognosis. Blood 1998;92(4):1150–9.

73. Wolfe JT, Chooback L, Finn DT, et al. Large-cell transformation following detection of minimal residual disease in cutaneous T-cell lymphoma: molecular and in situ analysis of a single neoplastic T-cell clone expressing the identical T-cell receptor. J Clin Oncol 1995;13(7):1751–7.

74. Wood GS, Tung RM, Haeffner AC, et al. Detection of clonal T-cell receptor gamma gene rearrangements in early mycosis fungoides/Sezary syndrome by polymerase chain reaction and denaturing gradient gel electrophoresis (PCR/DGGE). J Invest Dermatol 1994;103(1):34–41.

75. Agar NS, Wedgeworth E, Crichton S, et al. Survival outcomes and prognostic factors in mycosis fungoides/Sezary syndrome: validation of the revised International Society for Cutaneous Lymphomas/European Organisation for Research and Treatment of Cancer staging proposal. J Clin Oncol 2010;28(31): 4730–9.

76. Horwitz SM, Kim YH, Foss F, et al. Identification of an active, well-tolerated dose of pralatrexate in patients with relapsed or refractory cutaneous T-cell lymphoma. Blood 2012;119(18):4115–22.

77. Koch E, Story SK, Geskin LJ. Preemptive leucovorin administration minimizes pralatrexate toxicity without sacrificing efficacy. Leuk Lymphoma 2013; 54(11):2448–51.

78. Awar O, Duvic M. Treatment of transformed mycosis fungoides with intermittent low-dose gemcitabine. Oncology 2007;73(1–2):130–5.

79. Quereux G, Marques S, Nguyen JM, et al. Prospective multicenter study of pegylated liposomal doxorubicin treatment in patients with advanced or

refractory mycosis fungoides or Sezary syndrome. Arch Dermatol 2008;144(6):727–33.

80. Horwitz SM, Duvic M, Hsi ED. Clinical roundtable monograph. The management of aggressive T-cell lymphoma: a discussion on transformed mycosis fungoides. Clin Adv Hematol Oncol 2010;8(12):1–15.

81. Whittaker SJ, Demierre MF, Kim EJ, et al. Final results from a multicenter, international, pivotal study of romidepsin in refractory cutaneous T-cell lymphoma. J Clin Oncol 2010;28(29):4485–91.

82. Piekarz RL, Frye R, Turner M, et al. Phase II multi-institutional trial of the histone deacetylase inhibitor romidepsin as monotherapy for patients with cutaneous T-cell lymphoma. J Clin Oncol 2009;27(32):5410–7.

83. Akilov OE, Grant C, Frye R, et al. Low-dose electron beam radiation and romidepsin therapy for symptomatic cutaneous T-cell lymphoma lesions. Br J Dermatol 2012;167(1):194–7.

84. Mitteldorf C, Stadler R, Bertsch HP, et al. Folliculotropic mycosis fungoides with CD30+ large-cell transformation in a young woman: beneficial effect of bexarotene. Br J Dermatol 2007;156(3):584–6.

85. de Masson A, Guitera P, Brice P, et al. Long-term efficacy and safety of alemtuzumab in advanced primary cutaneous T-cell lymphomas. Br J Dermatol 2014;170(3):720–4.

86. Kennedy GA, Seymour JF, Wolf M, et al. Treatment of patients with advanced mycosis fungoides and Sezary syndrome with alemtuzumab. Eur J Haematol 2003;71(4):250–6.

87. de Masson A, Beylot-Barry M, Bouaziz JD, et al. Allogeneic stem cell transplantation for advanced cutaneous T-cell lymphomas: a study from the French Society of Bone Marrow Transplantation and French Study Group on Cutaneous Lymphomas. Haematologica 2014;99(3):527–34.

88. Duvic M, Donato M, Dabaja B, et al. Total skin electron beam and non-myeloablative allogeneic hematopoietic stem-cell transplantation in advanced mycosis fungoides and Sezary syndrome. J Clin Oncol 2010;28(14):2365–72.

89. Talpur R, Thompson A, Gangar P, et al. Pralatrexate alone or in combination with bexarotene: long-term tolerability in relapsed/refractory mycosis fungoides. Clin Lymphoma Myeloma Leuk 2014;14(4):297–304.

90. Zindanci I, Kavala M, Turkoglu Z, et al. A CD30(-) transformed mycosis fungoides case responding very well to systemic bexarotene and methotrexate. Int J Low Extrem Wounds 2014;13(2):127–9.

91. Kadin ME, Hughey LC, Wood GS. Large-cell transformation of mycosis fungoides - differential diagnosis with implications for clinical management: a consensus statement of the US Cutaneous Lymphoma Consortium. J Am Acad Dermatol 2014;70(2):374–6.

92. Kaye FJ, Bunn PA Jr, Steinberg SM, et al. A randomized trial comparing combination electron-beam radiation and chemotherapy with topical therapy in the initial treatment of mycosis fungoides. N Engl J Med 1989;321(26):1784–90.

Diagnosis and Management of Cutaneous B-cell Lymphoma

Lauren C. Pinter-Brown, MD

KEYWORDS

- Cutaneous B-cell lymphoma • Marginal zone lymphoma
- Primary cutaneous follicle center lymphoma • DLBCL, leg type • Primary cutaneous lymphoma

KEY POINTS

- A primary cutaneous B-cell lymphoma (CBCL) by definition is one in which the lymphoma involves no other tissue but skin at the time of diagnosis.
- Primary cutaneous follicle center lymphoma and diffuse large B-cell lymphoma, leg type, are unique clinicopathologic entities, not to be confused with nodal counterparts with similar names.
- The diagnosis of CBCL requires a 4-mm to 6-mm punch biopsy or incisional or excisional biopsy that includes the reticular dermis and subcutaneous fat.
- Along with histologic differences, the common CBCLs present on different parts of the body in different age groups.
- The treatment approach may vary widely between observation, local therapy, or systemic therapy depending on the histology and extent and area of skin involvement. Histology of the lesion determines prognosis.

INTRODUCTION

The skin is the second most common extranodal site involved by non-Hodgkin lymphomas (NHLs) after the gastrointestinal tract. By definition, the designation of a lymphoma as primary to the skin implies that there is no extracutaneous disease discovered at diagnosis. As such, the cutaneous B-cell lymphomas (CBCLs) make up 25% to 30% of all primary cutaneous lymphomas, with cutaneous T-cell lymphomas (CTCLs) being the more common subtype.[1]

Although the clinical presentation of CBCLs compared with CTCLs is more uniform, clinico-pathologic correlation is still important and, in the absence of features clearly suggesting a benign diagnosis, the evaluation of nonepidermotrophic or dermal lymphoid cutaneous infiltrate such as

seen in these cancers requires assessment of multiple parameters, including a good clinical history and physical examination.

The 3 most common histologic types of primary cutaneous lymphomas as designated in the World Health Organization (WHO) 2008 Classification of Tumors of Haematopoietic and Lymphoid Tissues are primary cutaneous follicle center lymphoma (PCFCL), extranodal marginal zone lymphoma (MZL) of mucosa-associated lymphoid tissue (MALT; previously called primary cutaneous MZL [PCMZL]), and primary cutaneous diffuse large B-cell lymphoma (PCDLBCL), leg type. The first and last of these are recognized as unique entities in the WHO 2008 classification.[2] Although they carry names and have some histologic similarities with nodal counterparts, there remain differences not only in presentation and histology but also in

The author has done consulting for Celgene, Pharmacyclics.
Department of Internal Medicine, Division of Hematology-Oncology, Geffen School of Medicine, University of California, Los Angeles, 2020 Santa Monica Suite 600, Santa Monica, CA 90404, USA
E-mail address: lpinterbrown@mednet.ucla.edu

Dermatol Clin 33 (2015) 835–840
http://dx.doi.org/10.1016/j.det.2015.05.003
0733-8635/15/$ – see front matter © 2015 Elsevier Inc. All rights reserved.

natural history, treatment, and outlook. PCMZL, however, is discussed within the general category of extranodal MZLs, which are frequently found in extranodal sites such as skin or stomach. Although both PCFCL and PCMZL are considered slow-growing or indolent diseases with an excellent outlook, PCDLBCL, leg type, is a more aggressive entity with behavior more similar to its nodal counterpart.

DIAGNOSIS AND STAGING

The diagnosis of a CBCL first requires a biopsy of these mostly papular or tumoral erythematous to violaceous skin lesions. To this end, a 4-mm to 6-mm punch biopsy or excisional or incisional biopsy that includes the reticular dermis and fat should be obtained.

After the diagnosis is confirmed, staging procedures in addition to history and physical examination should be performed to evaluate for extracutaneous disease and anticipate treatment. Groups such as the National Comprehensive Cancer Network (NCCN)[3] have suggested performance of complete blood count (CBC) with differential, a comprehensive chemistry panel, and lactate dehydrogenase level. If a lymphocytosis or immature cells are seen in the CBC, peripheral blood flow cytometry should be ordered to evaluate for a monotypic lymphoid population, which may signify blood involvement by the lymphoma. In the case of PCMZL, both a serum protein electrophoresis and quantitative immunoglobulins should be sent to evaluate for a paraprotein given the increased incidence of this finding in this specific entity. Serologic testing for hepatitis B and C, especially if systemic therapies such as rituximab, systemic steroids, or other immunomodulatory agents are being considered, and testing for *Borrelia burgdorferi* serologies should be considered. Although an association between *B burgdorferi* infection and CBCL has been made in several European countries, such a relationship has not been shown in North American patients and the strength of this association may relate in part to geographic diversity.[4]

In addition to laboratory testing, PET/computed tomography (CT) scanning or CT scanning with contrast of the chest, abdomen, and pelvis should be performed at diagnosis, but not routinely in follow-up unless clinical or laboratory parameters are concerning for extracutaneous progression. Bone marrow examination should be performed if the diagnosis is PCDLBCL, leg type, and considered if the diagnosis is PCFCL.

Although a TNM (tumor, node, metastasis) classification for cutaneous lymphomas other than MF/SS has been proposed,[5] unlike the larger group of NHLs, the histology of these diseases remains the main determinant of a patient's outcome. However, the TNM classification can be used effectively for the documentation of anatomic location and extent of disease involvement.[6]

The histology of primary cutaneous lymphomas is discussed in depth elsewhere in this issue, the clinical presentation and treatment of the 3 most common forms of CBCLs are discussed here separately. Other uncommon CBCLs, such as intravascular large B-cell lymphoma, a subtype of diffuse large B-cell lymphoma (DLBCL) that may present primarily in skin, and cutaneous immunodeficiency-associated lymphoproliferative diseases such as Epstein-Barr virus (EBV)–positive mucocutaneous ulcer are briefly discussed.

PRIMARY CUTANEOUS FOLLICLE CENTER LYMPHOMA

The most common type of primary CBCL, PCFCL, represents 60% of all cases. The median age of patients is 51 years, with a slight male predominance (1.5:1).[7,8] Lesions are firm, erythematous to violaceous nodules or plaques with a smooth skin surface; ulcerations are rarely observed. These lesions characteristically present as solitary or localized skin lesions on the scalp, head and neck, or trunk. Only 5% present on the leg and 15% are multifocal.[7,8]

In contrast with its nodal counterpart, follicular lymphoma, PCFCL does not necessarily have CD10 staining by immunohistochemistry, and may have negative or faint staining with bcl-2. When present, these positive stains raise suspicion for secondary rather than primary skin involvement. Surface immunoglobulin (Ig) G is usually negative in PCFCL, in contrast with follicular lymphoma. In addition, PCFCL is not graded as nodal follicular lymphoma in terms of number or proportion of large cells noted.[2]

Although the rate of cutaneous relapse with PCFCL reaches 30%, the condition has an excellent prognosis, with a 5-year survival of greater than 95%. Although some patients experience spontaneous regression, approximately 10% experience extracutaneous dissemination.[7,8]

EXTRANODAL MARGINAL ZONE LYMPHOMA OF MUCOSA-ASSOCIATED LYMPHOID TISSUE

Primary cutaneous MALT lymphomas are described in the WHO classification of 2008 as part of the general group of extranodal MZLs of MALT in which there is often a role described for a chronic antigenic stimulus to lymphomagenesis. Approximately 11% of MALT lymphomas involve the skin,[9] with gastrointestinal tract involvement being the most common extranodal site; MALT lymphomas of the skin represent approximately 7% of all skin lymphomas, either of B-cell or T-cell origin. Patients with PCMZL have a slightly higher median age of 55 years than PCFCL with a male predominance (2:1).[7,8] Lesions present as erythematous papules, nodules, or plaques, especially on the extremities and trunk.

MALT lymphomas as a group are distinguished from other B-cell lymphomas by having no specific associated marker. They may express IgM and show light chain restriction, distinguishing them from reactive lymphoid infiltrates. Although PCMZL is classified with other MALT lymphomas, it has distinctive features, including the finding of plasmacytic differentiation within the lymphocytic infiltrate, which is an especially common finding in the skin lesions. Overall, 30% of patients show a serum monoclonal protein.[10] The higher incidence of monoclonal proteins in PCMZL compared with other NHLs reflects the finding of concurrent plasmacytic differentiation or plasmacytosis. The finding of a monoclonal protein provides clinicians with another parameter with which to follow the patient's clinical course.

The 5-year survival is 100%, although recurrences are common and occur in up to half of patients.[11,12] Waxing and waning lesions, and occasional spontaneous remission, can be seen.

PRIMARY CUTANEOUS DIFFUSE LARGE B-CELL LYMPHOMA, LEG TYPE

In contrast with the previous CBCLs, PCDLBCL, leg type, is considered an aggressive lymphoma with a poor outcome. It represents 4% of all cutaneous lymphomas and 20% of all primary CBCLs,[1] and affects the elderly with a median age of 70 years. The predominant gender is female, with a 1:3 to 1:4 ratio.[13] The condition presents as red or violaceous tumors commonly arising on 1 or both legs, with 10% to 15% of cases involving other sites.[7,8,14] The lymphoma frequently disseminates to extracutaneous sites.

On histology, large transformed B-lymphocytes with frequent mitotic figures are seen. The cells show monotypic IgG, and have strong expression of bcl-2, IRF4/MUM-1, and bcl-6. Ten percent of cases lack bcl-2 or MUM-1. CD10 is usually negative. In this way, both immunohistochemistry and gene expression profiling have many similarities to nodal diffuse large B-cell lymphoma of the activated B-cell (ABC) phenotype, which has been shown to have a worse prognosis than other phenotypes of DLBCL, like the germinal center phenotype given therapies such as RCHOP. Fluorescent in situ hybridization may show both c-myc, bcl-6, and bcl-2 mutations, similar to the so-called triple-hit diffuse large B-cell lymphoma, which has a poor prognosis.[15]

In this elderly population of patients, presentation with multiple skin lesions at diagnosis seems to be an additional adverse risk factor. Overall, the 5-year survival is approximately 50%, which is far worse than the other CBCLs previously described.[13,16]

OTHER B-CELL LYMPHOMAS THAT PRESENT IN SKIN

Other lymphomas that have been described as presenting primarily in skin include intravascular large B-cell lymphoma, a rare form of extranodal lymphoma characterized by intravascular growth of large B cells, especially in small vessels and capillaries in brain and skin, a presentation that has been described in Western countries. This lymphoma primarily affects an older population with a median age of 67 years.[17] Skin lesions may look like livedo (with a reticular erythema), may resemble panniculitis, or may present as painful telangiectasia or nodules. Conventional staging often does not show extracutaneous disease because the lymphoma spares lymph nodes, although it may present in any other tissue. Some investigators have described a more indolent behavior of this usually fatal lymphoma in which only the skin is affected.[18]

T cell–rich B-cell lymphoma, a type of large B-cell lymphoma rich in T-cells in association with a limited number of scattered large malignant B cells[19] and plasmablastic lymphomas, have also been described as presenting primarily in skin; plasmablastic lymphomas often being seen in individuals infected with human immunodeficiency virus.[20]

Mucocutaneous ulcer represents an EBV-driven cutaneous lymphoproliferative disorder that is associated with immunodeficiency. It presents with sharply demarcated ulcers in skin or mucosa, largely in individuals with either immune senescence of age or iatrogenic immune suppression. These ulcers show spontaneous regression about 45% of the time.[21]

TREATMENT OF THE INDOLENT CUTANEOUS B-CELL LYMPHOMAS: PRIMARY CUTANEOUS FOLLICLE CENTER LYMPHOMA AND MUCOSA-ASSOCIATED LYMPHOID TISSUE LYMPHOMA

In general, treatment of these entities may vary depending on the presentation of disease, with patients presenting with a solitary lesion or lesions limited to a single anatomic site being approached differently from patients presenting with generalized or treatment-refractory disease or evidence of extracutaneous spread. Data supporting these forms of treatment are limited to small retrospective or case studies, and groups such as NCCN,[3] the European Organisation for Research and Treatment of Cancer, and the International Society for Cutaneous Lymphomas[22] have provided consensus opinions of a group of experts because of this lack of data in the literature.

Patients presenting with solitary lesions or lesions limited to a single anatomic site may be treated with localized electron beam radiotherapy or surgical excision. Typical radiation doses are at least 30 Gy, with a margin of 1 to 1.5 cm around the lesion. Selected cases may also be closely observed or treated with topical or intralesional steroids. These approaches may be particularly attractive when the site of involvement renders a surgical or radiotherapeutic approach less desirable because of poor cosmetic outcomes, as in hair-bearing areas of the body, large lesions, or involvement of the face. The use of cryotherapy has also been described.[23]

Patients with more generalized or refractory lesions may also be treated with similar approaches or with systemic treatments such as rituximab, a chimeric anti-CD20 antibody, with or without maintenance infusions, or radioimmunotherapy with an anti-CD20 antibody conjugate. Clinicians should be aware that case reports of localized edema or urticaria have been described in the CBCL skin lesions in these patients after systemic treatment with rituximab.[24,25]

Patients with the development of extracutaneous disease should be treated as patients with nodal follicular lymphoma.

TREATMENT OF PRIMARY CUTANEOUS DIFFUSE LARGE B-CELL LYMPHOMA, LEG TYPE

The treatment of patients presenting with a single lesion has been described with local radiation, a choice that may be especially attractive in this elderly patient population, or with the addition of systemic multiagent chemotherapy such as rituximab with CHOP (cyclophosphamide, adriamycin, vincristine, and prednisone). Patients with generalized lesions are likely to be treated as in nodal DLBCLs. As in the more indolent CBCLs, there are no randomized controlled data to guide treatment choices in this entity and treatment may proceed in keeping with individual and institutional experience. In the future, reports are anticipated of less toxic treatment alternatives that have

been or are being explored in nodal DLBCL, ABC phenotype, such as the use of nuclear factor kappa B inhibitors such as bortezomib,[26] immunomodulatory drugs such as lenalidomide with rituximab[27] (so-called R2), or newer drugs such as ibrutinib,[28] an oral Bruton tyrosine kinase pathway inhibitor that seems to have preferential activity in DLBCL of the ABC phenotype.

SUMMARY

The diagnosis of primary CBCL requires that the evaluation for a more widespread lymphoma has been negative. In contrast with the more common CTCLs, these lymphomas have a more consistent clinical presentation and, on histologic examination of representative skin biopsies, are not epidermotrophic, instead involving the dermis and subcutaneous tissue. Treatment may range from observation, to topical therapies, to systemic therapies, depending on the histology, degree and area of skin involvement, patient performance, and comorbidities, and may be influenced by individual practitioner and institutional experience and capabilities. Randomized, controlled data are lacking in the medical literature to direct optimal treatment of all CBCLs. The indolent types of CBCL, PCFCL and PCMZL of MALT lymphoma, have an excellent prognosis regardless of treatment selected. In the more aggressive and dire PCDLBCL, leg type, which affects older and perhaps more debilitated patients, published experience is anticipated with novel, more targeted agents and perhaps less toxic agents that show activity in the similar lymphoma, nodal DLBCL of ABC type.

REFERENCES

1. Willemze R, Jaffe ES, Burg G, et al. WHO-EORTC classification for cutaneous lymphomas. Blood 2005;105(10):3768–85.
2. Swerdlow SH, Campo E, Harris NL, et al. WHO classification of tumours of haematopoietic and lymphoid tissue. 4th edition. Lyon (France): IARC Press; 2008.
3. Zelenetz AD. Guidelines for NHL: updates to the management of diffuse large B-cell lymphoma and new guidelines for primary cutaneous CD30+ T-cell lymphoproliferative disorders and T-cell large granular lymphocytic leukemia. J Natl Compr Canc Netw 2014;12(5 Suppl):797–800.
4. Wood GS, Kamath NV, Guitart J, et al. Absence of *Borrelia burgdorferi* DNA in cutaneous B-cell lymphomas from the United States. J Cutan Pathol 2001;28(10):502–7.
5. Kim YH, Willemze R, Pimpinelli N, et al, ISCL and the EORTC. TNM classification system for primary

cutaneous lymphomas other than mycosis fungoides and Sezary syndrome: a proposal of the International Society for Cutaneous Lymphomas (ISCL) and the Cutaneous Lymphoma Task Force of the European Organization of Research and Treatment of Cancer (EORTC). Blood 2007;110(2): 479–84.

6. Senff NJ, Willemze R. The applicability and prognostic value of the new TNM classification system for primary cutaneous lymphomas other than mycosis fungoides and Sézary syndrome: results on a large cohort of primary cutaneous B-cell lymphomas and comparison with the system used by the Dutch Cutaneous Lymphoma Group. Br J Dermatol 2007;157(6):1205–11.

7. Senff NJ, Hoefnagel JJ, Jansen PM, et al. Reclassification of 300 primary cutaneous B-cell lymphomas according to the new WHO-EORTC classification for cutaneous lymphomas: comparison with previous classifications and identification of prognostic markers. J Clin Oncol 2007;25(12):1581–7.

8. Zinzani PL, Quaglino P, Pimpinelli N, et al, Italian Study Group for Cutaneous Lymphomas. Prognostic factors in primary cutaneous B-cell lymphoma: the Italian Study Group for Cutaneous Lymphomas. J Clin Oncol 2006;24(9):1376–82.

9. Thieblemont C, Bastion Y, Berger F, et al. Mucosa-associated lymphoid tissue gastrointestinal and non gastrointestinal lymphoma behavior: analysis of 108 patients. J Clin Oncol 1997;15(4):1624–30.

10. Wöhrer S, Streubel B, Bartsch R, et al. Monoclonal immunoglobulin production is a frequent event in patients with mucosa-associated lymphoid tissue lymphoma. Clin Cancer Res 2004;10(21): 7179–81.

11. Golling P, Cozzio A, Dummer R, et al. Primary cutaneous B-cell lymphomas-clinicopathological, prognostic and therapeutic characterisation of 54 cases according to the WHO-EORTC classification and the ISCL/EORTC TNM classification system for primary cutaneous lymphomas other than mycosis fungoides and Sezary syndrome. Leuk Lymphoma 2008;49(6):1094–103.

12. Hoefnagel JJ, Vermeer MH, Jansen PM, et al. Primary cutaneous marginal zone B-cell lymphoma: clinical and therapeutic features in 50 cases. Arch Dermatol 2005;141(9):1139–45.

13. Vermeer MH, Geelen FA, van Haselen CW, et al. Primary cutaneous large B-cell lymphomas of the legs. A distinct type of cutaneous B-cell lymphoma with an intermediate prognosis. Dutch Cutaneous Lymphoma Working Group. Arch Dermatol 1996; 132(11):1304–8.

14. Kodama K, Massone C, Chott A, et al. Primary cutaneous large B-cell lymphomas: clinicopathologic features, classification, and prognostic factors in a large series of patients. Blood 2005;106(7):2491–7.

15. Hallermann C, Kaune KM, Gesk S, et al. Molecular cytogenetic analysis of chromosomal breakpoints in the IGH, MYC, BCL6, and MALT1 gene loci in primary cutaneous B-cell lymphomas. J Invest Dermatol 2004;123(1):213–9.

16. Grange F, Bekkenk MW, Wechsler J, et al. Prognostic factors in primary cutaneous large B-cell lymphomas: a European multicenter study. J Clin Oncol 2001;19(16):3602–10.

17. Murase T, Yamaguchi M, Suzuki R, et al. Intravascular large B-cell lymphoma (IVLBCL): a clinicopathologic study of 96 cases with special reference to the immunophenotypic heterogeneity of CD5. Blood 2007;109(2):478–85.

18. Ferreri AJ, Campo E, Seymour JF, et al, International Extranodal Lymphoma Study Group (IELSG). Intravascular lymphoma: clinical presentation, natural history, management and prognostic factors in a series of 38 cases, with special emphasis on the 'cutaneous variant'. Br J Haematol 2004;127(2): 173–83.

19. Vezzoli P, Fiorani R, Girgenti V, et al. Cutaneous T-cell/histiocyte-rich B-cell lymphoma: a case report and review of the literature. Dermatology 2011; 222(3):225–30.

20. Corti M, Villafañe MF, Bistmans A, et al. Oral cavity and extra-oral plasmablastic lymphomas in AIDS patients: report of five cases and review of the literature. Int J STD AIDS 2011;22(12):759–63.

21. Dojcinov SD, Venkataraman G, Raffeld M, et al. EBV positive mucocutaneous ulcer–a study of 26 cases associated with various sources of immunosuppression. Am J Surg Pathol 2010;34(3):405–17.

22. Senff NJ, Noordijk EM, Kim YH, et al, European Organization for Research and Treatment of Cancer, International Society for Cutaneous Lymphoma. European Organization for Research and Treatment of Cancer and International Society for Cutaneous Lymphoma consensus recommendations for the management of cutaneous B-cell lymphomas. Blood 2008;112(5):1600–9.

23. Kuflik AS, Schwartz RA. Lymphocytoma cutis: a series of five patients successfully treated with cryosurgery. J Am Acad Dermatol 1992;26(3 Pt 2): 449–52.

24. Ingen-Housz-Oro S, Ortonne N, Chosidow O. Rituximab-related urticarial reaction overlying primary cutaneous follicle centre lymphoma: histological appearance and pathophysiological hypotheses. J Eur Acad Dermatol Venereol 2014;28(7):976–8.

25. Brunet-Possenti F, Franck N, Tamburini J, et al. Focal rituximab-induced edematous reaction at primary cutaneous follicle center lymphoma lesions: case report and literature review. Dermatology 2011; 223(3):200–2.

26. Dunleavy K, Pittaluga S, Czuczman MS, et al. Differential efficacy of bortezomib plus chemotherapy

within molecular subtypes of diffuse large B-cell lymphoma. Blood 2009;113(24):6069–76.

27. Ivanov V, Coso D, Chetaille B, et al. Efficacy and safety of lenalinomide combined with rituximab in patients with relapsed/refractory diffuse large B-cell lymphoma. Leuk Lymphoma 2014;55(11): 2508–13.

28. Young RM, Shaffer AL 3rd, Phelan JD, et al. B-cell receptor signaling in diffuse large B-cell lymphoma. Semin Hematol 2015;52(2):77–85.

Index

Note: Page numbers of article titles are in **boldface** type.

Dermatol Clin 33 (2015) 841–849
http://dx.doi.org/10.1016/S0733-8635(15)00117-5
0733-8635/15/$ – see front matter © 2015 Elsevier Inc. All rights reserved.

United States Postal Service

Statement of Ownership, Management, and Circulation
(All Periodicals Publications Except Requester Publications)

1. Publication Title	2. Publication Number									3. Filing Date
Dermatologic Clinics of North America	0	0	0	—	7	0	5			9/18/15

4. Issue Frequency	5. Number of Issues Published Annually	6. Annual Subscription Price
Jan, Apr, Jul, Oct	4	$365.00

7. Complete Mailing Address of Known Office of Publication (Not printer) (Street, city, county, state, and ZIP+4®)

Elsevier Inc.
360 Park Avenue South
New York, NY 10010-1710

Contact Person
Stephen R. Bushing
Telephone (Include area code)
215-239-3688

8. Complete Mailing Address of Headquarters or General Business Office of Publisher (Not printer)

Elsevier Inc., 360 Park Avenue South, New York, NY 10010-1710

9. Full Names and Complete Mailing Addresses of Publisher, Editor, and Managing Editor (Do not leave blank)

Publisher (Name and complete mailing address)

Linda Belfus, Elsevier Inc., 1600 John F. Kennedy Blvd., Suite 1800, Philadelphia, PA 19103

Editor (Name and complete mailing address)

Jessica McCool, Elsevier Inc., 1600 John F. Kennedy Blvd., Suite 1800, Philadelphia, PA 19103-2899

Managing Editor (Name and complete mailing address)

Adrianne Brigido, Elsevier Inc., 1600 John F. Kennedy Blvd., Suite 1800, Philadelphia, PA 19103-2899

10. Owner (Do not leave blank. If the publication is owned by a corporation, give the name and address of the corporation immediately followed by the names and addresses of all stockholders owning or holding 1 percent or more of the total amount of stock. If not owned by a corporation, give the names and addresses of the individual owners. If owned by a partnership or other unincorporated firm, give its name and address as well as those of each individual owner. If the publication is published by a nonprofit organization, give its name and address.)

Full Name	Complete Mailing Address
Wholly owned subsidiary of	1600 John F. Kennedy Blvd, Ste. 1800
Reed/Elsevier, US holdings	Philadelphia, PA 19103-2899

11. Known Bondholders, Mortgagees, and Other Security Holders Owning or Holding 1 Percent or More of Total Amount of Bonds, Mortgages, or Other Securities. If none, check box ☐ None

Full Name	Complete Mailing Address
N/A	

12. Tax Status (For completion by nonprofit organizations authorized to mail at nonprofit rates) (Check one)
The purpose, function, and nonprofit status of this organization and the exempt status for federal income tax purposes:
☐ Has Not Changed During Preceding 12 Months
☐ Has Changed During Preceding 12 Months (Publisher must submit explanation of change with this statement)

PS Form 3526, July 2014 (Page 1 of 3 (Instructions Page 3)) PSN 7530-01-000-9931 PRIVACY NOTICE: See our Privacy policy in www.usps.com

---

13. Publication Title		14. Issue Date for Circulation Data Below
Dermatologic Clinics of North America		July 2015

15. Extent and Nature of Circulation			Average No. Copies Each Issue During Preceding 12 Months	No. Copies of Single Issue Published Nearest to Filing Date
a. Total Number of Copies (Net press run)			528	461
b. Legitimate Paid and/Or Requested Distribution (By Mail and Outside the Mail)	(1)	Mailed Outside County Paid/Requested Mail Subscriptions stated on PS Form 3541. (Include paid distribution above nominal rate, advertiser's proof copies and exchange copies)	159	119
	(2)	Mailed In-County Paid/Requested Mail Subscriptions stated on PS Form 3541. (Include paid distribution above nominal rate, advertiser's proof copies and exchange copies)		
	(3)	Paid Distribution Outside the Mails Including Sales Through Dealers And Carriers, Street Vendors, Counter Sales, and Other Paid Distribution Outside USPS®	83	105
	(4)	Paid Distribution by Other Classes of Mail Through the USPS (e.g. First-Class Mail®)		
c. Total Paid and/or Requested Circulation (Sum of 15b (1), (2), (3), and (4))		▲	242	224
d. Free or Nominal Rate Distribution (By Mail and Outside the Mail)	(1)	Free or Nominal Rate Outside-County Copies included on PS Form 3541	60	70
	(2)	Free or Nominal Rate In-County Copies included on PS Form 3541		
	(3)	Free or Nominal Rate Copies mailed at Other classes Through the USPS (e.g. First-Class Mail®)		
	(4)	Free or Nominal Rate Distribution Outside the Mail (Carriers or Other means)		
e. Total Nonrequested Distribution (Sum of 15d (1), (2), (3) and (4))			60	70
f. Total Distribution (Sum of 15c and 15e)		▲	302	294
g. Copies not Distributed (See instructions to publishers #4 (page #3))		▲	226	167
h. Total (Sum of 15f and g)			528	461
i. Percent Paid and/or Requested Circulation (15c divided by 15f times 100)		▲	80.13%	76.19%

* If you are claiming electronic copies go to line 16 on page 3. If you are not claiming Electronic copies, skip to line 17 on page 3.

16. Electronic Copy Circulation	Average No. Copies Each Issue During Preceding 12 Months	No. Copies of Single Issue Published Nearest to Filing Date
a. Paid Electronic Copies		
b. Total paid Print Copies (Line 15c) + Paid Electronic copies (Line 16a)		
c. Total Print Distribution (Line 15f) + Paid Electronic Copies (Line 16a)		
d. Percent Paid (Both Print & Electronic copies) (16b divided by 16c X100)		

☐ I certify that 50% of all my distributed copies (electronic and print) are paid above a nominal price

17. Publication of Statement of Ownership
If the publication is a general publication, publication of this statement is required. Will be printed in the **October 2015** issue of this publication.

18. Signature and Title of Editor, Publisher, Business Manager, or Owner

[signature] Stephen R. Bushing

Stephen R. Bushing – Inventory Distribution Coordinator

Date September 18, 2015

I certify that all information furnished on this form is true and complete. I understand that anyone who furnishes false or misleading information on this form or who omits material or information requested on the form may be subject to criminal sanctions (including fines and imprisonment) and/or civil sanctions (including civil penalties).

PS Form 3526, July 2014 (Page 3 of 3)

Printed and bound by CPI Group (UK) Ltd, Croydon, CR0 4YY

03/10/2024

01040376-0001